Susan S. Aronson, MD, FAAP, Editor

Healthy Young Children

A Manual for Programs

Fifth Edition

National Association for the Education of Young Children
Washington, DC

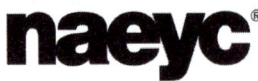

National Association for the Education of Young Children
1313 L Street NW, Suite 500
Washington, DC 20005-4101
202-232-8777 • 800-424-2460
www.naeyc.org

NAEYC Books

Chief Publishing Officer
Derry Koralek

Editor-in-Chief
Kathy Charner

Director of Creative Services
Edwin C. Malstrom

Senior Editor
Holly Bohart

Design and Production
Malini Dominey

Assistant Editor
Elizabeth Wegner

Editorial Assistant
Ryan Smith

Through its publications program, the National Association for the Education of Young Children (NAEYC) provides a forum for discussion of major issues and ideas in the early childhood field, with the hope of provoking thought and promoting professional growth. The views expressed or implied in this book are not necessarily those of the Association or its members.

Some of the information in this manual applies to specific conditions of individual children. It is not a substitute for the advice of a child's health care provider or a program's health consultant. The manual reflects current research and standards in the fields related to health and early childhood education. However, in rapidly changing fields new information constantly emerges. Be alert to such changes and check the websites of nationally credentialed organizations identified in the chapters of this book for the most current recommendations.

Primary Reference

This fifth edition of *Healthy Young Children: A Manual for Programs* aligns with and contains content adapted with permission from *Caring for Our Children: National Health and Safety Performance Standards; Guidelines for Early Care and Early Education Programs,* 3rd edition, by the American Academy of Pediatrics, American Public Health Association, and National Resource Center for Health and Safety in Child Care and Early Education (Elk Grove Village, IL: American Academy of Pediatrics; Washington, DC: American Public Health Association). References to the scientific evidence supporting the performance standards and guidelines contained in *Caring for Our Children* appear at the end of each of its chapters.

Caring for Our Children is available in print from the American Academy of Pediatrics bookstore at www.aap.org, from the National Resource Center for Health and Safety in Child Care and Early Education at www.nrckids.org, and from the National Association for the Education of Young Children bookstore at www.naeyc.org/store/. It is also available in PDF and HTML formats at www.nrckids.org/CFOC3/.

Credits

Copy editor: *Lisa Cook*
Contributing editor: *Darcie Vugrinovich*
Indexer: *Sherri Emmons*

Cover photographs: Copyright by Ellen B. Senisi

Illustrations: *Dilworth Design*

Editors of Past Editions
1st and 2nd editions: Abby Shapiro Kendrick, Roxane Kaufmann, and Katherine P. Messenger
3rd edition: Karen Sokal-Gutierrez, MD, MPH
4th (2002) edition: Susan S. Aronson, MD, FAAP, with Patricia M. Spahr

Healthy Young Children: A Manual for Programs, Fifth Edition

Copyright © 2012 by the National Association for the Education of Young Children. All rights reserved. Printed in the United States of America.

Library of Congress Control Number: 2012930709
ISBN: 978-1-928896-82-1
NAEYC Item #369

Acknowledgments

The first edition of this manual was funded through an intra-agency agreement between the Administration on Children, Youth and Families; the Division of Maternal and Child Health, U.S. Department of Health and Human Services; and the Massachusetts Department of Public Health, using federal Maternal and Child Health Block Grant funds to the Commonwealth of Massachusetts and to Georgetown University Child Development Center in Washington, DC.

Background

The origin of this manual was a handbook called *Health Power*, written by Hannah Nelson and Susan Aronson, MD, FAAP, for Head Start. Subsequently, Abby Shapiro (then Kendrick) adapted the material for use in Massachusetts and then collaborated with the Georgetown Child Development Center and NAEYC to adapt the material for a national audience. Further revisions and updates were the work of Karen Sokal (then Gutierrez), MD, MPH, and Susan Aronson, MD, FAAP, for the 1995 and 2002 editions respectively. These correspond with the publication of the first and second editions of *Caring for Our Children: National Health and Safety Performance Standards—Guidelines for Out-of-Home Child Care Programs* by the American Academy of Pediatrics and the American Public Health Association, funded by the Maternal and Child Health Bureau, U.S. Department of Health and Human Services, in 1992 and 2002.

> Any undertaking of this magnitude necessarily involves many people with expertise in different areas. NAEYC acknowledges the hundreds of people who have been involved in the preparation of previous editions of *Healthy Young Children*. The Association gratefully acknowledges the American Academy of Pediatrics for its cooperative efforts and permission to quote specified text from *Caring for Our Children*.

Contents

Preface   viii

Chapter 1. This Manual and the Integration of the Health Component into the Early Care and Education Program   2
  Major Concepts   2
  About This Manual   3
  The Purpose of the Child Care Health Component   3
  Suggested Activities   4

Chapter 2. Preventing Infections   6
  Major Concepts   6
  Reassuring Families   7
  Working Together to Reduce the Risk of Infectious Disease   7
  1. Prevent Infections from Spreading   7
  2. Require Certain Immunizations and Routine Health Supervision Services   13
  3. Report Some Illnesses   14
  4. Exclude Some Children and Staff Members for Illness   14
  5. Prepare—Don't Wait Until an Outbreak Occurs!   16
  Diseases Spread through the Respiratory Tract   17
  Diseases Spread through the Intestinal Tract   19
  Diseases Spread by Direct Contact or Contact with Surfaces with Germs on Them   21
  Infectious Diseases Spread through Blood   22
  Vaccine-Preventable Diseases   24
  Noncontagious Infectious Diseases   26
  Notification of Exposure to Communicable Diseases   27
  Controlling the Spread of Infection through Cleaning, Sanitizing, and Disinfecting   27
  The Role of Ventilation, Temperature, and Humidity in Resistance to Infectious Disease   31
  Staff/Child Turnover and Infectious Disease   32
  Suggested Activities   32

Chapter 3. Preventing Injuries   34
  Major Concepts   34
  Program Planning for Safety Inside the Facility   35
  Safety Beyond the Classroom   41
  Special Safety Tips for Infants and Toddlers   47
  Supervision   51
  Safety Education and Hazard Checks   51
  Suggested Activities   52

Chapter 4. Ready for Emergencies and Injuries   54
  Major Concepts   54
  Prepare for Emergencies   56
  Getting Help   57
  Emergency Evacuation   58
  Closings Due to Power Failure or Natural Catastrophe   59
  Security and Handling Persons Who Pose Security Risks   60
  Suggested Activities   62

Chapter 5. Promoting Health with Good Nutrition   64
  Major Concepts   64
  The Nutrition Consultant   65
  Obesity   65
  National Standards and Recommendations for Nutrition in Early Care and Education Programs   66
  General Approaches to Eating   67
  Feeding Infants   69
  Feeding Toddlers and Preschool-Age Children   74
  Feeding School-Age Children   75
  Basic Nutrition Facts   75
  Food Habits Are Learned: Nutrition Education   75
  Food Safety   78
  Activity and Physical Exercise Affect Appetite   79
  Common Nutritional Concerns   79
  Dietary Guidelines for Young Children   85
  Community Nutrition Resources   85
  Running a Food Service   85
  Storing Nonfood Supplies   87
  Cleaning and Caring for Equipment   87
  Insect and Rodent Control in Food Areas   87
  Suggested Activities   87

Chapter 6. Promoting Health with Physical Activity   88
  Major Concepts   88
  National Standards for Physical Activity for Children in Group Care   89
  Assessment of Children's Nutrition and Physical Activity   91
  Playing Outdoors   91
  Teachers' Views of Active Play   92
  Encouraging and Modeling Physical Activity   93
  Physical Activity for Children with Asthma   94
  Structured Physical Activities   94
  Suggested Activities   94

Chapter 7. Promoting Health through Oral Health, Mental Health, and Health Education   96
  Major Concepts   96
  Oral Health   97
  Mental Health   101

Health Education for Children, Staff Members, and Families   106
Suggested Activities   109

Chapter 8. Medical Care—Clinical Health Services for Children   110
Major Concepts   110
Health Care   111
Assessing Health Status   113
Tracking and Advocating for Preventive Health Care   120
Communicating with Families   123
Suggested Activities   124

Chapter 9. Staff Members and Consultants for Safe and Healthy Child Care   126
Major Concepts   126
Program Responsibilities of All Personnel   127
Health and Safety Concerns in Recruiting, Selecting, and Retaining Staff Members   127
Adult Health Needs—Occupational Risks   133
Infectious Disease Risks for Adults   135
When Not to Come to Work   135
Breaks   137
Child Care Health Consultants   138
Suggested Activities   143

Chapter 10. Facility Design and Support Services for Safe and Healthy Early Care and Education   144
Major Concepts   144
Space and Structural Design   145
Equipment and Furnishings   146
Air Quality, Ventilation, Heating, and Cooling   147
Lighting   147
Noise Levels   147
Electrical Items   147
Plumbing   148
Fire Warning and Safety Systems   149
Maintenance of the Facility   149
Transportation   153
Suggested Activities   157

Chapter 11. Caring for Children with Short-Term or Chronic Health Needs or Disabilities   158
Major Concepts   158
The Daily Health Check   159
Care of the Mildly Ill Child   160
Setting Policies for Care of Ill Children   162
Special Considerations for Programs That Do Not Exclude Mildly Ill Children   162
Giving Medication in a Child Care Program   163
Common Illnesses and Chronic Health Conditions   165
Suggested Activities   169

Chapter 12. Inclusion of Children with Special Needs   170
Major Concepts   170
Inclusive Care   171
Benefits of Inclusion   171
How Is Inclusion Carried Out?   173
Inclusive Education: The Individuals with Disabilities Education Act   173
Preparing to Care for Children with Special Needs   175
Modifying an Early Education Program to Accommodate Children with Special Needs   176
Medical Procedures   178
Emergency Planning Considerations for Children with Special Needs   179
Resources to Plan Care for Children with Special Needs   180
Suggested Activities   181

Chapter 13. Child Maltreatment (Abuse and Neglect) and Administration of the Health Component   182
Major Concepts   182
Child Maltreatment (Abuse and Neglect)   183
How Programs Can Help Abused Children and Stressed Families   185
Preventing Maltreatment in Programs for Young Children   187
Administration of the Health Component   190
Suggested Activities   193

Appendices   195
Appendix A. Forms and Checklists   196
Appendix B. Acronyms Used in This Book   230
Appendix C. Links to Internet Resources in This Book   231
Appendix D. Crosswalk of *Healthy Young Children* and NAEYC Early Childhood Accreditation Criteria   233

References   239

Index   240

List of Figures

2.1 Hand Hygiene: The First Line of Defense Against Infectious Diseases, 9
2.2 Handwashing Poster, 10
2.3 Procedure for Changing Diapers, Disposable Training Pants, and Soiled Underwear, 12
2.4 Deciding When a Mildly Ill Child Can Stay, 15
2.5 Conditions/Symptoms Not Requiring Exclusion, 16
2.6 Conditions for Which Temporary Exclusion Is Recommended, 18
2.7 Preventing Exposure to Blood and Body Fluids, 23
2.8 Daily Sanitizing and Disinfecting Solutions, 28
2.9 Clean, Sanitize, Disinfect: What Are the Differences?, 30

3.1 Using Playdough and Other Manipulative Art or Sensory Materials, 40
3.2 How to Choose Art Supplies, 41
3.3 Basic Playground Safety Rules, 42
3.4 Minimum Compressed Loose-Fill Surfacing Depths, 43
3.5 Safe Sleeping for Infants, 49

4.1 Emergency Medical Procedures, 56
4.2 Inventory for First Aid Kits and Emergency Supplies, 57

5.1 Categories of Food Offered, 68
5.2 Guidelines for Storing Human Milk, 71
5.3 Ideas for Nutritious Snacks, 76
5.4 Sources for Nutrition Education, 78
5.5 Dietary Sources of Calcium, 82
5.6 MyPlate Mini-Poster, 84

6.1 Physical Activity Guidelines, 90

7.1 Dental Referral Criteria, 100
7.2 Pyramid Model for Promoting Social and Emotional Competence in Infants and Young Children, 105

8.1 What Early Educators Can Do to Help Families Use a Medical Home, 112

9.1 *Caring for Our Children* Training Standards, 132
9.2 Wise Moves to Avoid Injury in Child Care, 134
9.3 Protect Your Back, 136
9.4 Child Care Health Consultants, 140

10.1 Transportation Safety Rules, 154

11.1 Items to Include in the Daily Health Check, 159
11.2 How to Take a Child's Temperature, 166

12.1 Examples of ADA Information Available, 172

13.1 What Is Child Abuse and Neglect?, 184

A.1 Diapering, 196
A.2 Selecting an Appropriate Sanitizer or Disinfectant, 197
A.3 Routine Schedule for Cleaning, Sanitizing, and Disinfecting, 199
A.4 Sample Letter to Families about Exposure to Communicable Diseases, 201
A.5 Safety Checklist for Active Play Areas, 202
A.6 Incident Report Form, 209
A.7 Emergency Telephone List, 210
A.8 Recommended Daily Meal Patterns for Breakfast and Lunch/Supper, 211
A.9 Weekly Meal Pattern for Regular Snacks, 212
A.10 Behavioral Data Collection Sheet, 213
A.11 Special Care Plan for a Child with Behavioral Issues, 214
A.12 Developmental Health History, 216
A.13 Observation and Symptom Record, 218
A.14 Situations that Require Medical Attention Right Away, 219
A.15 Medication Administration Skills Checklist, 220
A.16 Care Plan for a Child with Special Needs in Child Care, 222
A.17 Adaptive Equipment for Children with Special Health Care Needs, 223
A.18 Recognizing Child Abuse and Neglect: Signs and Symptoms, 225
A.19 Conceptual Model of Child Neglect, 229

Preface

Here, in one convenient manual, you will find answers to many questions about keeping young children healthy when they participate in group programs.

- What are the most effective methods of preventing the spread of disease?
- How do we create a safe and healthful environment to prevent injury and illness?
- What is recommended for routine preventive care for children, and why is it so important?
- How do we help children develop healthful eating habits?
- How do we ensure that children have the amount and type of physical activity they need to prevent obesity and keep their bodies healthy?
- What do we do to prepare for the types of emergencies that might occur?
- How do we inform families about possible exposure to contagious diseases?
- How do we include children with special needs?
- When do we exclude children or adults who are ill from the program? When can they return?
- How do we promote the well-being of adults who are involved with the program?
- How do we prevent and handle suspected maltreatment of children?
- How do we integrate the activities for the health component with all the other tasks involved in operating a quality program?

Healthy Young Children is a manual for teachers, directors of early care and education programs, health professionals who work with programs that care for children in group settings, and other individuals who give technical assistance to early education professionals. The manual is not only a tool for those who work in group care settings but also a guide for those who are preparing to enter the field. It may be used as a textbook to support coursework on this topic. Using the manual will help implement national standards and guidelines for the health component. For those working on accreditation of a center or family child care home, the manual provides information related to compliance with health and safety criteria.

Healthy Young Children: A Manual for Programs was first published by NAEYC in 1988 and has been extensively reviewed and updated. This, the fifth edition, reflects the most current recommendations from health professionals available at the time of writing for keeping children healthy and safe in group care. In many places in the manual, the reader will find links to information posted on the internet. Be sure to use these links, as the internet provides information on companion documents for this manual that may be updated more frequently than print material.

Healthy Young Children is one of a set of resources that early educators will find helpful in integrating health and safety effectively with the child development, administrative, and other components of the program. The manual is compatible with and is an implementation tool for *Caring for Our Children: National Health and Safety Performance Standards; Guidelines for Early Care and Education Programs,* 3rd edition, published in 2011. *Caring for Our Children* is more than a compendium of detailed requirements for care of children in center- and home-based group settings. Its standards document procedures for protecting health and safety, the rationale and implementation strategies for each requirement, and the references to the scientific literature that justify the standard. The extensive appendices provide many useful forms, handouts, and tools.

Caring for Our Children is published collaboratively by the American Academy of Pediatrics (AAP), the American Public Health Association, and the National Resource Center for Health and Safety in Child Care. The work involves many contributors. The National Resource Center is funded by the Maternal and Child Health Bureau of the Health Resources and Services Administration of the U.S. Department of Health and Human Services. The authoring organizations and NAEYC offer the print publication for sale in their respective bookstores. In addition, PDF and HTML versions are available on the website of the National Resource Center for Health and Safety in Child Care and Early Education (www.nrckids.org). Updates to the standards and clarifying comments will appear on this website. Be sure to check the site periodically for notices of updates.

Healthy Young Children contains some information taken directly from *Caring for Our Children*. The fifth edition of *Healthy Young Children* is being published around the same time as the third edition of *Caring for Our Children* so that readers can use these two publications together.

Other tools that will help meet the standards in *Caring for Our Children* include the following:

- A six-videotape series called *Caring for Our Children,* videotaped in 1995 in center- and home-based child care programs across the United States, shows what child care looks like when it meets national standards. Because the series is based on the second edition of *Caring for Our Children,* a few items illustrated in the videos have changed since its publication. For example, new vaccines have been added to the routinely recommended schedule of immunizations that all children and teachers should have. Also, putting infants down to sleep on their backs without soft bedding or toys in their cribs is now required in order to help prevent sudden infant death syndrome (SIDS). Although some new standards and updates are not shown in the video series, most of the information is still useful and appropriate.

- To help programs implement the standards for written health and safety policies in *Caring for Our Children,* the Pennsylvania Chapter of the American Academy of Pediatrics (PA AAP) publishes *Model Child Care Health Policies*. These policies originated from best practice submissions of policies from many child care programs. The Early Childhood Education Linkage System-Healthy Child Care Pennsylvania is the program of the PA AAP that updates this document from time to time. The fill-in-the-blank policy statements provide an easy starting point for programs to customize policy statements to serve their needs. After adapting the model policies that meet national standards to fit a specific facility's characteristics, the site-specific written policies become a useful tool to orient staff members and parents and describe expectations for program operation. At the time of this writing, *Model Child Care Health Policies* is being updated to be released in its fifth edition. It will correspond with standards for written policies in the third edition of *Caring for Our Children*. For online access to the most current edition and ongoing updates of *Model Child Care Health Policies,* go to www.ecels-healthychildcarepa.org.

- To help early educators know how to deal with infectious diseases in group care, the American Academy of Pediatrics publishes *Managing Infectious Diseases in Child Care and Schools: A Quick Reference Guide*. The most recent update of this book, the second edition, was published in 2009. It is based on the AAP's widely used health professional reference book on infectious diseases in children called *The Red Book*. Infectious disease is the most common cause of illness among young children. *Managing Infectious Diseases in Child Care and Schools* demystifies medical jargon and dispels widespread, strongly held misperceptions about what causes these illnesses, how to prevent them, and how to manage them when they occur among children in group care.

The book is largely made up of a set of one- or two-page Quick Reference Sheets about specific types of infectious illnesses. You may photocopy individual sheets to share with parents and staff members when needed. Each Quick Reference Sheet contains a brief description of the condition, the signs and symptoms, the incubation and contagious periods, how the illness is spread, how to control it, the roles of the teacher and the family in managing the illness, when/whether exclusion from group care is needed, when readmission is appropriate if the child is excluded, and comments that provide additional information. The information is in parent- and educator-friendly language.

In addition to the Quick Reference Sheets, the book includes chapters about keeping children healthy, how infection spreads, measures to control infection, teacher health, recognizing a child's illness, the health consultant's role, immunization schedules, outbreaks/epidemics and other infectious disease emergencies, sample letters and forms, and a glossary of terms. The book is available in both e-book and print form from the AAP bookstore (www.aap.org).

- Determining whether records of children's and staff members' vaccines and other health services are up-to-date is a tedious and complex but essential task. Staff members must check records against the recommended schedule for the individual's age and special conditions. Several tools are available to accurately evaluate records. The Centers for Disease Control has tools to look at an individual child or adult record at www.cdc.gov/vaccines. The PA AAP developed a software tool called WellCareTracker™ to track children's preventive care records for both vaccines and routinely recommended screening tests. This tool is described more fully in Chapter 8. To view a demonstration of how it works, go to www.wellcaretracker.org.

These tools are helpful to all who work with children in group care settings—whether full-day or part-day, full-year or part-year; whether in child care centers, preschools, family child care homes, Head Start programs, before- and after-school programs, or other types of group care where families share the responsibility of care and education for their children with trusted teachers.

Note: Throughout this manual, various terms are used interchangeably to refer to programs serving young children ages birth to 8, including *early childhood programs, early care and education programs, child care centers,* and *group care settings.* These and other terms used refer to any program in which young children are cared for and educated in a group setting, including family child care homes.

The term *teacher* is used in this manual to refer to any adult responsible for the direct care and education of a group of children in any early childhood setting. Included are not only classroom teachers but also infant/toddler caregivers, family child care providers, assistants, and specialists in other disciplines who fulfill the role of teacher. The terms *director* and *administrator* are used to refer to professionals with oversight responsibilities for programs.

For Your Convenience

You may copy any part of this manual for staff members, families, health consultants, or community agencies, but be sure to acknowledge the source of the material each time you use it.

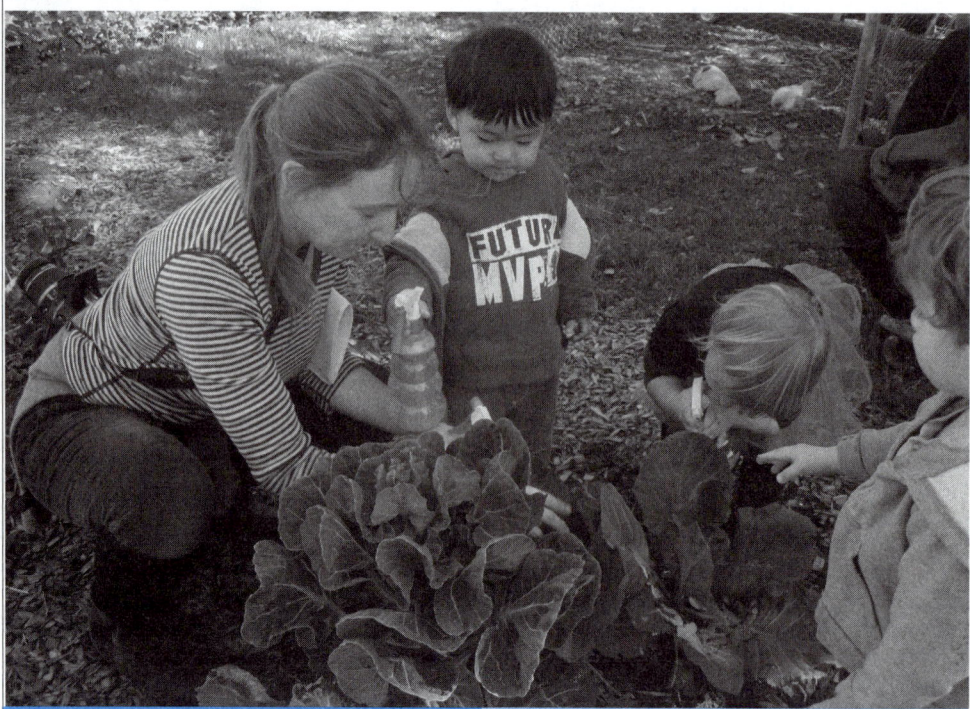

This Manual and the Integration of the Health Component into the Early Care and Education Program

MAJOR CONCEPTS

- Young children need warm, positive, continuous relationships for healthy brain development—the core of service in quality care.
- The role of early childhood educators working in group care programs (center- and home-based) includes prevention of harm to children from known risks and promotion of children's health. This is achieved by ensuring that facilities are safe and healthful and by following practices that meet the physical, medical, nutritional, oral, and social-emotional (mental) health needs of the children and adults involved in the program.
- The highest risks of physical harm to children in group care settings are from injury and infectious disease.
- The health component of child care programs must be carefully planned and integrated with other aspects of the program. Competent performance is facilitated by using written health policies and procedures developed from up-to-date recommendations and use of community resources.
- All staff members and families must understand and work on implementing the child care program's health policies and practices.
- The experiences of children and families in a group care program can lay the foundation for lifelong personal health practices and well-being.

As a program director, teacher, student studying to be a teacher, or other professional working with child care facilities, you must be able to protect and promote the health and well-being of the young children, staff members, and families in the program. You can achieve major health gains by taking simple steps. For example, diligently following hand hygiene procedures (appropriate handwashing or proper use of alcohol-based hand sanitizers) and keeping everyone—children and adults—up-to-date with required vaccines are two strong defenses against the spread of infectious disease. Supporting sustained breastfeeding through at least the first year of life is a preventive health measure now known to have lifelong benefits. Including toothbrushing in the daily routine teaches children a good habit that will protect their teeth throughout life. Frequent safety checks of the site, with corrective actions when necessary, can prevent injuries. Careful, regular observations of children may reveal physical health and social-emotional difficulties that respond best to early treatment. You will find specific information, procedures, and recommendations on each of these topics, as well as on many others, in this manual.

About this manual

This manual is based on national standards. From its first writing through each update, both health professionals and early childhood professionals have reviewed it. The manual is intended as a guide to facilitate collaboration among early childhood educators, health consultants, and family members for implementing currently accepted health and safety standards. The primary reference for this manual is *Caring for Our Children: National Health and Safety Performance Standards; Guidelines for Early Care and Education Programs,* 3rd edition (American Academy of Pediatrics et al. 2011). These guidelines describe the conditions and practices for which sound evidence exists that following the standards will reduce an unacceptable risk of harm. If you find it challenging to meet some of the standards in your program, implement what you can do now. Set targets to address the standards you cannot currently meet. Assess your priorities for avoiding significant risks; don't expect to change everything overnight. To increase the likelihood of changes being successful, plan carefully and thoroughly, involving those who are affected, those with authority, and those with expertise related to the situation.

Some recommendations in *Healthy Young Children* may differ from those in other credible sources. Materials are published and updated in different time periods, drawing on a changing base of information. Also, within the medical and scientific community, some experts differ on specific approaches. When there is a conflict, seek the *rationale* for the recommendations. Sometimes the different approaches are equally acceptable alternatives. Other times, you will have to make the best decision you can after exploring the basis for the differing points of view. If the issue involves technical information, you may want to consult a trusted local expert with the appropriate scientific background. Your state or local department of public health may be able to provide guidance or suggest where to get the help you need.

Healthy Young Children has been used both as a textbook and a guide. To use this manual effectively, read it through at least one time so you become familiar with the contents and grasp the scope of what you need to do to ensure a safe and healthful program. If you are using the manual as a textbook, use the chapters as convenient units, noting that each chapter starts with Major Concepts and ends with Suggested Activities that may help adult learners apply the concepts to real-world experience. There are other published textbooks that are intended for coursework and reference by early educators or by parents. These may be useful if they draw on up-to-date, broadly reviewed expert sources. When such a publication would be particularly helpful on a topic, it is mentioned in the text.

The purpose of the child care health component

Childhood is a unique period of life when physical, intellectual, emotional, and social growth all occur simultaneously and interactively. Children's bodies and minds are constantly learning how to meet challenges in their environment. Research shows that development of the brain (intellectual, cognitive, social-emotional) and children's physical, nutritional, and oral health depend on the quality of early experiences. Children need protection from injury and infection, both of which can lead to discomfort, disability, or death. They also need activities that promote healthy growth and development. Many practices in group care enable learning, promote the development of strong bodies that resist disease, foster brain growth, and support desired behavior simultaneously. Here are some examples:

- Developing warm, positive, continuous relationships between children and caring adults and among children while doing gross motor activities

- Following recommended nutritional practices, such as offering children opportunities to choose among healthful food and beverage choices; involving children in practicing safe and sanitary practices to store, prepare, and serve food; presenting food so children learn to serve themselves and eat appropriate portions; and eating at appropriate times

- Providing sufficient developmentally appropriate and vigorous structured and unstructured physical activity that promotes fitness and enables children to focus better on subsequent learning activities
- Checking and tracking preventive health care services for children and staff members, including:
  - Ensuring that they receive all recommended immunizations to control vaccine-preventable illness so children can be present in the program for learning
  - Obtaining timely recommended screenings to detect and manage health problems to limit disability that can impair learning
  - Maintaining a continuing and trusted relationship with a provider of well and sick health care to reduce illness that can affect health status throughout life
- Following oral health practices to prevent dental illness that can be painful, interfere with speech and nutrition, and reduce social competence

Early educators should plan and implement the health component of their programs to respond to the predictable developmental patterns of young children. As children progress from young infants to toddlers to preschool children to school-age children and then to self-sufficient older children, their needs at each developmental stage will differ. At each developmental level, early childhood professionals must simultaneously function as protectors, role models, and teachers for the children in their care. In addition, they play an important role in children's development by supporting the families of children in their program.

The many hours of contact that teachers have with children can be very influential. Many children remember throughout life their early care and school experiences as well as elements of family life. Children are always learning, growing, and developing, even when they sleep. Healthful routines in the early childhood program can promote this growth and development.

Health and safety are not external patches or optional aspects of programs. Regardless of the limits imposed by funding, staffing, physical, or curricular constraints, the health component should be an integrated part of daily program activity. The health component involves risk management and anticipatory learning for the group. A completely risk-free and infection-proof program is neither possible nor desirable: Children need to experience challenge. Risk *management* involves making choices and finding acceptable alternative approaches so children can experience challenges without significant adverse consequences. While compromise is necessary, usually it is possible to meet the seemingly conflicting objectives of risk management and risk taking.

Suggested activities

- Do a self-assessment of your own health-related behavior. When you are in a hurry or distracted or just busy, do you take risks that you would not consider acceptable if you gave more thought to them? What are those risks? What practices would you change?
- Look at the table of contents for this manual. To which aspects of a child care health component have you given the most attention? To which could you give more consideration? Are there areas that you avoid or emphasize because you find them more or less appealing? Which are these, and why are they more or less appealing to you?
- What references and resources inform your work on health and safety in child care settings? How current are they? How can you determine whether they are authoritative and up to date? Who in your community can you consult as an expert on physical health, nutrition, oral health, and mental health issues?

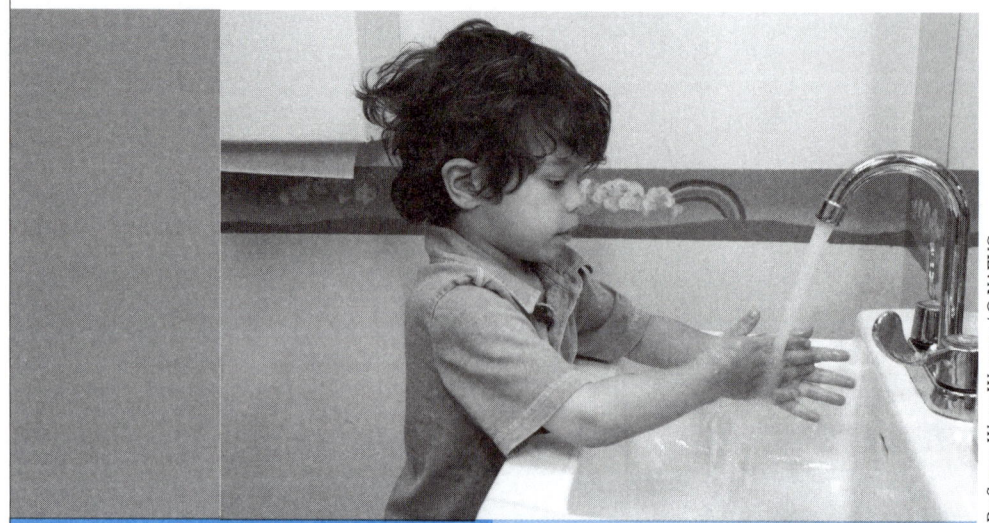

Preventing Infections

MAJOR CONCEPTS

- Child care programs must establish detailed policies to prevent and manage infectious illness.
- Infections are spread by one of three mechanisms: 1) by germ-laden droplets that are carried in the air or left on touched surfaces; 2) by direct contact with body fluids such as saliva and mucus from the mouth, nose, or eyes, urine, feces, blood, and wounds on body surfaces; or 3) through openings made in the body by insects, such as ticks or mosquitoes, or objects that pierce body tissues.
- Always treat body fluids from children, adults, and animals, as well as surfaces that may have been in contact with body fluids, as possibly infectious. You must handle and clean up body fluids carefully.
- Check the health records of children and adults involved with group care upon entry into the program, using the currently recommended vaccine schedules to be sure everyone is up-to-date. Continue to track the records to be sure everyone stays up to date as additional vaccines come due.
- Despite your best efforts, children and adults will get sick; infectious illness is an expected part of life. The early educator's role is to identify illness by carrying out daily health checks during the transition from home to the program and whenever the child seems to be acting ill during the program day, and to take action that will prevent adverse consequences.
- Use the current guidelines from the American Academy of Pediatrics to decide when mildly ill children should or should not be temporarily excluded from group care.
- Take active steps to educate staff members, families, and children about infectious illnesses, techniques to prevent their spread, and proper care of ill children.
- Practice good hand hygiene and cleaning of materials and surfaces. Sanitize and disinfect materials and surfaces in the facility as required to prevent the spread of disease.
- Some necessary sanitation procedures for diapering and toileting in child care settings differ from what parents do at home.
- To keep everyone mindful of needed sanitation and hygiene, someone in the program should be responsible for regular observations of infection control routines to identify opportunities for improvements.

Infectious diseases are illnesses caused by invasion of the body by germs—viruses, bacteria, fungi, or parasites. Some germs are helpful or harmless and only rarely cause disease. Others are more commonly responsible for significant illness. Infectious means capable of causing an infection. Contagious or communicable diseases are infectious diseases that can spread from one person to another.

Concern about infectious disease in child care is an everyday challenge for teachers, parents, and health professionals. When children become ill in a group setting, they may require more attention. They may pass their illnesses on to other children, to adults who work in the program, and to families of other children and workers. Having an infected child is costly and burdensome to families who need group care and for their employers. Family members may miss work days to care for sick children. They may need to arrange for an appointment with health care professionals for diagnosis and treatment. Sometimes parents seek antibiotics or use over-the-counter medicines that are not appropriate in the belief that these drugs might hasten the child's return to group care.

Early educators must follow state regulations about actions to take when a child is ill. However, because regulations may be based on obsolete information, educators may have to manage conflicts between the regulations and current recommendations of national health experts or of the ill child's health care professional.

Reassuring families

At enrollment, families should be informed about the likelihood that their children will have a few more common illnesses than they would if they were cared for at home without contact with other children. (Similarly, siblings in large families have more common illnesses than children who have no siblings.) Every family needs a backup plan to use when the child is too ill to participate or to be cared for in the child's usual group program. As discussed later in the chapter, however, not every child who is ill must be excluded from care. Teachers should advise families that many parents feel guilty about their choice to use group care, especially when their children become ill. This guilt may be aggravated by comments some people make, such as "Your children might not get sick so much if you stayed home to take care of them." While research does show that infants and toddlers have somewhat more frequent infections when they participate in group care, not every infection is attributable to participation in the group care setting. In fact, participation in group care adds only a few episodes to the usual number of illnesses that very young children experience. Families often hear, and are troubled by, comments from health care providers and others suggesting that a particular illness is attributable to group care exposure. Since the germs in the child care setting are the same as those in the community, it is rarely possible to say where the exposure to germs that caused a particular illness occurred.

Illness-causing germs are on surfaces at the grocery store, on restroom door handles, and in many other places. Most of the infectious illnesses they cause are mild, require no medication, and clear up in a short time. Reassure families with young children that the frequency of illness steadily decreases as children grow older. In addition, children build immunity from their experience with minor infectious illnesses. By kindergarten age, those who have been in group care since infancy have fewer illnesses than children cared for only at home.

Exclusion guidelines that apply when children and staff members are ill are discussed in item 4 later in this chapter, as well as in Chapter 9. (See also Standards 3.6.1.1 and 3.6.1.2 of *Caring for Our Children*.)

Working together to reduce the risk of infectious disease

Much can be done to reduce the risk of transmission of infectious disease in group care settings. Teachers, families, and health care providers need to work together to help children avoid preventable illnesses. Occasionally, outbreaks of serious diseases may occur. If precautions are not taken, these serious diseases can spread quickly. Contact the local health department for any condition that might pose a threat to the group or is reportable according to state regulations for infectious disease. (See item 3 later in this chapter.) Sometimes programs receive what seem to be conflicting opinions from different health care providers about how to address a particular health issue. Usually these conflicts are best resolved with the help of the program's child care health consultant. For reportable infectious disease, the health department has the legal authority to make final determinations about what the program must do.

Recommended health practices and policies are essential tools in the management of illness. Written program policies should describe expectations for staff members and families. Even with clear and appropriate written policies, practices must be regularly monitored to ensure that they are followed.

1. Prevent infections from spreading

The germs that cause infections and contagious diseases are spread in three main ways:

> **The Teacher's Five Commandments for Infectious Disease Control**
>
> 1. Prevent infections from spreading with measures that focus on people, germs, and places.
> 2. Require certain immunizations and routine health supervision services.
> 3. Report some illnesses.
> 4. Exclude some children and staff members for illness.
> 5. Prepare—don't wait until an outbreak occurs!

- By germ-laden droplets that are carried in the air or left on touched surfaces
- By direct contact with body fluids such as saliva and mucus from the mouth, nose, or eyes; urine; feces; blood; and wounds on body surfaces
- By insects, such as ticks or mosquitoes, or objects that pierce body tissues

The presence of disease-causing germs does not cause illness in everyone. Infectious diseases occur when vulnerable *people* (hosts) succumb to disease-causing *germs* (agents) in the *places* (environment) where there are enough germs to overcome barriers to infection. The principles involved in reducing the risk of infection thus focus on modifying the hosts, agents, and environment:

- Increase people's resistance to disease-causing germs through measures that foster health and well-being, such as immunization, nutrition, good sleep habits, and physical fitness activity
- Reduce the number of disease-causing germs by ventilating spaces and by cleaning, sanitizing, and disinfecting surfaces and materials
- Modify the places people occupy to reduce their contact with illness-causing germs

Put these principles into action with the following steps.

Increase people's resistance. Use health promotion practices that make children and adults stronger, with better body defenses.

For infants: Encourage breastfeeding of infants enrolled in the program. Although participating in group care settings increases the risk of infections for infants, breastfeeding protects against this increased risk. Any amount of breast milk helps, although exclusive feeding of milk from the mother's breast until 6 months of age is the most beneficial. Therefore, everyone involved with families with infants should encourage and support continued breastfeeding of infants to any extent the mother is willing and able to provide throughout infancy, preferably at least until 1 year of age. Standard 1.1.2.1 in *Caring for Our Children* recommends that, when possible, families with infants wait to enroll their infants in group care until they are at least 3 months of age, for the following reasons: the increased risk of infection to young infants' immature immune systems; the desirability of breastfeeding; and the likelihood that keeping the infant only with the parents during this early period will promote parent-child attachment. The standard expresses a generally desirable goal for minimum age of entry into group care that may not be appropriate for all families. If your program enrolls children younger than 3 months of age, be extra-diligent about practicing infection control, supporting breastfeeding, and fostering parent-child attachment.

Up-to-date immunizations for everyone: Ensure that all adults and children have received the vaccines listed in the national recommendations for their age, condition, and situation. (See item 2 in this chapter.)

Healthful practices: Encourage adults and children to follow practices that help their bodies resist infections. For example,

- Drink enough water, avoid beverages containing sugar, and eat foods and portions recommended for good nutrition. This helps the whole body resist infection better.
- Promote healthy skin through good nutrition, adequate rest, and skin care. Healthy skin and mucous membranes help prevent germs from entering the body, while cracked skin and dry mucous membranes allow entry of germs. Using lotion after handwashing keeps moisture in the skin and reduces cracking, which can result from frequent handwashing.
- Get enough sleep every day to allow time for body tissues to repair, and get recommended amounts and types of exercise.
- Have children practice oral hygiene to keep their teeth healthy and reduce their chances of developing caries (cavities). Teachers should look after their own oral health, too. Caries are the result of an infection by a specific type of bacteria in the mouth, which make acid that destroys the surfaces of the teeth. A parent or teacher usually transmits these germs to a child by kissing the child on the mouth or sharing objects contaminated with the adult's saliva. These germs thrive with frequent eating, especially when foods contain sugar. Oral hygiene helps remove the food that feeds these bacteria and the substance called plaque that the bacteria build up at the gum line. Plaque holds large numbers of bacteria in the mouth. (See Chapter 7 for more about oral health.)

- Be especially vigilant about practicing infection control for those who have special health needs that may make them more vulnerable to infection.

Reduce the number of disease-causing germs. Germs transmit disease to people in three main ways: by droplets carried in the air; by direct contact with surfaces where there are germs; and by insects or objects that pierce the skin, putting germs into the body.

Sneezing and coughing: Teach children and staff members how to sneeze and cough into a tissue, elbow, or shoulder to reduce the spread of their germs carried in the air; (Tissues are rarely handy when a sneeze or cough occurs.) If you see visible body fluid from a cough or sneeze, wash the area and do what you can to prevent others from contact with the fluid until you can launder a fabric article or disinfect a hard surface. When a sneeze or cough is caught by a tissue or by hands, wash those contaminated hands before they touch anything or anyone. Do not save used tissues. Throw the tissue and the germs it contains away!

Spacing children for resting/napping: Most respiratory droplets expelled during breathing, coughing, or sneezing fall out of the air onto surfaces within three feet of the person. Therefore, spacing children at least three feet apart while they rest or sleep helps to reduce the number of germs passed from one child to another. Research shows that a three-foot separation of children and young adults who are sleeping in group settings reduces the spread of infection. A shorter distance is not effective.

Hand hygiene: Hand hygiene at appropriate times is a key tool for controlling the spread of infection by direct contact. Ensuring proper practice of hand hygiene procedures for adults and children reduces both respiratory and diarrhea/vomiting diseases. (See Figure 2.1 for situations in which hand hygiene is necessary.) Handwashing removes soil and germs from the skin that would be transferred into children's or adults' mouth, nose, eyes, or other body openings by touching surfaces that other people have touched and then putting the germs into their body openings with their hands. Antibacterial soap is not necessary and may remove only the weaker germs, making it easier for the more troublesome ones to flourish. Even after wearing gloves to change a diaper or to handle other contaminated materials, hand hygiene is still necessary. Wearing gloves reduces the germ contamination of the skin, but it does not eliminate it. (For details about hand hygiene standards and rationale for procedures, see *Caring for Our Children* Standards 3.2.2.1 through 3.2.2.5. See Figure 2.2 for a handwashing poster to put up over every sink. Keep in mind that lathering the soap helps to loosen soil from surfaces. Finger-nails should be kept short, with no artificial nails or extenders. Jewelry should be simple and kept to a minimum.)

Handwashing is essential for hand hygiene if there is visible soil on the hands. However, as an alternative to handwashing, children over 24 months of age and adults may use alcohol-based hand sanitizers if their hands are visibly clean. Hand sanitizers that do not contain 60–95 percent alcohol are not recommended. When using hand sanitizer, be sure to use the amount recommended by the manufacturer. Rub both hands together to distribute the sanitizer on all hand and finger surfaces. Then let the hands air-dry. Keep the hand sanitizer out of the eyes, nose, and mouth. Supervise children very closely when they are using hand sanitizers and limit children's independent access to containers of this toxic, flammable chemical. Follow the instructions in *Caring for Our Children* Standard 3.2.2.5 for the maximum size and safe placement of hand sanitizer dispensers in

---

Figure 2.1.

Hand Hygiene: The First Line of Defense Against Infectious Disease

Everyone should wash hands at the following times:

a. Upon arrival for the day, after breaks, or when moving from one child care group to another

b. Before and after:
  1. Preparing food or beverages
  2. Eating, handling food, or feeding a child
  3. Giving medication or applying a medical ointment or cream in which a break in the skin (e.g., sores, cuts, or scrapes) may be encountered
  4. Playing in water (including swimming) that is used by more than one person
  5. Diapering*

c. After:
  1. Using the toilet or helping a child use a toilet
  2. Handling bodily fluid (mucus, blood, vomit) from sneezing, wiping and blowing noses, from mouths, or from sores
  3. Handling animals or cleaning up animal waste
  4. Playing in sand, on wooden play sets, and outdoors
  5. Cleaning or handling the garbage

*or changing disposable training pants (such as Pull-Ups) or soiled underwear

Source: Standard 3.2.2.1, *Caring for Our Children*. Reprinted with permission.

Figure 2.2.

Handwashing Poster

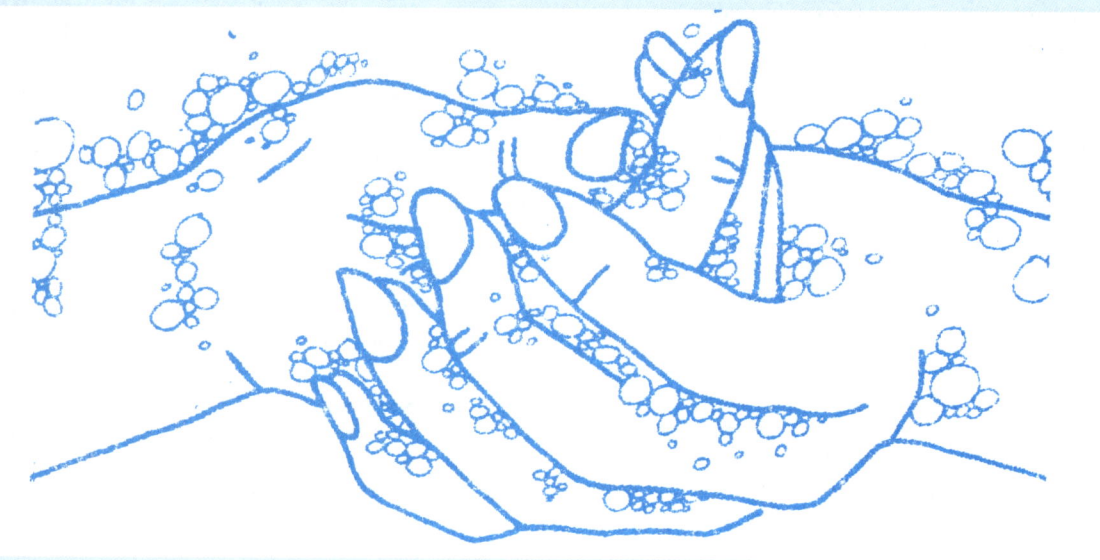

How to wash your hands or children's hands

- Wet hands with clean, running water (warm or cold) and apply liquid or powdered soap.
- Rub your hands together to make a lather and rub them well. Be sure to rub the backs of your hands, between your fingers, and under your nails.
- Try to continue rubbing your hands for at least 20 seconds. Sing a song such as "Happy Birthday" or "Row, Row, Row Your Boat" from beginning to end twice.
- Rinse hands well under running water.
- Dry hands using a fresh paper towel or a single-use cloth towel, or air-dry them.
- If the water does not shut off automatically, leave it running until you can turn it off with the towel used for drying hands.
- Apply hand lotion to prevent excessive drying or cracking of the skin if needed.
- Use the towel or cloth to turn off the water and to open any door that must be touched to leave the sink area.

Notes:
- Do not use antibacterial soap.
- Keep nails short and jewelry simple. No artificial nails.
- You can sing alternate lyrics to the melody of "Row, Row, Row Your Boat": "Wash, wash, wash your hands; sing this handy song. Scrub and rub, rub and scrub. Germs go down the drain!"

child care facilities.

Pre-moistened disposable cleansing cloths do not effectively clean hands. There are only two allowable situations when these disposable cleaning cloths can be used as a substitute for hand hygiene with soap and running water or an alcohol-based hand sanitizer: 1) When changing diapers, disposable training pants, or soiled underwear, you may use a disposable wipe for your hands and the child's hands when all soiled materials have been discarded, and before putting a clean diaper or underwear and clothing on the child. (Hand hygiene with soap and water or alcohol-based hand sanitizer must still be done for the child before returning the child to the group, and for the teacher, after completing the disinfecting step for the changing surface.) 2) If you are out on a trip and handwashing sinks are not available, you can use some pre-moistened disposable cleansing cloths to remove visible soil and then apply hand sanitizer. Follow up with a handwashing sink as soon as one is available.

Animals and vermin: Limit exposure to pets, insects, wild mice, rats, and other vermin that may transmit disease-causing germs to people. Practice Integrated Pest Management (see Chapters

5 and 10) to reduce the risk of exposure to pests using minimally toxic methods. Some pets are not appropriate for early care and education settings because they or their habitat have disease-causing germs that pose risks for young children. Check with a veterinarian or look on the website of the Centers for Disease Control and Prevention (CDC) before bringing any animal into the setting, even just for a visit. (You can browse animal-related diseases at **www.cdc.gov/healthypets/**.)

Insect bites: *Caring for Our Children* Standard 3.4.5.2 addresses the issues related to prevention of insect bites. Some insects transmit infections when they bite. Reducing the risk of insect bites is the first line of defense. When possible, stay indoors at dawn and dusk because these are times of day when disease-carrying insects are most active. Use screens on windows. Eliminate from children's play areas any standing water, fruit trees, and open trash because they attract biting and stinging insects. When children do get insect bites, the swelling of body tissues or scratching may lead to secondary infection by bacteria on the skin. This is a common cause of impetigo—superficial, crusty infections of the skin. In areas where the risk of insect-borne illness is significant, a child's health care professional or public health authorities may recommend use of an insect repellent. DEET (N,N-diethyl-3-methylbenzamide) is the most effective insect repellent; it is safe when used properly, even for very young children. With written parental consent, apply DEET to exposed skin or clothing, but not to skin covered by clothing, following the manufacturer's instructions. The American Academy of Pediatrics (AAP) recommends using concentrations of DEET of not more than 30 percent, and using it only for children over 2 months of age. Concentrations as low as 10 percent are just as effective as 30 percent and typically last two hours. Do not use aerosol products because they produce an easily breathed mist. Handwashing should always be done when returning indoors from outdoors. It will reduce the germs picked up during outdoor play, as well as any insect repellent on adults' and children's hands.

Fresh air: Ventilate all rooms with fresh outdoor air as much as possible. Outdoor air dilutes the germs that are put into the indoor air by individuals who are using the space. If the facility has operable windows, open them whenever the weather permits. Whatever the weather, routinely open the windows to air out the room whenever the room is not being used. Make sure that a certified heating, ventilation, and air conditioning (HVAC) contractor checks the facility's systems to be sure they supply the required amount of outdoor air at recommended temperatures and humidity to each room. (See The Role of Ventilation, Temperature, and Humidity in Resistance to Infectious Disease later in this chapter for further information, and *Caring for Our Children* Standards 5.2.1.1 through 5.2.1.15 for HVAC requirements.) These requirements specify the amount of air circulation per person and the acceptable range of temperature and humidity. The purpose is to maintain environmental conditions that make it easiest for people to resist disease-causing germs.

Safe food handling: Be sure all food is wholesome and is prepared and served using recommended methods to prevent food poisoning. (See Chapter 4.)

Exclusion when it matters: Perform daily health checks and exclude children from the setting when doing so will actually reduce the risk of exposure of others to illness-causing germs. (See Chapter 11 for instructions on performing a daily health check and item 4 later in this chapter.)

Modify the places people occupy to reduce their contact with illness-causing germs. Design, organize, and maintain the setting's space and furnishings to reduce the ways people are likely to be contaminated by disease-causing germs.

Sufficient space for the group: *Caring for Our Children* Standard 5.1.2.1 requires a minimum of 42 square feet of usable floor space (exclusive of space occupied by furnishings) per child. Although many state regulations and NAEYC accreditation criteria specify 35 square feet per child, research-based recommendations are that 42 to 54 square feet per child is best to foster child development, minimize challenging behavior, and reduce infectious diseases (e.g., Olds 2001).

Separate areas: To decrease the spread of germs from one group to another, separate groups of children with full walls that minimize contact between the groups. Separate children in sleeping spaces by three feet, the distance required to prevent the airborne spread of germs when people are lying down. Provide storage that keeps clothing and bedding used by one person from contact with those of another person. Bedbugs and skin infections spread when personal items are improperly stored. If cubbies are too small to completely contain personal articles, hang a bag in each child's cubby to hold them. Provide more than several arm's lengths of distance between food preparation/handling areas and areas and surfaces used for toileting/diapering.

Each room in which diapers, disposable training pants, or soiled underwear are changed should have its own changing area adjacent to a handwashing sink, even when there is a hand sanitizer dispenser. Changing areas should not be shared by more than one group of children to prevent sharing of disease-causing germs across groups.

Skill, practice, and a good setup make it possible to follow the healthful practices recommended for sanitary changing while also using the opportunity to interact with each child one-to-one, fostering warm, positive relationships. Keep supplies off the changing surface, but have them neatly and accessibly stored on open shelves nearby. Occasionally, some extra supplies are needed during the change. They should be in a location that does not require opening cabinet doors to reach them. Everything touched, such as cabinet doors, door handles, and supply containers, will need to be cleaned and disinfected along with the changing surface. (See Figure 2.3. For a tri-fold poster that illustrates the changing-procedure steps, go to **www.ecels-healthychildcarepa.org** and search for "diapering poster." Figure A.1 in Appendix A shows a small-scale version of this poster.)

Choose surfaces wisely: When installing surfaces, carefully select those that people will touch. They should be easy to clean and disinfect.

Recommended cleaning, sanitizing, and disinfecting routines: Use the guidelines in Figures A.2 and A.3 in Appendix A to implement best practices for the maintenance of surfaces in the facility. These routines are discussed later in this chapter.

Art and sensory materials: Follow Standard 5.2.9.8 in *Caring for Our Children,* which specifies appropriate procedures when using handmade or purchased manipulative art and sensory materials.

Figure 2.3.

Procedure for Changing Diapers, Disposable Training Pants, and Soiled Underwear

Step 1: Get organized. Before bringing the child to the diaper changing area, with clean hands, gather and bring the following supplies to the diaper changing area:

a. Non-absorbent paper liner large enough to cover the changing surface from the child's shoulders to beyond the child's feet

b. Unused diaper or clean underwear (and clean clothes if you think you'll need them)

c. Number of wipes needed for cleaning skin, so the wipes container is not on the changing surface and will not be touched during the change

d. A plastic bag for any soiled clothes or cloth diapers

e. Disposable gloves, if you plan to use them (put gloves on before handling soiled clothing or diapers and remove them before handling clean diapers and clothing)

f. If the child uses it, a thick application of any diaper cream (e.g., zinc oxide ointment), when appropriate, removed from the container to a piece of disposable material such as facial or toilet tissue

Step 2: Carry the child to the changing surface, keeping soiled clothing away from you and any surfaces you cannot easily clean and disinfect after the change. Decide whether you intend to change the child lying down or standing up. Changing a child standing up makes the caregiver assume an awkward position. Also, it is difficult to control contamination and clean the child's skin in a standing position.

a. Always keep a hand on the child.

b. If the child's feet cannot be kept from contact with soiled skin or materials during the changing process, remove the child's shoes and socks so the child does not contaminate the shoes and socks with stool or urine during the change.

c. To avoid contaminating the child's clean clothes, push the clothing up well above the child's waist. If possible, have the child hold the shirt, sweater, etc. up during the change. This keeps the child's hands busy and allows the caregiver/teacher to know where the child's hands are during the changing process.

Step 3: Clean the child's buttocks and genitalia with wipes.

a. Unfasten the diaper, tear open the sides of soiled Pull-Ups, or carefully remove soiled underwear. For a supine diaper change, leave the soiled diaper under the child.

b. If safety pins are used, close each pin immediately once it is removed and keep pins out of the child's reach. (Never hold pins in your mouth.)

c. Lift the child's legs as needed to use disposable wipes to clean the skin on the child's genitalia and buttocks and prevent recontamination from any soiled surface. Remove stool and urine from front to back and use a fresh wipe each time you swipe. Put the soiled wipes into the soiled diaper or directly into a plastic-lined, hands-free covered can.

Step 4: Remove the soiled materials without contaminating any surface not already in contact with stool or urine.

a. Fold the soiled diaper, Pull-Ups, or underwear inward.

b. Put soiled disposable diapers or Pull-Ups in a covered, plastic-lined, hands-free covered can. If reusable cloth diapers or cloth underwear is involved, put the soiled cloth items and their contents (without

2. Require certain immunizations and routine health supervision services

All children and adults in your program should be immunized against vaccine-preventable diseases recommended for their age unless they are exempted because of a contraindication for a health condition or another legal exemption. Information about which vaccines children and adults have received should appear on their health assessment information from their health care provider. (See Chapter 8 for a discussion of routine preventive care for children. See Chapter 9 for a discussion of routine information that child care programs should have on hand for adults who work in the facility. A suggested Child Care Staff Health Assessment form appears in both *Model Child Care Health Policies* and Appendix E of *Caring for Our Children*.)

Annually, the CDC, the AAP, and the Academy of Family Practice jointly publish a new schedule of recommended vaccines on the CDC website (**www.cdc.gov/vaccines**). Health exemptions to certain vaccines include having an immune deficiency condition as a congenital disease, as the result of an infection such as AIDS, or as a side effect of immunity-suppressing medications used for cancer treatment or to prevent rejection of a tissue transplant. Some vaccines are not recommended during pregnancy or during the time someone is moderately to severely ill. Legal exemptions vary from state to state. In addition to contraindication for a health condition, in some states, legal exemptions

---

emptying or rinsing) in a plastic bag or into a plastic-lined, hands-free covered can to give to parents/guardians or laundry service.

c. If gloves were used, remove them using the proper technique (and put them into a plastic-lined, hands-free covered can).

d. Whether or not gloves were used, use one disposable wipe to clean the surfaces of the caregiver/teacher's hands and another wipe to clean the child's hands, then put the wipes into the plastic-lined, hands-free covered can. If hand sanitizer is used, allow sanitized hands to dry completely before proceeding.

e. Check for spills under the child. If there are any, use the paper that extends under the child's feet to fold over the soiled area so a fresh, unsoiled paper surface is now under the child's buttocks.

Step 5: Put on any diapering cream (if used), then the clean diaper, Pull-Ups, or underwear, and dress the child.

a. Use a facial or toilet tissue or wear a clean disposable glove to apply any necessary diaper creams, discarding the tissue or glove in a covered, plastic-lined, hands-free covered can.

b. Note and plan to report any skin problems such as redness, skin cracks, or bleeding.

c. Fasten the diaper or pull on new Pull-Ups or underwear. If pins are used for a diaper, place your hand between the child and the diaper when inserting the pin.

Step 6: Wash the child's hands with soap and running water and return the child to a supervised area.

a. Use soap and warm water, between 60° F and 120° F, at a sink to wash the child's hands, if you can. If the child cannot safely wash hands at a sink, then use a paper towel wet with soap and water, followed by a paper towel wet with water, then another dry towel to perform the child's hand hygiene.

Step 7: Clean and disinfect the changing surface.

a. Dispose of the disposable paper liner used on the changing surface in a plastic-lined, hands-free covered can.

b. If clothing was soiled, securely tie the plastic bag used to store the clothing and send it home.

c. If there is any visible soil on the changing surface, remove it with a disposable paper towel saturated with water and detergent, and then rinse the surface with water.

d. Wet the entire changing surface with a disinfectant that is appropriate for the surface material you are treating. Follow the manufacturer's instructions for use.

e. Put away the disinfectant. Some types of disinfectants may require rinsing the changing table surface with fresh water afterward.

Step 8: Perform hand hygiene and record the diaper or underwear change in the child's daily log.

In the daily log, record what was in the diaper, Pull-Ups, or soiled underwear and any problems (e.g., a loose stool, an unusual odor, blood in the stool, or any skin irritation), reporting as necessary.

Source: Adapted from Standards 3.2.1.4 and 3.2.1.5, *Caring for Our Children*. Reprinted with permission.

may include religious or philosophical objections to immunization.

Staff members and volunteers who do not have a health exemption should be immune by vaccination or show evidence of immunity by prior infection or laboratory testing. People who choose not to receive recommended vaccines place not only themselves at increased risk of significant disease but also others around them who are underimmunized by age or health condition. Individuals who are not immunized or who are underimmunized gain protection from having most of the others around them fully immunized. Young children require multiple doses at specified intervals of many vaccines to achieve sufficient levels of protective immunity; until they receive every dose, they are among those who must rely on full immunization of the people around them. Recommended vaccines protect a high proportion of, but not all, people who receive them. Some people still get the disease, but their illness is less severe than it would be otherwise. A small number of people do not respond to a particular vaccine sufficiently to be protected. Protection from vaccines often wanes as people grow older. That is why booster doses are important. For more details about specific vaccines, see the section about Vaccine-Preventable Diseases later in this chapter.

3. Report some illnesses

Every state has laws requiring early childhood programs to report the occurrence of certain infectious diseases to the state's public health authorities. The CDC and state health departments maintain a list of "notifiable diseases." Sometimes called "reportable diseases," these are conditions for which public health authorities need timely information when someone has the health problem so they can institute measures to prevent and control disease. The list of notifiable diseases varies from state to state. Contact your local health department for the current list. *Be sure to include this list and a reporting procedure in your facility's health policy.* Even though the health care facility that makes the diagnosis is required to report to the state, group care programs should report to the state promptly when a child has a disease on the state's list to make sure that public health authorities can take appropriate action to protect others in the group.

For some diseases (e.g., hepatitis and meningitis), any occurrence must be reported to health authorities. Other diseases must be reported when an *outbreak* occurs—that is, when two or more children or adults involved in the program become ill. Generally, an *epidemic*—a large number of cases in a short period—should be reported, even if the disease is not on the list of notifiable diseases. For example, outbreaks of flu, mononucleosis, the rapid spread of severe conjunctivitis, or pneumonia should be reported promptly so public health authorities can offer advice about preventing additional cases. All programs should have a written plan for seasonal and pandemic influenza that includes: approaches for coordination among program staff members, families, and public health authorities; infection control policies and procedures; communication procedures; and maintenance of child learning and program operations.

Special reporting requirements usually exist for illnesses caused by consumption of contaminated food. Food-borne illness is very common. Data collected by federal agencies show that, annually, one in every six people becomes sick enough from contaminated food to generate a public health report. The number of unreported cases is probably much higher. Suspect food contamination if a number of staff members and children experience stomach cramps, vomiting, diarrhea, and/or dizziness, and report the situation to your local health department.

4. Exclude some children and staff members for illness

Contrary to popular belief and practice, only a *few* illnesses require sick children and staff members to be sent home ("excluded") to protect other children and staff members. Children and adults in group care settings are exposed to one another all the time. The signs and symptoms of illness usually appear only after the germs causing the illness have been shed for days before the person seems sick. So before someone has any symptoms, other people have already been exposed to that person's disease-causing germs. With few specific exceptions, programs do not need to exclude a mildly ill child with normal behavior who is able to participate and does not need excessive attention that would interfere with the care of the other children. (See Figure 2.4 for criteria to determine whether an ill child can stay. See Figures 2.5 and 2.6 for lists of illnesses that do not require exclusion and that do require it.)

The criteria for exclusion depend on the circumstances that staff members assess. Families should know that the staff members have the final say about whether a child may be included or must be excluded from the group.

With the same exceptions that apply to children, staff members who are well enough to perform their role as expected do not need to be excluded. As with the decisions regarding exclusion of children, someone should be designated to decide when a staff member who wants to work needs to be excluded for illness. For guidelines about when those who are excluded for illness may return, see Chapter 11.

Early childhood programs should avoid unnecessary exclusion of mildly ill children whenever possible. Exclusion of ill children forces parents to make alternative arrangements on short notice; many take their ill children to work or leave them in make-do arrangements. These alternate arrangements may be less appropriate than the ill child's group care setting. As indicated above, for many illnesses, children have already exposed others before becoming obviously ill and therefore do not need to be excluded because of the risk of contagion. However, when a child's illness meets the criteria for exclusion, then the family will need to use a preplanned, alternative care arrangement.

When the child comes to the program each day, use the daily health check procedure described in Chapter 11 to quickly gather information on the child's health status and, if necessary, decide whether the child should remain. If the child develops symptoms after the parent leaves, then a new health check is necessary to make the decision about what to do and to tell the parent about the change in the child.

The most common symptoms that young children experience are those of the respiratory tissues: runny nose; cough; eye irritation; and difficulty breathing. Fever and diarrhea occur much less frequently than respiratory symptoms. With the exception of untreated lice and ringworm, for which exclusion for treatment is not required until the end of the day, the specific conditions listed in Figure 2.6 require that parents be asked to remove the child from care as soon as possible. In the meantime, the ill child should receive appropriate care in an area where the child will not expose individuals not already exposed.

Become familiar with Appendix A: Signs and Symptoms Chart in *Caring for Our Children* and the Quick Reference Sheets in *Managing Infectious Diseases in Child Care and Schools: A Quick Reference Guide* (Aronson & Shope 2009). Each of the Quick Reference Sheets gives a succinct, easy-to-understand summary for a specific symptom or diagnosis. The book gives permission to copy the Quick Reference Sheets and distribute them to families and staff members. These resources make clear not only when to exclude a child or staff member, but also when the child can return based on symptoms, treatment, or evidence that the child is no longer contagious. Also see Figure A.13 for a sample form that programs can use to document children's symptoms and any care the child received at home or in the child care facility.

In general, most conditions do not require a doctor's note to return. Doctors determine when the child is able to return by asking whether the parent thinks the child is acting normally. A doctor's note is useful to provide instructions when the child or adult needs continued special care or arrangements while in the group

> **Figure 2.4.**
> **Deciding When a Mildly Ill Child Can Stay**
> A mildly ill child does **NOT** need to be excluded from the setting if all of these criteria are met:
> 1. The child is behaving normally.
> 2. The illness does not prevent the child from participating comfortably in the program's activities, as determined by the teacher.
> 3. The illness does not cause a greater need for care than the teachers can manage without compromise to the care of other children in the group.
> 4. The child does not have a specific condition that is likely to expose others to a communicable disease. (See list of excludable conditions/diseases.)

setting, or when the individual has a type of bacterial diarrhea for which a report of negative cultures must be obtained from a clinician before the child or adult returns.

Programs should have a plan for the care of a child who is ill while the child remains in the program. For more detailed discussion about what programs need to do to care for ill children, see Chapter 11.

Sound science provides the rationale for why some conditions that were commonly reasons for excluding children in the past do not actually require exclusion. For example, pink eye—or conjunctivitis—may be caused by allergies, irritants, a scrape injury of the eye, bacteria, or viruses. By far the most common cause is that the lining or membrane of the eye, called the conjunctiva, is irritated by a viral infection in the same way that the lining of the nose can be irritated. The irritated membrane drips fluid that changes to a thick discharge as the body sheds the secretions and debris from the body's fight to get rid of the infection. Use good hand hygiene to help prevent spread of this type of infection. The common cold and most episodes of conjunctivitis will get better without antibiotic treatment. Children with pink eye generally feel less ill than those with a cold. Programs do not exclude for the common cold and do not need to exclude for pink eye unless the other general criteria for exclusion are met. Unless the child cannot participate or requires an amount of care that precludes appropriate care for the other children, children who have pink eye with thick green or yellow discharge may remain in care. One form of viral conjunctivitis, caused by an adenovirus, can cause epidemics. If two or more children in a group care setting develop conjunctivitis in the same period, seek the advice of the program's health consultant.

Children who are carriers of viral illnesses such as cytomegalovirus (CMV), hepatitis B, or HIV infection

Figure 2.5.

Conditions/Symptoms Not Requiring Exclusion

- Common colds, runny noses (regardless of color or consistency of nasal discharge)
- A cough not associated with an infectious disease (such as pertussis) or a fever
- Watery, yellow, or white discharge or crusting eye discharge without fever, eye pain, or eyelid redness
- Yellow or white eye drainage that is not associated with pink or red conjunctiva (i.e., the whites of the eyes)
- Pink eye (bacterial conjunctivitis) indicated by pink or red conjunctiva with white or yellow eye mucus drainage and matted eyelids after sleep. Parents/guardians should discuss care of this condition with their child's primary care provider, and follow the primary care provider's advice. Some primary care providers do not think it is necessary to examine the child if the discussion with the parents/guardians suggests that the condition is likely to be self-limited. If two unrelated children in the same program have conjunctivitis, the organism causing the conjunctivitis may have a higher risk for transmission, and a child health care professional should be consulted.
- Fever without any signs or symptoms of illness in children who are older than six months regardless of whether acetaminophen or ibuprofen was given. Fever (temperature above 101° F [38.3° C] orally, above 102° F [38.9° C] rectally, or 100° F [37.8° C] or higher taken axillary [armpit] or measured by an equivalent method) is an indication of the body's response to something, but is neither a disease nor a serious problem by itself. Body temperature can be elevated by overheating caused by overdressing or a hot environment, reactions to medications, and response to infection. If the child is behaving normally but has a fever of below 102° F per rectum or the equivalent, the child should be monitored, but does not need to be excluded for fever alone.
- Rash without fever and behavioral changes
- Lice or nits (exclusion for treatment of an active lice infestation may be delayed until the end of the day)
- Ringworm (exclusion for treatment may be delayed until the end of the day)
- Molluscum contagiosum (do not require exclusion or covering of lesions*)
- Thrush (i.e., white spots or patches in the mouth or on the cheeks or gums)
- Fifth disease (slapped cheek disease, parvovirus B19) once the rash has appeared
- Methicillin-resistant Staphylococcus aureus, or MRSA, without an infection or illness that would otherwise require exclusion. Known MRSA carriers or colonized individuals should not be excluded.
- Cytomegalovirus infection
- Chronic hepatitis B infection
- Human immunodeficiency virus (HIV) infection
- Asymptomatic children who have been previously evaluated and found to be shedding potentially infectious organisms in the stool. Children who are continent of stool or who are diapered with formed stools that can be contained in the diaper may return to care. For some infectious organisms, exclusion is required until certain guidelines have been met. Note: These agents are not common and teachers will usually not know the cause of most cases of diarrhea.
- Children with chronic infectious conditions that can be accommodated in the program according to the legal requirement of federal law in the Americans with Disabilities Act. The act requires that child care programs make reasonable accommodations for children with disabilities and/or chronic illnesses, considering each child individually.

Source: Standard 3.6.1.1, *Caring for Our Children*. Reprinted with permission.

*At the time of this printing, the AAP recommends that lesions be covered by clothing or bandage when possible.

---

should not be excluded. These diseases can be present without symptoms, so the precautions for handling body fluids to prevent the spread of these diseases must be used for everyone all the time.

See Chapter 11 for how to handle situations when your program allows mildly ill children to attend. See Chapter 9 for more about staff health.

5. Prepare—Don't wait until an outbreak occurs!

Do some advance planning. Use the following summary to review necessary steps:

- Help families plan ahead for how they will handle illnesses that will inevitably arise.
- Review inclusion/exclusion criteria with families,

clarifying that program staff members will make the final decision about whether ill children whose families want them to remain at the facility may do so.

- Develop procedures for handling child illness, including care plans and establishing designated individuals who will use the inclusion/exclusion criteria to make final decisions.

- Insist that staff members learn and follow guidelines for hand hygiene, cleaning/disinfection, and ventilation all the time, but especially during spring, fall, and winter, when illness seems more common.

- At least annually, provide creative, attention-getting reminders for all staff members, children, and families about hand hygiene, cough and sneeze control, and the need to obtain influenza vaccine each fall.

- Choose a health consultant who knows about infectious disease in early childhood settings.

- Prominently post telephone numbers of local and state departments of public health.

- Make sure children's immunizations are up-to-date before you admit them. Keep track of when children are due for their next immunization and remind families to get these important protections. If an outbreak of a vaccine-preventable disease does occur, you will need to be able to immediately identify children who are fully immunized and those who are not protected—either because they are not old enough to have received all their doses or because their families have not obtained the recommended vaccines for them.

- Staff members also should be up-to-date on their immunizations to protect themselves and the children. Keep track of staff members' protection from vaccine-preventable disease just as you do for the children.

- Make sure families recognize their responsibility for obtaining advice about their sick child from their usual source of health care and for reporting a contagious illness to you. Do not assume that parents will read all the material you give them. Review health procedures orally at enrollment in addition to sending an annual letter to all families. Describe each of your health policies and ask parents to do the following:
  - Call or email your program when a child is ill.
  - Call or email if a clinician makes a specific diagnosis (e.g., strep throat) or provides a specific treatment.
  - Tell your program *immediately* if the child is hospitalized or treated for a serious infection, such as *Haemophilus influenzae* type b (Hib) or meningococcal disease.
  - Keep the child at home if she has an excludable illness, until the exclusion criteria no longer apply. Require a note from a health professional only if the child has a need for special care in the facility or there is a genuine concern about whether the child's condition poses a risk to others. A note from a health professional to readmit a child who seems well to the parents is not necessary otherwise.
  - Call and discuss whether their children should attend when they have mild illness.
  - Inform the program of any changes in emergency numbers where parents can be reached promptly at any time during the day.

- *Be watchful!* Learn to look for signs of infectious disease. Call or send a note home if you suspect a health concern.

- Inform staff members and parents of any contagious disease to which they or their children might have been exposed so they can watch for symptoms and alert their own health care professionals about the exposure.

Diseases spread through the respiratory tract

Respiratory tract diseases include the common cold, pink eye, sore throat, croup/laryngitis, bronchiolitis/bronchitis, and pneumonia. They are spread through microscopic infectious droplets of the nose, eyes, or throat. Most droplets are shared via hand contact of infected individuals, who get their infected fluids on their hands and then touch surfaces that uninfected people subsequently touch. Some germs are spread by airborne droplets from infected people's sneezes and coughs. These droplets infect a healthy person through contact with mucus membranes of the eyes, nose, and mouth. With few exceptions (e.g., chickenpox), most germs can travel on airborne droplets that fall onto nearby surfaces within three feet. This may be why separating children by three feet for sleeping reduces the spread of infection. Having fewer than three feet between resting children, using partitions that are not floor-to-ceiling, or putting solid crib ends against each other does not stop this airborne spread.

People touch their hands to their mouths, noses, and eyes all day long—usually without washing first. Each time they touch their mucus membranes with contaminated hands, they allow the germs they have picked up from touched surfaces to invade their bodies. Diseases that enter the body through the respiratory tract range from mild (e.g., viral colds and strep throat) to life threatening (e.g., bacterial meningitis).

Some diseases are more common or more frequent in children than in adults. For example, while the common cold affects people of all ages, infants and toddlers cared for only at home usually have six to eight of these viral respiratory infections per year, and those in group care have seven to nine. Among adults, the average is four colds per year.

Figure 2.6.

Conditions for Which Temporary Exclusion Is Recommended

Temporary exclusion is recommended when the child has any of the following conditions:

- The illness prevents the child from participating comfortably in activities.
- The illness results in a need for care that is greater than the staff can provide without compromising the health and safety of other children.
- An acute change in behavior—this could include lethargy/lack of responsiveness, irritability, persistent crying, difficult breathing, or having a quickly spreading rash
- Fever (temperature above 101° F [38.3° C] orally, above 102° F [38.9° C] rectally, or 100° F [37.8° C] or higher taken axillary [armpit] or measured by an equivalent method) and behavior change or other signs and symptoms (e.g., sore throat, rash, vomiting, diarrhea). An unexplained temperature above 100° F (37.8° C) axillary (armpit) or 101° F (38.3° C) rectally in a child younger than four months should be medically evaluated. Any infant younger than two months of age with any fever should get urgent medical attention.
- Diarrhea is defined by watery stools or decreased form of stool that is not associated with changes of diet. Exclusion is required for all diapered children whose stool is not contained in the diaper and toilet-trained children if the diarrhea is causing soiled pants or clothing. In addition, children with diarrhea should be excluded if the stool frequency exceeds two or more stools above normal for that child, because this may cause too much work for the teachers. Readmission after diarrhea can occur when diapered children have their stool contained by the diaper (even if the stools remain loose) and when toilet-trained children are continent. Special circumstances that require specific exclusion criteria include the following:
    - Toxin-producing *E. coli* or *Shigella* infection, until stools are formed and the test results of two stool cultures obtained from stools produced twenty-four hours apart do not detect these organisms
    - *Salmonella* serotype Typhi infection, until diarrhea resolves. In children younger than five years with *Salmonella* serotype Typhi, three negative stool cultures obtained with 24-hour intervals are required; people five years of age or older may return after a 24-hour period without a diarrheal stool. Stool cultures should be collected from other attendees and staff members, and all infected people should be excluded.
- Blood or mucus in the stools not explained by dietary change, medication, or hard stools
- Vomiting more than two times in the previous twenty-four hours, unless the vomiting is determined to be caused by a non-infectious condition and the child remains adequately hydrated
- Abdominal pain that continues for more than two hours or intermittent pain associated with fever or other signs or symptoms of illness
- Mouth sores with drooling unless the child's primary care provider or local health department authority states that the child is noninfectious
- Rash with fever or behavioral changes, until the primary care provider has determined that the illness is not an infectious disease
- Active tuberculosis, until the child's primary care provider or local health department states child is on appropriate treatment and can return
- Impetigo, until treatment has been started
- Streptococcal pharyngitis (i.e., strep throat or other streptococcal infection), until twenty-four hours after treatment has been started
- Head lice until after the first treatment (note: exclusion is not necessary before the end of the program day)
- Scabies, until after treatment has been given
- Chickenpox (varicella), until all lesions have dried or crusted (usually six days after onset of rash)
- Rubella, until six days after the rash appears
- Pertussis, until five days of appropriate antibiotic treatment
- Mumps, until five days after onset of parotid gland swelling
- Measles, until four days after onset of rash
- Hepatitis A virus infection, until one week after onset of illness or jaundice if the child's symptoms are mild or as directed by the health department. (Note: immunization status of child care contacts should be confirmed; within a fourteen-day period of exposure, incompletely immunized or unimmunized contacts from one through forty years of age should receive the hepatitis A vaccine as post exposure prophylaxis, unless contraindicated.) Other individuals may receive immune globulin. Consult with a primary care provider for dosage and recommendations.
- Any child determined by the local health department to be contributing to the transmission of illness during an outbreak

Source: Standard 3.6.1.1, *Caring for Our Children*. Reprinted with permission.

Young children do not wash their hands before and after touching their nose, eyes, or mouth. They have constant physical and oral contact with objects around them, increasing opportunities for the spread of disease. As a result, respiratory tract diseases spread easily when they are in group settings.

How to stop spread of respiratory tract diseases

- Handwashing, use of alcohol-based hand sanitizers, and hygiene measures that reduce the number of germs on surfaces are essential to stop the spread of all respiratory tract diseases.
- Do not allow children to share food while eating.
- Follow the requirements in *Caring for Our Children* Section 3.2 and in Figure A.3 in Appendix A to determine which objects must be cleaned only or, when clean, sanitized or disinfected. Figure A.2 in Appendix A explains the definitions of sanitizing and disinfecting and gives some helpful instructions about selection and necessary use of chemicals that are least toxic yet effective. *Caring for Our Children* Appendix L gives specific instructions for what to do when cleaning up body fluids.
- Wash eating utensils carefully in hot soapy water; then sanitize and air-dry them. Whenever possible, clean and sanitize utensils and other food service items in a dishwasher that uses a chemical or hot-water sanitizing method. Hot-water sanitizing methods are relatively inexpensive, easy to use, and generally effective. However, they require using a booster heater to raise the temperature of water from safe handwashing temperatures to sanitizing temperatures. The exposure to heat may make some equipment wear out faster. The time required for hot-water sanitizing depends on the temperature of the water: immersion for at least 30 seconds at 170° F (77° C); a final rinse temperature of 165° F (74° C) in single tank, single temperature dishwashing machines; and 180° F (82° C) for other machines. Many state regulations require a utensil surface temperature of 160° F (71° C), measured by an irreversible registering temperature indicator in the dishwashing machine.
- Use disposable paper cups whenever possible. The environmental impact and labor cost of using disposables compares favorably with using reusable cups that must be cleaned and sanitized after each use. Paper cups are sanitary and more environmentally friendly than plastic or foam disposables.
- Air out the rooms daily with fresh, outdoor air, even in winter. Have a heating and ventilation contractor check to see whether any closed, filtered air exchange system is turning over the recommended volumes of air per hour for the type of activity and occupancy in each space. Open windows whenever possible to maximize ventilation.
- Allow children to play outdoors as often as possible. The concentration of germs outdoors is much less than in closed spaces.
- Because coughs and sneezes often come too quickly to cover the mouth and nose with a tissue, teach children and staff members to cough or sneeze toward their shoulder or elbow. If someone sneezes or coughs into a tissue or hand, properly dispose of the tissue and wash hands.
- Wipe runny noses and eyes promptly, dispose of the used tissue, and wash hands afterward.
- Use disposable towels and tissues. If your program prefers single-use cloth towels and handkerchiefs, these will need to be laundered (which will have a consequent labor and environmental impact).
- Dispose of towels or tissues contaminated with nose, throat, or eye fluids in a hands-free covered container with a plastic liner. Keep waste cans away from food and classroom materials. Teach children to drop tissues into the waste receptacle and not to poke around in waste cans.

Diseases spread through the intestinal tract

These diseases are caused by viruses, bacteria, or parasites that multiply in the intestines and pass out of the body in the stool. Anyone can catch these diseases, and some can be caught repeatedly. Programs that care for children in diapers or children who are not able to successfully use a flushing toilet all the time are especially at risk because staff members and children get some fecal material on their hands. When infectious stool gets on hands or objects, people who fail to wash before touching other surfaces, their mouths, or food swallow the germs or transfer the germs to others who swallow them. Swallowing as few as 10 *Shigella* or *Giardia* germs can cause intestinal tract illness. *Salmonella* and *Campylobacter* germs must be swallowed in larger quantities to cause illness. Other bacteria, viruses, and parasites that cause diarrhea enter the body when an individual touches contaminated surfaces and then gets the germs into food or directly into the mouth.

Pinworms are commonly occurring, small threadlike worms that live in the large intestine and cause itching and irritation around the anal and vaginal area. They are not dangerous, but they can easily spread in families and group care settings. Pinworms are spread by eggs on shared toys, bedding, clothing, toilet seats, and other touched surfaces. The eggs remain viable for two to three weeks outside the body. The eggs that an infected person leaves on surfaces can infect or reinfect others. Keeping children's personal items separated helps prevent diseases like pinworms from spreading. If storage spaces are not large enough for this separation, use a hanging bag to contain each child's articles.

Children or staff members with disease-causing germs in their stool may not act or feel sick or have diarrhea. Laboratory tests are the only way to tell if a particular stool has these germs. Tests are sometimes done as part of an effort to control an outbreak of disease, but they are not routine when a child is ill with diarrhea or vomiting.

In cases of infectious diarrhea, or infections with hepatitis A, notify parents, staff members, and the program's health consultant. Be sure to notify your local health department about infectious diarrhea from reportable types of germs and hepatitis A, too. (Refer to your local reporting requirements.)

How to stop spread of intestinal tract diseases

Because children and staff members who have intestinal tract diseases don't always feel sick or have diarrhea, the best method for preventing the spread of disease is to have a constant prevention program in place. Take these precautions:

- Insist on frequent, thorough hand hygiene for both staff members and children before any activity that involves food or touching the mouth, and whenever contact with stool may have occurred. Handwashing is best, but staff members and children over 24 months of age may use alcohol-based hand sanitizers if their hands are visibly clean (see Figures 2.1 and 2.2).

- Insist on general cleanliness and sanitizing. (See detailed information on hygiene, cleaning, sanitizing, and disinfecting, including procedures for diapering and changing soiled underclothing, in Sections 3.2 and 3.3 of *Caring for Our Children*.)

- Separate children into three groups whenever possible—infants, older diapered children, and children who use the toilet reliably. Try to have a staff member work with only one group to avoid carrying germs from group to group. (Note: Because this type of grouping may not meet a particular program's administrative or child development needs, directors often consider a variety of factors when grouping children and assigning staff. If mixing staff members and child groups is necessary, minimize the number of people involved and emphasize careful hand hygiene when moving from group to group and within mixed groups.)

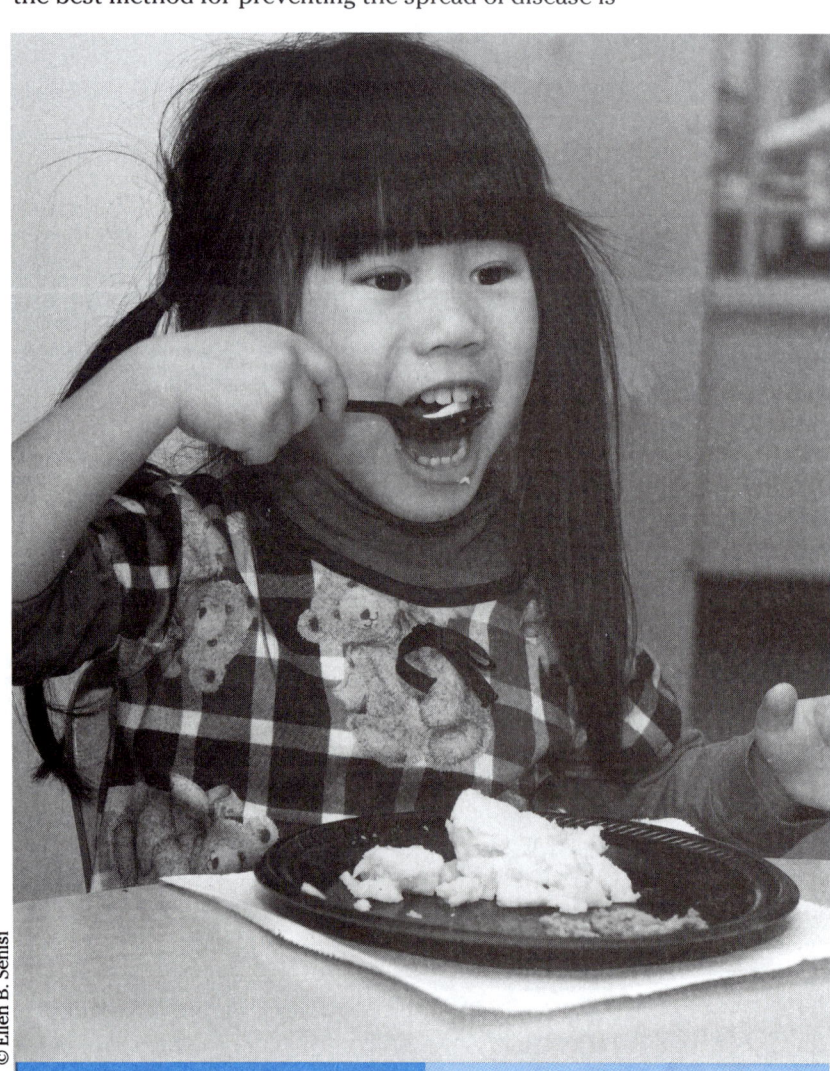

© Ellen B. Senisi

Infectious diarrhea—*Giardia, Shigella, Salmonella, Campylobacter,* and viruses and parasites

People have diarrhea when they have more frequent stools than normal for them and their stools are loose, watery, and unformed. Diarrhea can occur from non-infectious causes, such as drinking excessive amounts of fruit juice, eating more than usual amounts of certain foods, having a disease that makes it difficult for the body to absorb nutrients (e.g., a food allergy or food intolerance), toxins in spoiled foods, or using some medications. Note that infants who are not yet eating solids normally have unformed and frequent stools.

The only sure way to tell whether diarrhea is infectious is by a stool culture. Routine stool cultures identify bacterial causes. Cultures for viruses are usually done only in the investigation of outbreaks or special studies.

In general, stool cultures are done when diarrhea is *bloody* or *persistent* (lasting more than four or five days). If a child or adult has diarrhea that is bloody or persistent, or more than one person in a group develops diarrhea at the same time, the health care providers of the involved children and adults, and the public health department, should be asked to investigate the cause and advise the program about whether the diarrhea is infectious.

Special precautions for diarrhea

- *Strictly enforce* all hand hygiene, diapering, toileting, and cleaning procedures.
- *Exclude* children with diarrhea that is not explained by a change of diet or use of medication and who have 1) two or more stools above their normal frequency or 2) diarrhea not contained in the diaper or toilet without accidents. The rationale for excluding children who have two or more stools above their normal frequency is that such frequent need to be changed or use the toilet may cause more work for the staff members than they can provide while maintaining sanitary conditions.

How to stop spread of infectious diarrhea

- Follow hand hygiene and surface sanitation procedures.
- Keep track of the number of cases of diarrhea, and when *two or more* people in the program have diarrhea, ask the health department or your health consultant to determine what additional steps are necessary.

Diseases spread by direct contact or contact with surfaces with germs on them

Superficial infections and skin infections—impetigo, ringworm, scabies, and head lice—are caused by bacterial, viral, or fungal infections or parasites. They are common and usually are not serious. They are spread by direct contact with infected secretions, infected skin areas, or infested items. Because young children constantly touch their surroundings and their teachers, these infections can spread easily among children and teachers. The direct-contact method of disease spread is illustrated in these examples:

- A child with oozy sores on her arm brushes against a playmate. A small amount of ooze gets on the playmate's arm and into a cut or scratch on his skin.
- Two children huddle over a project. A louse on the head of one child crawls onto the head of the other child.
- A child with a runny nose handles a toy. Another child later handles the toy, rubs his eyes, and puts his finger into his nose or mouth. The second child develops a runny nose, cough, and eye discharge.

How to stop spread by direct contact or contact with surfaces with germs on them

Follow these hand hygiene, cleaning, and sanitation guidelines:

- Make sure staff members and children thoroughly wash their hands and/or use alcohol-based hand sanitizer after contact with any possible infectious material. (See Figure 2.1.)
- Always use disposable tissues or towels for wiping and washing. Single-use cloth towels are acceptable as long as they are placed in a hands-free container after they are used and then laundered before being used again. The environmental impact of doing that much laundry should be weighed against that of using disposable paper towels.
- Never use the same tissue or towel for more than one child.
- Dispose of used tissues and paper or single-use cloth towels in a lined and covered hands-free container that is stored away from food and classroom materials. Be sure children do not go into the container to retrieve objects.
- Clean all toys and other surfaces and objects (e.g., toys, tables, counters, floors, linens, etc.) following the guidelines in Figure A.3 in Appendix A; then sanitize or disinfect those surfaces for which the extra step is required.

Each child should have his own crib or mat and never switch unless all surfaces are cleaned first. Sheets and mats should be kept clean and stored so that sleeping surfaces do not touch each other.

Do not allow children to share personal items, such as combs, brushes, blankets, pillows, hats, or clothing, without cleaning them before use by another child. Do not allow children's stored clothing or bedding to touch. If storage cubbies or hooks are too small or too close together, use a large laundry bag to store each child's articles separately. Store each child's dirty clothing separately in plastic bags and send it home for laundering. Plastic bags should be inaccessible to children to avoid suffocation.

Promptly wash and cover sores, cuts, and scrapes. Report rashes, sores, and severe itching to the child's parents so they can consult their child's usual source of health care.

Cytomegalovirus (CMV), herpes simplex virus (HSV), human papilloma virus (HPV), and sexually transmitted diseases (STDs), such as human immunodeficiency virus (HIV)

These infections are caused by direct contact. CMV is transmitted by contact with saliva and urine. HSV, HPV, and STDs are most commonly spread through skin and mucous membranes. People with these infections may experience no symptoms, mild illness (e.g., cold sores or skin warts), or a total body illness. Anyone can get these infections and can carry the germs in their body secretions for months or years and not experience symptoms. Transfer occurs when germs get on skin that is broken, cut, or scraped, or on mucous surfaces such as the inside linings of the mouth, eyes, nose, rectum, or sex organs. A mother can pass on infection to her newborn infant.

How to stop the spread of these infectious diseases

Assume that all body secretions are potentially contagious and take these preventive actions:

- Insist that staff members and children practice proper procedures for hand hygiene, especially after any contact with blood, saliva, urine, stool, skin sores, or genital secretions.
- Make sure that staff members and children place disposable items that are contaminated with body secretions (e.g., diapers, tissues, bandages, paper towels) in a hands-free, covered container lined with a disposable plastic bag and kept away from food and other materials. Children should not retrieve objects from or touch the inside of the waste container.
- Store clothing and other personal items contaminated with body secretions separately in plastic bags, and send them home for laundering.
- Wash and disinfect all surfaces contaminated with body secretions or blood. Clean mops, rags, and towels properly. Disinfect or dispose of them after contact with blood.
- Do not allow sharing of personal items (e.g., toothbrushes, washcloths, teething rings).

Infectious diseases spread through blood

Hepatitis B and HIV/AIDS are two serious viral infections that can be spread when infected blood comes in contact with a broken surface of a mucus membrane (such as the inside lining of the mouth, eyes, nose, rectum, or sex organs). This can also happen when the skin is accidentally or intentionally punctured by a contaminated needle. An infected mother can pass on a virus to her child during pregnancy or childbirth or by breastfeeding. Once these viruses enter a body, they may stay for months or years. An infected person may appear to be healthy but can spread the virus.

How to stop the spread of infectious diseases transmitted through contact with blood and other potentially infectious body fluids

Although the spread of disease does not always occur on contact with blood or body fluids, *you should treat all contact with blood and body fluids as if these fluids might cause infection*. People can be infected by contaminated materials or contact with body fluids, such as nasal discharge, feces, blood, drainage from sores or wounds, and urine on materials such as tissues, toilet paper, soiled diapers, bandages, soiled clothing, and surfaces in the facility. Cuts and scrapes are the usual sources of blood spills in child care settings. Biters do not usually have bleeding gums that can transfer blood to someone they are biting. When one child bites another, it rarely draws blood from the bitten child into the mouth of the biter. If bleeding occurs, it usually happens after the biter's mouth is no longer in contact with the bitten child. No case of transmission of HIV by biting in child care has been reported. Hepatitis B spread by biting is unlikely because most children have received the hepatitis B vaccine.

Teachers are subject to OSHA regulations for handling anything that might involve contamination with blood. OSHA uses the term "Universal Precautions" to describe the measures that the CDC calls "Standard Precautions." OSHA can impose heavy fines on any employer who fails to comply with OSHA regulations. These regulations include having written policies, procedures, and training about the procedures to manage exposure to blood-borne pathogens, and steps to make sure staff members follow the procedures. Compliance with all of these requirements must be documented. Regional OSHA offices can provide interpretation of the requirements. Find your regional OSHA office at **www.osha.gov/html/RAmap.html/** or in the telephone directory with other federal offices.

Cleaning up of body fluids needs to be done carefully. Because you cannot know what germs are in any fluid from any person, be sure that as few people as possible handle contaminated items. Do all you can to separate people and places involved with handling body fluids and those associated with handling food. Follow the Standard Precautions described in Figure 2.7. (See also Appendix L: Cleaning Up Body Fluids in *Caring for Our Children*.)

Do *not* rinse or wash soiled cloth diapers or clothing at the child care facility. Place the soiled items in a plastic bag, close it tightly, label it with the child's name, keep it out of the reach of children, and ask the family

Figure 2.7.

Preventing Exposure to Blood and Body Fluids

Child care facilities should adopt the use of Standard Precautions developed for use in hospitals by the Centers for Disease Control and Prevention (CDC). Standard Precautions should be used to handle potential exposure to blood, including blood-containing body fluids and tissue discharges, and to handle other potentially infectious fluids.

In child care settings:

a) Use of disposable gloves is optional unless blood or blood-containing body fluids may contact hands. Gloves are not required for feeding human milk, cleaning up of spills of human milk, or for diapering.

b) Gowns and masks are not required.

c) Barriers to prevent contact with body fluids include moisture-resistant disposable diaper table paper, disposable gloves, and eye protection.

Caregivers/teachers are required to be educated regarding Standard Precautions to prevent transmission of blood-borne pathogens before beginning to work in the facility and at least annually thereafter. Training must comply with requirements of the Occupational Safety and Health Administration (OSHA).

Procedures for Standard Precautions should include:

a) Surfaces that may come in contact with potentially infectious body fluids must be disposable or of a material that can be disinfected. Use of materials that can be sterilized is not required.

b) The staff should use barriers and techniques that

1) Minimize potential contact of mucous membranes or openings in skin to blood or other potentially infectious body fluids and tissue discharges.

2) Reduce the spread of infectious material within the child care facility. Such techniques include avoiding touching surfaces with potentially contaminated materials unless those surfaces are disinfected before further contact occurs with them by other objects or individuals.

c) When spills of body fluids, urine, feces, blood, saliva, nasal discharge, eye discharge, injury or tissue discharges occur, these spills should be cleaned up immediately, and further managed as follows:

1) For spills of vomit, urine, and feces, all floors, walls, bathrooms, tabletops, toys, furnishings and play equipment, kitchen countertops, and diaper-changing tables in contact should be cleaned and disinfected as for the procedure for diaper changing tables in Standard 3.2.1.4, Step 7.

2) For spills of blood or other potentially infectious body fluids, including injury and tissue discharges, the area should be cleaned and disinfected. Care should be taken and eye protection used to avoid splashing any contaminated materials onto any mucous membrane (eyes, nose, mouth).

3) Blood-contaminated material and diapers should be disposed of in a plastic bag with a secure tie.

4) Floors, rugs, and carpeting that have been contaminated by body fluids should be cleaned by blotting to remove the fluid as quickly as possible, then disinfected by spot-cleaning with a detergent-disinfectant. Additional cleaning by shampooing or steam-cleaning the contaminated surface may be necessary. Teachers should consult with local health departments for additional guidance on cleaning contaminated floors, rugs, and carpeting.

Before using a disinfectant, clean the surface with a detergent and rinse well with water. Facilities should follow the manufacturer's instruction for preparation and use of disinfectant. For guidance on disinfectants, refer to Appendix J: Selecting an Appropriate Sanitizer or Disinfectant.

If blood or bodily fluids enter a mucous membrane (eyes, nose, mouth), the following procedure should occur. Flush the exposed area thoroughly with water. The goal of washing or flushing is to reduce the amount of the pathogen to which an exposed individual has contact. The optimal length of time for washing or flushing an exposed area is not known. Standard practice for managing mucous membrane(s) exposures to toxic substances is to flush the affected area for at least fifteen to twenty minutes. In the absence of data to support the effectiveness of shorter periods of flushing, it seems prudent to use the same fifteen-to twenty-minute standard following exposure to blood–borne pathogens.

Source: Standard 3.2.3.4, *Caring for Our Children*. Reprinted with permission.

to launder the items at home. Keep changes of clothing handy. Place soiled disposable diapers in a tightly covered, hands-free lidded container that is lined with a disposable plastic bag.

As indicated in Figure A.3 in Appendix A, the program needs to have a routine to clean (wash and rinse) and sanitize all mouthed toys before they pass from one child to another. One easy way to manage mouthed toys is to put a soiled toy into a dishpan labeled SOILED on a counter when the child is no longer using it. Use a diluted solution of dishwashing detergent and water for soaking. These toys should be thoroughly cleaned and sanitized by the end of the day. If toys are dishwasher-safe, use a dishwasher that meets the requirements of the public health authorities as explained in *Caring for Our Children* Standard 4.9.0.11. Other toys can be washed by hand, rinsed, and sanitized by spraying them with or soaking them in a bleach solution. (See Controlling the Spread of Infection through Cleaning, Sanitizing, and Disinfecting in this chapter for concentration of bleach for different applications.)

Because of the time required for household/domestic dishwashers to complete a full wash, rinse, and dry cycle, these dishwashers are recommended for centers that do only one load of dishes after a snack or meal. Some centers may be required by the local regulatory health agency to use commercial dishwashers. These wash in a few minutes, operate at low water temperatures (140–150° F) to be energy efficient, and are equipped with automatic detergent and sanitizer injectors. When choosing a dishwasher, consult the local health authority or the program's nutrition consultant to ensure that the equipment and procedures meet requirements.

Group care programs should not own anything that cannot be washed in a dishwasher, by hand, or in a laundry machine. Allow such an item only if it is a child's personal belonging that will not be shared. Adequate numbers of toys should be available to correspond with the washing frequency.

Label all toothbrushes and children's personal items. Make sure they are used only by their owners and that objects such as toothbrush bristles do not touch any surface other than the child's mouth.

Avoid carpets in areas used by children. While carpets can help reduce the level of noise, they absorb moisture from infectious body fluids and are difficult to clean and sanitize. Where rugs are needed, use those with nonslip backing that are of a size that staff members can remove and wash often. Do not use carpets or rugs in toilet, diaper-changing, or food-handling areas. Follow the procedure for cleaning carpets that are contaminated by body fluids outlined in Appendix L of *Caring for Our Children*. Routinely shampoo or steam-clean wall-to-wall rugs at least every six months or when otherwise soiled.

Vaccine-preventable diseases

Before specific immunization programs were instituted, diseases such as measles, mumps, rubella, polio, pertussis (whooping cough), diphtheria, tetanus, Hib, chickenpox, pneumococcus, and rotavirus-caused infant/toddler diarrhea were major causes of severe illness. While it is true that many people caught and recovered from some of these now vaccine-preventable diseases, experiencing only some discomfort, others suffered permanent complications or died. Prior to the development of the corresponding vaccines, many people thought getting these diseases was inevitable.

Some people believe that these diseases are no longer a problem in the United States and that children cannot get them anymore. Others worry about children having to receive so many vaccines. However, these diseases still occur, particularly in non-immunized or inadequately immunized children and adults. The amount of exposure to the material in the vaccine is minuscule compared with the amount of foreign material in the environment to which the body is exposed every day. Vaccines enable people to make protective antibodies that prevent severe disease when the body encounters the germs after being immunized. When skeptical parents withhold vaccines from their children, the incidence of these diseases predictably increases.

Group programs are especially at risk because some children may be too young to be fully immunized and because the close contact occurring in the group allows easy spread of any infectious disease. Programs with staff members born after the late 1950s are at particular risk because this age group does not have natural immunity from having caught some of the diseases during childhood. Immunity wanes without boosters from exposure to the germ in the environment or vaccine boosters. So, throughout life, people need immunization to help their bodies respond to an exposure that, without a vaccine, would make them sick.

How to stop spread of vaccine-preventable diseases

Make sure all children and adults who are involved with group care in any way are immunized as completely as possible for their age. Detailed up-to-date information about immunization schedules and individual vaccines is available at **www.cdc.gov/vaccines**.

Among the recommended vaccines for children from birth to 7 years of age are those that prevent tetanus, diphtheria, pertussis (whooping cough in children, bronchitis in adults), deep tissue infections (e.g., meningitis, cellulitis, and abscess) from Hib bacteria, pneumococcal bacteria (e.g., ear infections, meningitis, and pneumonia), polio, hepatitis B, rotavirus (diarrhea in infants), varicella (chickenpox), measles, mumps, rubella, and influenza. Children 7 to 18 years of age need catch-up and booster doses for some vaccines given at younger ages. In addition, the meningococcal vaccine and human papilloma virus vaccine are recommended for children 11 to 12 years of age. Thereafter, people of all ages should continue to receive annual influenza vaccine and booster doses of certain vaccines.

Two vaccines deserve special emphasis, pertussis (whooping cough) and influenza. All adolescents and adults should receive Tdap, a vaccine in use since 2005. In addition to boosting immunity to diphtheria and tetanus, Tdap vaccine protects the recipient and the children with whom they come in contact against pertussis infection. The pertussis germ causes prolonged bronchitis in adults and whooping cough in children. Pertussis is highly contagious, even before any symptoms appear. People who have the pertussis germ in their airways easily spread the germ to young children, causing severe and sometimes fatal cases of whooping cough. All adults should receive a dose of the Tdap vaccine, even if they recently received a tetanus and diphtheria vaccine booster.

Influenza vaccine is especially important for those who are involved in group care (although the vaccine is recommended for everyone) because young children not only share the disease-causing virus with their peers in group care but also with their families and others in their community. Influenza is a debilitating and potentially lethal disease. It can sicken people for months and kills thousands every year, even people who keep themselves fit and otherwise healthy. Group care programs are a key source of spread of influenza throughout the community. The yearly modified influenza vaccine protects not only the person who receives it but also infants younger than 6 months of age. Although these young infants are among those most likely to get severe influenza, they must wait to receive influenza vaccine until 6 months of age when their immune systems mature sufficiently to benefit from this immunization. After 6 months of age and until 8 years of age, children need two doses the first time they receive flu vaccine to get a sufficient response from their immune systems. Thousands of deaths from influenza occur annually that could have been prevented by use of the vaccine. The CDC reports that, each year, an average of 20,000 children younger than 5 years of age are hospitalized because of flu-related complications. Modern influenza vaccine may cause mild illness in a few recipients. However, it is much better to get the vaccine than the disease.

Some vaccines that were once optional are recommended for everyone now. Therefore, some adults may lack immunity to vaccines that all young children receive routinely. For example, all young children should receive hepatitis B and hepatitis A vaccine. OSHA requires that employers offer hepatitis B vaccine at no cost to anyone who is not already immune and who, as part of a work role, may have contact with someone else's blood. Teachers of young children are expected to provide first aid for minor bloody injuries, so they should receive hepatitis B vaccine.

Too often, immunization schedules are delayed or disrupted because of illness or missed appointments for well-child checkups. Such children must receive makeup immunizations. Those who start immunization after 12 months of age follow a special schedule that may involve fewer doses, with specified intervals between doses. Consider the risk of exposure to the other children in the group when you accept a child into the program or allow participation by an adult who is not immunized as recommended. Misperceptions about the safety of vaccines have been promoted widely by people whose claims are not backed by medical research. Some parents believe these false claims and choose not to give their children some or all of the recommended vaccines. A program that does not exclude children or adults who have not received nationally recommended vaccines by choice rather than because of a medical contraindication may have legal liability if someone in the program develops a vaccine-preventable disease. Check with an attorney before you accept this risk. For their own protection, children or adults who lack vaccines for medical reasons should be excluded from the facility if an outbreak of that disease occurs in the group care. Note how *Caring for Our Children* handles this sensitive topic in Standard 7.2.0.2:

> The parent/guardian of a child who has not received the age-appropriate immunizations prior to enrollment and who does not have documented medical, religious, or philosophical exemptions from routine childhood immunizations should provide documentation of a scheduled appointment or arrangement to receive immunizations. This could be a scheduled appointment with the primary care provider or an upcoming immunization clinic sponsored by a local health department or health care organization. An immunization plan and catch-up immunizations should be initiated upon enrollment and completed as soon as possible...."
>
> Comments: ... Vaccine Safety and Parental Choice—Some parents/guardians question the safety of routinely recommended vaccines. Sometimes they choose not to have their children fully vaccinated or to delay particular vaccinations. Unfortunately, this leaves the unimmunized child at risk for serious diseases and puts other children and teachers who spend time with the unimmunized child at risk. Illness and death from vaccine-preventable diseases, including whooping cough and measles, have occurred in communities where there are unimmunized children who spread these diseases.

Vaccines are tested to establish safety and effectiveness before they are licensed by the U.S. Food and Drug Administration (FDA). The ACIP, a non-Federal advisory committee, makes evidence-based recommendations to the Centers for Disease Control and Prevention (CDC) following review of all data before a new vaccine is recommended. ACIP is one of many reputable sources of information. The Committee on Infectious Diseases makes evidence-based vaccine recommendations to the board of directors of the AAP. There are biased, inaccurate sources of vaccine information which are not based on evidence and often can confuse parents. . . .

Three sources of accurate information about immunizations are shown below. Each of the sites provides additional sources of information.

a. **www.aap.org/immunization/about/ programfacts.html**—CISP provides education and resources for parents/guardians and pediatricians on immunizations.

b. **www.cdc.gov/vaccines/**—This CDC site provides information for health care professionals and parents/ guardians about all aspects of immunization including vaccine recommendations, understanding vaccines and their purpose, vaccine misconceptions, and answers to commonly asked questions about vaccines.

c. **www.immunizationinfo.org**—The mission of the National Network for Immunization Information (NNii) is to provide the public, health care professionals, policy makers, and the media with up-to-date, scientifically valid information related to immunization to assist with understanding the issues so that informed decisions can be made.

Because the national schedule of recommended vaccines for children and adults is complex, using a software program or other tool will help educators keep track of vaccine records accurately. The CDC has online tools at **www.cdc.gov/vaccines** to look at an individual's record. (Scroll to the box titled Tools/Software, then select Instant Childhood Scheduler or Adult Immunization Scheduler.) Remember that the current online CDC Adult Immunization Scheduler may not take into account some vaccines recommended for adults who work in group care settings for children. Check with the public health authorities in your area to find out what vaccines are currently recommended for adult child care workers. Some states have tools that use the dose-counting method to assess childhood vaccine records. These tools may not be consistent with the current national schedule because they include only the vaccines that the state pays for, because their updating of regulations lags behind updated recommendations from national experts, or because they fail to account for the needs of a child who did not receive vaccines exactly according to the recommended schedule.

Because children need many vaccines in early childhood, a child who is up-to-date when he is admitted to group care may become due or overdue for vaccines later. In addition to checking at admission, tracking for necessary vaccine updates must be done throughout the period a child remains enrolled. Although this is a tedious task, it is necessary to ensure the safety of children in group care. Checking and tracking up-to-date status in education settings will continue to be necessary until there are community-wide vaccine-tracking registries that have follow-up capacity. These exist in some areas of the country now.

Computer software is available that uses the current recommended schedule for vaccines and screening test recommendations, and takes into account all the variations in intervals between vaccines and age at starting a particular vaccine series. Because the recommended schedules are complex, using computer software is more accurate than using dose-counting to check vaccine records or trying to use the national routine recommended schedule for well-child services to check records by hand. Educators need to determine whether a child should be referred to a health care provider to fill gaps in the child's care. Any such software program must be kept up to date as recommendations change.

The Pennsylvania Chapter of the American Academy of Pediatrics (PA AAP) developed a software tool called WellCareTracker™ to reduce the burden on programs of assessing the preventive care records of all the children in the group—both for vaccines and for routinely recommended screening tests. If screening tests are not administered as recommended, undetected conditions can make a child more vulnerable to infections. To learn more about WellCareTracker and view a demonstration of how it works, go to **www.well caretracker.org**.

Commercial software programs for use by early educators may claim to check health record data. However, they usually require software to be installed on the user's computer and lack built-in automatic, no-cost updates that compare preventive care records against currently recommended national schedules. (For more discussion about assessment of preventive health services for screening evaluations in addition to vaccines, see Chapter 8.)

Noncontagious infectious diseases

Some infectious diseases caused by bacteria, viruses, fungi, or parasites do not spread easily from person to person. Two of these noncontagious infections—otitis media (middle ear infection) and candida (yeast infection)—occur in young children. Tick-borne and mosquito-borne infections also can occur. Rocky Mountain spotted fever and Lyme disease are both caused by ticks that are now found in most of the United States. Infectious diseases that are carried by mosquitoes cause types of illness specific to a region of the country.

Otitis media (middle-ear infection)

Otitis media is an infection of the part of the ear behind the eardrum. There is a small passageway (the eustachian tube) from inside the throat to this middle ear. Bacteria and/or viruses can travel from the throat area through the eustachian tube to the middle ear and cause an infection. When infection occurs, pus develops, pushes on the eardrum, and causes pain and often fever. Sometimes the pressure is so great that the eardrum bursts, and the pus drains out into the ear canal. Although this can frighten a parent, the child feels better when the ear drains, and the hole in the eardrum usually will heal.

The biggest problem from otitis media is the potential for hearing loss. Fluid may remain in an ear for as long as six months after an infection is gone. This is called serous otitis media. Research suggests that children who have short-term hearing loss related to ear infections do not suffer long-term cognitive delays. Nevertheless, being unable to hear well is socially and intellectually challenging for children. The child's doctor will test the child's hearing and decide when it is necessary to remove the fluid.

Ear infections are less frequent among children who have received the pneumococcus vaccine. The majority of ear infections are caused by viruses that are not affected by antibiotics at all. Overuse of antibiotics has led to antibiotic-resistant infections—sometimes life-threatening ones. When an ear infection occurs in infants or young toddlers, health care professionals may prescribe antibiotics. For older children, watchful waiting with use of pain medication may resolve the problem in the same amount of time as would occur with antibiotics, with the added benefit of avoiding antibiotic therapy that contributes to the development of antibiotic-resistant germs.

Because ear infections themselves are not contagious, there is no reason to exclude a child with one unless she cannot comfortably participate in the program or requires more care than staff members can offer without compromising the care of the other children.

Special care notes to prevent ear troubles

- Never use cotton swabs or put anything smaller than your finger into a child's ear. Do not allow the child to do so, either.
- Do not bottle-feed or feed solids to infants who are lying on their backs. In that position, it is easier for the food or milk (along with mouth germs) to come in contact with the opening of the passageway from the throat to the ear (eustachian tube) and cause a middle-ear infection.
- Be especially alert for any sign of hearing or speech issues. If one is suspected, refer the child to the child's usual source of health care or to the local early intervention program.

Special care notes for children who have ear tubes

- An ear tube creates a hole in the eardrum so fluid and pus may drain out and not build up. The tube usually stays in for three to six months before the problem resolves and the tube falls out.
- Because pus can drain out, water from the outside (which has germs in it) can also run into the middle ear. Therefore, be very careful that children with tubes do not get water in their ears. This usually means no swimming unless the child uses special precautions to prevent water from getting into the ear and a doctor has granted permission for swimming.
- Watch for any sign of hearing or speech issues.

Notification of exposure to communicable diseases

Inform staff members and families about exposure to communicable diseases. Figure A.4 in the Appendix provides a sample letter to families. Use it with the Quick Reference Sheets about specific types of infectious diseases from *Managing Infectious Diseases in Child Care and Schools*. If there is no Quick Reference Sheet for a particular condition or diagnosis, have a health professional—preferably your child care health consultant—obtain the information for your program to complete the form as needed. Make this information available to staff members as well. One online source for up-to-date fact sheets about infectious diseases (not specific to the child care setting) is **www.cdc.gov**.

Controlling the spread of infection through cleaning, sanitizing, and disinfecting

Many programs for young children cannot totally control their environment. Some spaces are rented and were not designed to meet children's needs. Even so, there are ways to improve the space. As you work toward ideal conditions, establish policies to control the spread of infectious diseases and maintain a healthier environment.

This manual repeatedly emphasizes the importance of cleaning to remove visible soil with detergent and water, rinsing with water, and then sanitizing or disinfecting surfaces and objects with a recommended household bleach solution (see Figure 2.8) or a sanitizer or disinfectant registered by the Environmental Protection Agency (EPA). Except as specified in the Routine Schedule for

Figure 2.8.

Daily Sanitizing and Disinfecting Solutions

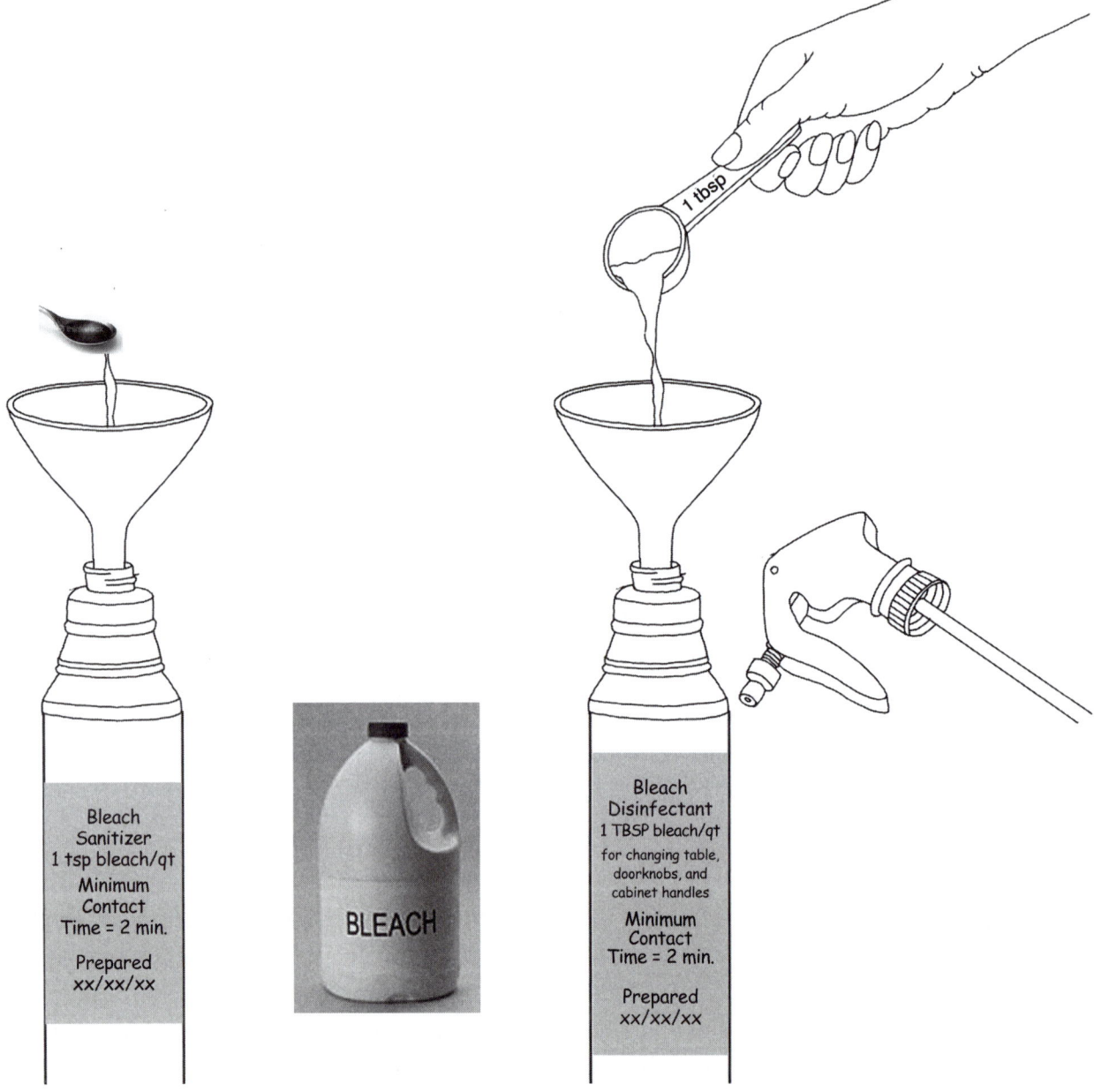

Sanitizing solution:
1 teaspoon per quart
(1 tablespoon per gallon),
mixed fresh daily

Disinfecting solution: 1 tablespoon per quart (1/4 to 3/4 of a cup per gallon), mixed fresh daily

Cleaning, Sanitizing, and Disinfecting (see Figure A.3 in Appendix A) and when there is a blood or body fluid spill, surfaces that are visibly clean do not need to be cleaned before they are sanitized. (See Figure 2.9 for definitions of *clean, sanitize*, and *disinfect*. See Figure A.2 for guidance on selecting appropriate sanitizers and disinfectants.)

Look for an EPA registration number on the product label that tells consumers they can rely on these products to reduce or destroy germs. The EPA registration label describes the product as a cleaner, sanitizer, or disinfectant. Use the least toxic product for the particular job. Products that are labeled as "green" sanitizers and disinfectants should be EPA-registered. The EPA has an industry-government collaboration program called Design for the Environment that permits the DfE label to appear on products that EPA scientists agree perform well, are cost effective, and are safer for the environment than other products in their class (see **www.epa.gov/dfe/**). All products must be used according to the manufacturer's instructions. Be sure the program follows the legally required protective measures for use of chemicals described in *Caring for Our Children* Standard 5.2.9.3:

> Employers should provide staff with hazard information, including access to and review of the Material Safety Data Sheets (MSDS) as required by the Occupational Safety and Health Administration (OSHA), about the presence of toxic substances such as formaldehyde, cleaning and sanitizing supplies, insecticides, herbicides, and other hazardous chemicals in use in the facility. Staff should always read the label prior to use to determine safety in use. For example, toxic products regulated by the Environmental Protection Agency (EPA) will have an EPA signal word of CAUTION, WARNING, or DANGER. Where nontoxic substitutes are available, these nontoxic substitutes should be used instead of toxic chemicals. If a nontoxic product is not available, caregivers/teachers should use the least toxic product for the job. A CAUTION label is safer than a WARNING label, which is safer than a DANGER label.

Generally, sanitizers and disinfectants do not work well to remove visible soil and are not effective if visible soil is present. Clean first to remove visible soil, and then sanitize or disinfect as required in Figure A.3. Cleaning is most easily done with a detergent followed by rinsing with water. Unless the product to be used requires pre-cleaning with detergent/soap and then rinsing with water, surfaces that are visibly clean may be sanitized or disinfected without pre-cleaning. Household bleach is inexpensive and safe to use as a sanitizer and disinfectant if diluted according to the recommended recipes for use of this product in early care and education settings. For details, see Controlling the Spread of Infection Through Cleaning, Sanitizing, and Disinfecting later in this chapter. Alternatively, you may use one of the many antimicrobial products registered by the EPA. (See Figures A.2 and A.3.) These chemicals are usually more expensive than bleach.

The *Caring for Our Children* national standard for sanitizing with bleach in child care programs is to use a bleach solution applied with a spray bottle, using a heavy spray rather than a fine mist. Make up the sanitizing solution (see Figure 2.8) by adding one teaspoon of household bleach to a quart of water or one tablespoon to a gallon. This more diluted solution is acceptable for sanitizing. For disinfecting, use one to three tablespoons added to a quart of water or 1/4 to 3/4 of a cup to a gallon. These bleach solutions must be made fresh daily. The solutions are effective if sprayed on a surface until the entire surface is glistening and then left in contact with the surface for at least two minutes. (When applying bleach, hold the spray container close to the surface to make sure the bleach gets on the surface and not into the air.) After a day, the solution becomes too diluted due to evaporation and breakdown of the chlorine, so it is no longer strong enough to kill germs on surfaces in typical child care facilities. Bleach solutions for dipping mops, rags, or sponges must be more concentrated. Follow the instructions on the bleach container that is labeled as an EPA-registered disinfectant, pesticide, or germicide to make up solutions for this type of application.

At the recommended dilution, few people have a problem with household bleach. Many swimming pools are chlorinated to control bacteria and have other chemicals added to stabilize the sanitation chemicals. Some adults with asthma or lung disease have difficulty when they swim in treated pools, but most do not. Ordinary household bleach that is available in groceries and other retail stores is a safe chemical to store in facilities that serve children. Even though full-strength household bleach is quite irritating, it will not cause lethal poisoning.

Many EPA-registered hospital-grade germicides are available and can be used on surfaces in group care if the manufacturer's instructions are followed. However, a large number of these are toxic and must be rinsed off surfaces after they are used. Be cautious about using any toxic chemical around children. Programs should avoid using toxic chemicals, if possible, or should use the least toxic product if no nontoxic alternatives are available. Before purchasing any of the EPA-registered products, read the Material Safety Data Sheets to learn about their toxicity and what is required to use the products correctly.

Use the appropriate solution to sanitize or disinfect items and surfaces. The surfaces routinely requiring disinfection at the end of the day include door and cabinet handles, and surfaces in toilet and changing areas for diapering or soiled underwear (this includes tables, countertops, toilets, diaper pails, potty chairs, sinks, faucets, and floors).

Hand hygiene

Hand hygiene is the first line of defense against infectious disease. Numerous studies show that hands are the primary carriers of infections. When and how often you practice hand hygiene is important. Ensure that staff members and children practice proper hand hygiene at the times described in Figure 2.1. You may want to display a handwashing poster near every sink as a reminder. There are several sources for free handwashing posters in addition to the one provided in Figure 2.2. Find handwashing posters on the CDC website (**www.cdc.gov**), or search the Internet to turn up several others that work well in child care settings. Switch out posters periodically to catch the attention of everyone about this important procedure. Review all the procedures for hand hygiene with everyone—and monitor staff members and children to ensure that the procedures are followed. There are five important handwashing components:

- Use running water that drains—not a stoppered sink or container. Using a common container of water spreads germs.
- Use liquid soap for children and preferably for adults, too. Bar soap gathers germs from the users.
- *Caring for Our Children* and many public health professionals recommend rubbing your hands together for at least 20 seconds. Aim for 20 seconds, but do not settle for less than 10 seconds of rubbing. The point is to rub long enough to loosen any adherent soil on the skin before rinsing. Friction helps remove soil that holds germs. Use the lather time to teach math, music, or poetry. (To count off the seconds, children can either chant twice "Bubble one, bubble two, bubble three, bubble four… bubble ten" or sing a song. Children can sing the ABC song once or sing one of the following songs twice: "Happy Birthday," "Row, Row, Row Your Boat," or [to the tune of "Row, Row, Row Your Boat"] "Wash, wash, wash your hands; sing this handy song. Scrub and rub, rub and scrub. Germs go down the drain!")
- Rinse hands, fingertips down, from wrists to nails, under running water until all soil and soap are gone.
- If the faucet does not turn off automatically, turn off the faucet with a paper towel. A hands-free faucet is best. Because dirty hands turn on a faucet, consider a faucet to be dirty at all times. Avoid contaminating clean hands. Ideally, throw the paper towel into a lined, covered, hands-free trash container.
- Have hand lotion available for staff members to apply to their hands and to use (with parental consent) with children after their hands have been washed. Lotion prevents dry or cracked skin. Dry skin traps germs, so using lotion is not only for comfort, but also for germ control.

Sinks should be located near all diapering, toileting, and food areas. If you are renovating or building new space, consider installing a sink with a hands-free faucet. Electric-eye faucets are more sanitary and are not much more expensive than conventional faucets when installing a new sink. Even where plumbing is not possible, you can use adequate alternatives. Portable sinks with one water tank for fresh water and another to receive soiled water are available. Moving the sink around to fill and drain it and keeping the supply tanks sanitary is a challenge, so a permanently placed sink with conventional plumbing is best. Some portable sinks come with water warmers, hands-free faucets, and soap dispensers. Automatic soap dispensers are unnecessary and costly if they use refill cartridges. Refillable soap dispensers must be regularly cleaned and sanitized. Search the internet using the term "portable sink" to discover many options that cost less than installing new plumbing. A sink should be a priority piece of equipment for every child area in the facility.

The critical features of the sink are:

- Clean *running* water—not a common basin
- Water temperature between 60–120° F (water between 80–100° F is comfortable and may encourage washing)

Figure 2.9.

Clean, Sanitize, Disinfect: What Are the Differences?

Task	Purpose
Clean	To physically remove all dirt and contamination. The friction of cleaning removes most germs and exposes any remaining germs to the effects of a sanitizer or disinfectant used later.
Sanitize	To reduce germs on inanimate surfaces to levels considered safe by public health codes or regulations.
Disinfect	To destroy or inactivate most germs on any inanimate object, but not bacterial spores.

Source: Standard 3.3.0.1, *Caring for Our Children*. Reprinted with permission.

- Collection of contaminated water out of the children's reach
- A system safe for children
- Readily available liquid soap and single-use (disposable or cloth) towels

When handwashing with running water is impossible, such as on a field trip, use disposable wet wipes to clean visible soil and then, for children over 24 months of age, use an adult-supervised application of an alcohol-based hand sanitizer. Disposable items such as paper towels, diaper table covers, wet wipes, gloves, and hand sanitizers are expensive. Consider buying in bulk from medical or paper supply companies. Use centralized buying whenever possible. If the program is not part of a system or large agency, ask other programs to join in bulk purchases. It is worth it!

Disposable gloves

Gloves can provide a protective barrier that significantly decreases exposure of the wearer's skin to germs that cause infections. However, they do allow some germs to get through to the skin. They are optional for diaper-changing unless contact with blood is expected. Wearing gloves while changing diapers, disposable training pants, or soiled underwear reduces the amount of skin contact between the teacher and the diaper's contents. Gloves do not need to be used when handling or cleaning up spilled breast milk unless the teacher has open skin wounds on her hands.

Always wear disposable gloves in these situations:

- When contact with blood or blood-containing fluids is likely (such as when providing first aid or changing a diaper with bloody diarrhea), particularly if the teacher's hands have open cuts or sores
- When cleaning surfaces that are contaminated with blood or body fluids (such as large amounts of vomit or feces)
- When cleaning an aquarium
- When changing the diaper of a child with diarrhea or a diagnosed gastrointestinal disease

First aid kits should contain disposable gloves. Try to use disposable gloves made of latex-free vinyl or nitrile to protect staff members who might become or are already allergic to latex. However, if using latex gloves, choose the powder-free gloves with reduced protein content. Remove and dispose of gloves properly after handling infectious material and each time they are used in food handling. There is a proper technique for removing used gloves. See Appendix D: Gloving in *Caring for Our Children* for an illustrated poster showing how this is done. After removing the gloves, you still need to wash your hands. In addition, any skin surfaces that are contaminated by blood or other body fluids should be washed immediately and thoroughly. *Remember: Wearing gloves is never a substitute for hand hygiene.*

You may wear reusable utility gloves for cleaning and disinfecting toilet equipment. After use, wash them with soapy water, and then dip them in disinfectant solution up to the wrist. Allow the gloves to air-dry.

Never inflate gloves to use them as a toy. Children can bite through the glove and, as with a balloon, have a piece of latex blow into their airway and choke them.

The role of ventilation, temperature, and humidity in resistance to infectious disease

Wherever people gather in groups, they put their germs into the communally breathed air. Exchanging indoor air with outdoor air reduces the density of infectious particles in the air. Even in winter, some form of ventilation is necessary to assure sufficient air exchange. The easiest and least expensive approach is to open the windows at least once a day. *Caring for Our Children* Standard 5.2.1.1 specifies that the rate at which outdoor air must be supplied to each room within the facility ranges from 15–60 cubic feet per minute per person (cfm/p), depending on what types of activities normally take place in each room. Air circulation is essential to clear infectious disease agents, odors, and toxic substances. Competent contractors for HVAC systems use levels of carbon dioxide as an indicator of the quality of ventilation. Adjust air circulation with a properly installed and adjusted HVAC system and by using fans and open windows. *Caring for Our Children* Standard 5.2.1.2 references standards from the American Society of Heating, Refrigerating and Air-Conditioning Engineers (ASHRAE) that define the conditions that air conditioning, dehumidification, heating, and humidification systems should maintain for group care. ASHRAE-certified heating and cooling contractors can measure air exchange and give advice on how to achieve healthful levels with mechanical ventilation.

For more information, contact ASHRAE, the EPA's Public Information Center, the American Gas Association (AGA), the Edison Electric Institute (EEI), the American Lung Association (ALA), the United States Consumer Product Safety Commission (CPSC), and the Safe Building Alliance (SBA).

Room temperature and humidity

In winter

Low indoor humidity occurs in cold weather because cold outdoor air holds very little water. When the dry air is brought inside and warmed, it can hold much more water. Unless some method is used to put an appropriate amount of moisture into the air, the dry air will pull moisture from anything that has available water—people, plants, rugs, clothing. When air is excessively dry, it draws water from mucus membranes. The loss of fluid from the membranes interferes with the protective functions of the mucus barrier. Keeping rooms too warm when outdoor temperatures are low makes it more difficult to maintain humidity at the healthful comfort level. When you get static shocks from walking across the floor, there is too little moisture in the air. In winter, an indoor, draft-free temperature between 68–75° F at 30–50 percent relative humidity is required. During naptime, put a sleeper garment over infants' clothing and a warm blanket over older children to keep them comfortable.

In summer

Humidity can be excessive in summer. High humidity can lead to growth of mold and dust mites in fabrics—a problem for many children with allergies. Children with allergic irritation of their respiratory tract are more likely to pick up infectious diseases. Dehumidification and cooling of air in summer may be necessary. The room temperature should be 74–82° F at 30–50 percent relative humidity during the warmer months.

Staff/child turnover and infectious disease

Aside from the obvious social-emotional and cognitive development benefits to children of having low turnover among staff members and children, there are also health benefits. High turnover constantly introduces new infections. New staff members need orientation and training to reliably practice the hygiene and sanitation routines required in group care. Because of the number of comings and goings, large programs (those with 50 or more children) that are open more than eight hours a day may be at greater risk for spreading infectious diseases. Such centers should be particularly careful to follow preventive health routines.

Do not enroll new children during an outbreak of a serious infectious disease. Consult with local health authorities and the program's child care health consultant about an appropriate waiting period to reopen enrollment for each infectious disease. While delaying enrollment can be a costly business decision, having an epidemic is an event that causes significant stress and public relations problems from which it is challenging for a program to recover.

Suggested activities

- Observe handwashing behaviors in a child care program. How many people wash their hands at the proper times? How many follow the correct procedure? Does the facility have the right setup to facilitate correct hand hygiene procedures? (See *Caring for Our Children* Section 3.2.2 and Standard 5.4.1.10.)

- Observe diaper-changing and/or toileting routines in a child care program. Make a checklist for your observation. Be sure the required technique and equipment are part of your checklist. What common problems in technique for preventing the spread of infection do you see? What would make following the routines easier? (See *Caring for Our Children* Section 3.2.1, Standards 5.4.1.1 through 5.4.1.9, and Standard 5.2.7.4.)

- Check the vaccine records of a group of children in group care against the current recommended schedule. Are the children up to date? How hard is it to work with the schedule? How hard is it for families to make sure their children are current? How hard is it for teachers to share responsibility for tracking immunizations of children and staff members with health care providers?

- Check adult vaccine records against the current recommendations for adults in general, and against the recommendations for those who have contact with young children. Are the adults up to date? What routine practices does the program use to ensure everyone in the facility is protected from vaccine-preventable disease? What barriers to this exist? How might these barriers be overcome?

- What are the points of view involved in implementing an exclusion policy? Whose interests are in conflict? How can these conflicts be lessened?

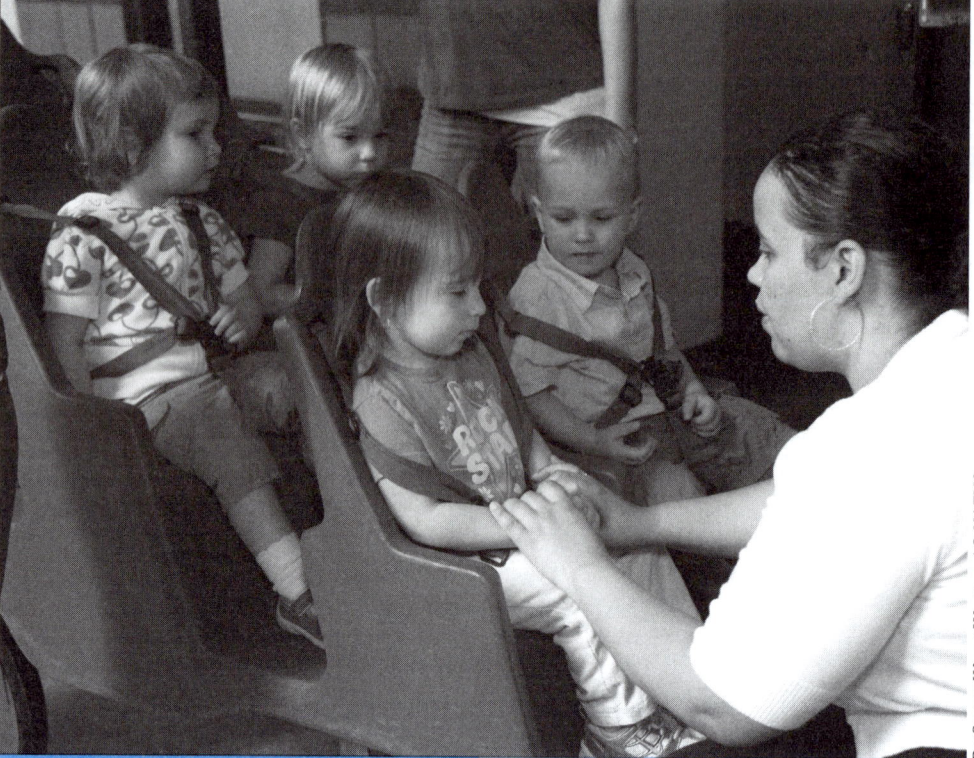

Preventing Injuries

MAJOR CONCEPTS

- Early childhood is the time of life when people are most likely to be injured.
- Most injuries can be prevented.
- Regular safety checks of the indoor and outdoor environment are necessary; hazards should be corrected immediately.
- Specific types of equipment and practices are known to be more likely to cause significant injury to children.
- Infants and toddlers require special safety precautions, including measures to prevent sudden infant death syndrome (SIDS) and shaken baby syndrome.
- Child care operators should provide safety education for staff members, children, and families.
- Safety rules stated as "dos" rather than "don'ts" help children and staff members make safe choices that lessen risk taking.

Children are more likely to be injured during certain situations and times of the day. Injuries are more likely:

- In late morning and late afternoon, especially in the spring and fall—times when children are more likely to be involved in gross motor activity, trying to do new or unpracticed activities
- When another child becomes ill or injured, and the routine is disrupted
- When staff members are absent or busy
- When children are not engaged in a planned activity, or they are tired or hungry (e.g., immediately before lunch)
- When hazards are too attractive to children
- When staff members are not aware of what children's abilities allow them to do safely or do not anticipate what children are likely to do
- When there are new places to explore and safety rules may be forgotten (e.g., on field trips)

Program planning for safety inside the facility

To be licensed, child care programs must follow certain safety standards and practices. Local building, sanitary, and fire safety codes must be observed. Create a safe environment by carefully following these additional basic guidelines:

- Be alert to hazards both indoors and outdoors, and eliminate or avoid them.
- Look at the world through the eyes of a young child—it is colorful, mysterious, and has new places and objects to experiment with and explore. Get down on your hands and knees to see what a child sees. You may be surprised at what you find!
- Conduct regular safety checks, varying the person who does them. Each room and the outdoor play area should be checked at least once a month. When checking the facility and surrounding areas, use the Health and Safety Checklist[1] from *Model Child Care Health Policies* (*MCCHP*), which is found on the ECELS-Healthy Child Care Pennsylvania website (**www.ecels-healthychildcarepa.org**).

    Of course, no checklist can include *all* potential hazards to children or identify *every* health and safety factor specific to a particular site. The items included on the *MCCHP* checklist are the ones most commonly associated with significant injury. Look for these on a regularly scheduled basis to promote the health and safety of children and staff members.

- Whenever a hazard is found, fix it immediately if you can. If you cannot fix it, make a note of it, place the hazard off-limits with easy-to-see barriers, and follow up with plans to get it fixed. Some features need to be checked daily, others weekly or monthly. Encourage all staff members to participate in conducting the checks and planning ways to deal with hazards. Families and older children can help, too. Different people using the same checklist will notice different hazards that need correction. Having staff members, parents, and school-age children participate in using the checklist will educate them about what is hazardous, identify more hazards, and engage everyone in being more safety-conscious.
- Know what you're buying or what is being donated to the child care program. Do not accept materials for which you cannot obtain manufacturer's instructions. Contact the manufacturer of every used and new product to see if it has been recalled. Read labels and instructions carefully. If you have any questions or complaints about the safety of a product, call the Consumer Product Safety Commission (CPSC) toll-free at 1-800-638-2772.

Foot traffic

- Make sure there is enough space for all furniture and equipment and for traffic around them.
- Bolt top-heavy furniture (e.g., cubbies) to the wall or floor.
- Experiment with different equipment and furnishing arrangements until you find one that best suits the needs of the children and your program, making sure that you have allowed space for rest areas. Adapt furnishings you need to move with glides or other devices so they can be moved safely.
- Place chairs and other furniture away from windows, cabinets, and shelves to prevent children from climbing or reaching hazards.
- Keep aisles free of toys, furniture, and other tripping hazards, such as spilled water. Break up long aisles to discourage children from running.

Indoor gross motor play

- Fun, vigorous, and safe indoor activities help children get the physical activity they need to help them learn from more sedentary activities. Examples include dancing, skipping, rolling a ball, crawling, crab-walking through a path, and jumping at floor level. Try to avoid activities in which a child has to wait and then has just a short opportunity for movement.

---

[1] At the time of this writing, the ECELS website has two Health and Safety Checklists. The checklist that appears in *Model Child Care Health Policies* on the site is intended for general use by staff members, families, and even older children. The other is intended for use by directors and child care health consultants. For each item on this checklist, references are given from *Caring for Our Children* and other relevant established requirements. Choose the checklist that works best for your situation.

- Head bumps matter. Traumatic brain injury can occur even without loss of consciousness and cause long-term learning problems. Falls are the most common cause of injury in child care settings. Children's heads are heavy relative to the rest of their bodies, so falling headfirst is common.

- Provide an impact-absorbing surface under indoor climbers, just as you would for outdoor climbers. The surfacing material should be warranted by the manufacturer to meet the play surface safety standards of ASTM International (formerly the American Society for Testing and Materials) to cushion a fall from the highest point on the equipment to which children could climb. Tumbling mats *do not* provide a safe surface under climbers. The manufacturer and installer of any surfacing material should be required to warrant that the material as installed meets or surpasses the ASTM playground surfacing test for the maximum fall height of the equipment. Many materials do not meet the ASTM test or are installed incorrectly. (For more information on ASTM standards, go to **www.astm.org**.)

    A study conducted by Indiana University found that one year after installation, many surfaces were not installed according to the manufacturer's recommendations. Playgrounds with loose-fill engineered wood fiber had the most deficiencies. Rubber tile and poured-in-place rubber surfaces had the highest level of firmness and stability. Indoor surfaces need to be just as safe as outdoor surfaces. A ceramic or other hard tile floor, including carpeted, concrete, or wood, is not suitable for any type of climbing. The more expensive surfaces that are appropriate for the intended use usually require less maintenance and last longer, making up for the difference in the initial cost of installation in a few years.

- Cover the entire fall zone. If the equipment is movable, move and install the surfacing wherever you put the equipment. ASTM is considering issuing new standards for equipment intended for use indoors in child care settings. In the meantime, do not purchase or use equipment for which the manufacturer does not provide a warranty that states it is safe if set up where and how you intend to use it.

- Do not use trampolines. They can cause very serious injuries. Even the popular trampolines that have a net enclosure around the jumping surface are not safe. They are particularly likely to cause injury when more than one child uses them at one time. Trampolines should be viewed as gymnastics equipment that requires close one-on-one supervision and training in the sport. They are not appropriate for group care settings.

- Teach children how to use all available equipment correctly and safely.

- Involve the children in setting rules to limit unsafe running, pushing, and other such behaviors. Enforce these rules consistently. Compliment children on safe play behavior.

- Plan and use positive transitions for children when they enter the program or begin new routines or activities within the program. Standard 2.1.1.6 in *Caring for Our Children* points out that planning for such transitions not only supports children's social-emotional health but also is necessary for safety.

Doors

Young children need to be in safe spaces secured by doors or barriers. As they develop mobility, their options should be limited by adults to safe alternatives. Since young children lack experience to judge danger, they can get into trouble quickly. They are likely to use an open door to go exploring unnoticed. Finger-pinch injuries and bumps from doors being opened onto children are common problems in child care. To avoid these problems, take the following steps:

- Use doors with full vision panels so you can see at child height on both sides of the door.

- Install finger-pinch protection devices that are available commercially. For the hinge gap area on the door, you can use a strip of durable and flexible material such as indoor-outdoor carpeting held by molding strips screwed onto the door and door jamb.
  - Install devices that slow the door as it closes, giving extra time for a person to enter or exit without body parts getting caught in the door.
  - Hardware stores carry simple devices to fit over doorknobs that keep children from opening doors while still allowing adults to open them easily. Alternatively, if lever handles are installed, they should be placed high enough to be out of the reach of young children.

Kitchen facilities and cooking

- Cooking and preparing foods are key learning activities for young children. During these activities, make sure that children do not have access to sharp or hot cooking utensils without one-on-one adult supervision. Children should not be in the kitchen unless you can provide constant and individual adult supervision.

- Be sure cleansers, sanitizing agents, and other toxic chemicals are not accessible to children and that they are stored in a way that prevents contamination of food.

- Place cooking facilities or food preparation equipment (e.g., hot plates, toaster ovens, microwave ovens, slow cookers used to warm infant bottles, and other types of bottle warmers) out of the reach of children unless they are doing a cooking activity under close supervision, and then only with equipment and utensils that are safe for them to use.

- Use only cookware and utensils intended for food preparation. Avoid heating foods in plastic containers. Some decorative and some plastic bowls, pots, and utensils contain toxic materials.

- Microwave energy heats food unevenly and continues heating the food for a few minutes after the oven stops. Some portions of the food can reach a scalding temperature while other parts remain cool. Microwave ovens *should not* be used to warm infant bottles or infant food. If you heat other foods in a microwave oven, allow the food to sit in the microwave oven for three–five minutes after the microwave oven stops, and then remove the food carefully to prevent spilling or spattering. Be sure to stir the food thoroughly to mix hot and cool portions before serving it.

- Secure electrical and extension cords so that children cannot reach them, they do not dangle, and they do not present trip hazards.

- Turn the handles of pots and pans toward the back of the stove.

- Keep hot foods or liquids out of rooms being used by children.

- Place hot items away from the edge of a counter or table. Do not use a tablecloth that could be pulled down by a child.

- Prevent scalds by keeping tap water temperature no higher than 120° F.

Electrical wiring

- Outlets that are adapted to be child-resistant are widely available. If this type is not installed, cover unused outlets with cover plates that have spring-loaded devices that put a blank over the opening when the outlet is not in use, or use similar safety mechanisms. Avoid using removable, individual plastic plugs; they may be attractive to young children, are choking hazards, and are apt to be left out after an outlet is used. Cover outlets that stay in use with appropriate screw-in plug covers, especially near sinks and where young children can reach them. All outlets near water sources should be of the ground-fault protected type. Many types of child-resistive shock guards and outlet covers are available in hardware and baby equipment stores.

- Use extension cords only when absolutely necessary, and be sure they are labeled UL (Underwriter's Laboratory) approved. This label identifies that nationally recognized electrical safety standards have been met. Place extension cords so they run along the wall, behind furniture, to reduce the chance of tripping. Never run an extension cord underneath a carpet or rug; it may become worn or frayed and cause a fire. Never run cords through doorways or walls instead of using proper electrical wiring. Do not nail appliance or extension cords to the wall. Extension cord guards are commercially available to reduce tripping hazards and keep cords out of the reach of infants and toddlers. Young children may bite on cords, getting electric shock and mouth burns.

Choking hazards

Choking receives considerable attention in *Caring for Our Children*. Nearly all fatal choking (90 percent) occurs in children younger than 4 years of age.

- Children younger than 4 years of age should not have any of the high-risk foods that have been associated with choking. These are foods that are round, hard, small, thick and sticky, smooth, compressible or dense, or slippery. Examples of these foods are hot dogs and other meat sticks (whole or sliced into rounds), raw carrot rounds, whole grapes, hard candy, nuts, seeds, raw peas, hard pretzels, chips, peanuts, popcorn, rice cakes, marshmallows, spoonfuls of peanut butter, and chunks of meat larger than can be swallowed whole. (Raisins have not been reported to be associated with choking injuries.) To prevent choking, cut food for infants into pieces 1/4 inch or smaller, and cut food for toddlers into pieces 1/2 inch or smaller.

- Children should not be allowed to eat or drink while walking, running, playing, lying down, or riding in vehicles. They should always be seated when eating to reduce choking hazards. When eating, they should be closely observed by an adult who sits with them, not only to have social interaction and promote a pleasant mealtime but also to monitor the size of food and to watch for stuffing or squirreling of food. A slumping posture promotes choking; having a foot rest for children whose feet cannot reach the floor helps them adjust their body position and avoid choking.

- Objects smaller than 1¼ inch in diameter and shorter than 2¼ inch in length should not be accessible to children who mouth items. No object should be small enough to completely fit into a child's mouth (e.g., LEGO pieces, beads, coins, small wads of paper, paper clips, safety pins, loose buttons, and small electrical outlet safety plugs).

- Check toys and equipment regularly for small parts that may break off (e.g., eyes and noses on stuffed animals, buttons on doll clothes, plastic hats or shoes on miniature people, Styrofoam parts). Remove or securely attach these items.

- Latex balloons and gloves blown up like balloons are choking hazards. When a child mouths either one, the latex fragment can blow into the child's airway. Bandages that are small enough for children to put into their mouths are also hazardous. With a breath, these can be sucked into a position that blocks the child's airway.

- Plastic bags and Styrofoam objects should not be accessible to children younger than 4. Pieces of these items can break off and block part of the airway.
- Soft bedding and other soft objects should not be allowed where infants sleep.

First aid

Learn proper first aid techniques for a choking infant or child. In 2010, the approach to managing a blocked airway was merged with and became identical to the instructions for cardiopulmonary resuscitation, or CPR. Learning CPR does not require taking a separate CPR course. Demonstration of CPR skills should be included as part of pediatric first aid training. Learning to perform CPR has been made easy, inexpensive, and effective with the CPR Anytime® Kits available from the American Heart Association. Two separate kits are available to learn the skills required: one for infant CPR, and the other for child and adult CPR. The kits include a step-by-step video and an inflatable manikin on which to practice. The learning activity with a kit requires 20–30 minutes. Programs can purchase and keep the kits on hand to use when new staff members are hired or as a skill refresher. Go to **www.heart.org** to learn more about these materials.

Staff members should be able to demonstrate mastery of CPR skills during preservice training and periodic continuing education in pediatric first aid. Every adult who is involved in providing direct care for children in group care settings should have this training. The 2010 C-A-B sequence (chest compressions, airway, and breathing) for unresponsive infants and children is as follows:

- For infants younger than 1 year of age, have someone call 911 while you give five back slaps alternating with five chest thrusts until an object is dislodged or the infant becomes unresponsive. If the infant is unconscious (unresponsive) or has stopped breathing, start 30 chest compressions at a rate of 100 per minute. Then, tilt the head and chin to open the airway. Look for an object you can see and remove with a finger sweep (no blind finger sweeps). Then give two breaths one second apart with your mouth over the infant's mouth and nose. Repeat cycles of 30 compressions with two breaths. Be sure someone calls 911 as soon as possible.
- For children 1–8 years of age, have someone call 911 while you perform the Heimlich maneuver: Use upward thrusts of a fisted hand placed just above the navel while you hold the child's back firmly against your abdomen and chest. If the child becomes unresponsive or stops breathing, start 30 chest compressions at a rate of 100 per minute. Then, tilt the head back and lift the chin forward to open the airway to check if you can see an object that you can sweep out with your finger. Then give two breaths into the child's mouth with the nose pinched. Continue cycles of 30 chest compressions to two breaths until the object is expelled or an emergency responder takes over. Be sure someone calls 911 as soon as possible.

Many sources of pediatric first aid training are available. Be sure that the course is approved by a recognized national organization and that the instructor includes all the required topics listed in *Caring for Our Children* Standard 1.4.3.2. Independent instructors who have the necessary background to teach pediatric first aid can be credentialed by the American Academy of Pediatrics (AAP) to teach the PedFACTs course (Pediatric First Aid for Caregivers and Teachers) after satisfactory completion of online training provided by the AAP. For more information about PedFACTs, to locate a PedFACTs instructor in your area, or for information on how to become a PedFACTs instructor, go to **www.pedfactsonline.com**.

Toys

Check that all toys are appropriate for the age and developmental level of the children who will use them, and that they can be easily cleaned. Most toys will pose a danger only if they are misused. Balls are for throwing and kicking, blocks are not. Choose hard-surface toys that can be washed in a dishwasher many times without damage. Select cloth toys that can go through the laundry without falling apart. Have some safe disposable toys for children to use when they are ill. Follow the manufacturer's age recommendations. If, for example, a toy is labeled "Not for children younger than 3 years of age," do not allow a younger child to play with it.

- Carefully examine toys for sharp, splintered, or jagged edges and small pieces that can be easily broken off. Tug at different parts to test for strength. Pull on the heads and limbs of dolls to make sure they won't come off and expose sharp wires.
- Check toys frequently and do minor repairs whenever necessary.
- Cover hinges and joints of toys to prevent fingers from being pinched or caught.
- Destroy projectile toys, such as darts, because they are not appropriate for children.
- Cut off or shorten toy pull strings that are long enough to wrap around a child's neck.
- Bend plastic toys to test for brittleness. Cheap, hard plastic breaks easily, leaving sharp edges.
- Look for the nontoxic label on all painted toys and play equipment.
- Keep wooden toys smooth and free of splinters.
- Check seams on cloth toys regularly for tearing and weak threads. Look for the flame-retardant label on

cloth toys. Some flame retardants have been found to be made from toxic chemicals—for example, polybrominated dipheylethers (PBDE). Scientific study of flame retardants suggests that many of these chemicals are polluting the environment. It is unclear which ones are safe. Because the fire safety afforded by using these chemicals in toys is limited, avoid toys whose labels show they have been treated with fire retardants.

- Do not use toys hung across cribs or mobiles in cribs. Children should not be left in cribs when they are awake, so these toys should be used elsewhere.
- Be extra vigilant when using toys for water play. Do not leave any water toys on the walking surface; they can trip a child or make the surface slippery.
- Teach children how to play safely and to put toys away immediately after playing.
- Be sure that riding toys (e.g., tricycles) used inside or outdoors are stable and well balanced. Helmets must be worn for riding any wheeled toy. Everyone, including the youngest children, should wear helmets that cover the top of the head and the forehead. The chin strap should fit so that no more than a single adult finger can be inserted between the strap and the child's skin. The helmet should not move around on the head or slip over the eyes when it is properly fitted. Children should remove their helmets when getting off the riding toy so that the helmet does not pose a hanging hazard by catching on other objects while they play.
- Comment positively on children's safe play behavior. Tell those who are using a toy in a way that could lead to injury how to play with it, rather than how not to use it.

Toy chests

Toy chests are inappropriate for groups of children. Store toys on low, open shelves or in a sturdy, open box or basket to limit toy breakage and make it easier for children to choose a toy.

Poisons

You probably think first of cleaning products and medicines when you think of poisons, but many other things could be harmful if eaten or sucked. You must always be prepared to call a regional poison control center in poison emergencies. A country-wide number (1-800-222-1222) will automatically connect you to the regional poison control center nearest you. Learn more about these centers and their educational and emergency services at **www.aapcc.org/dnn/default.aspx**. These centers can also advise about risks for materials you are considering bringing into the program.

Art materials

Always read labels on art materials and select products that are appropriate for the ages of the children who will use them. Watch children closely during art projects to stop them from mouthing paintbrushes, fingers, crayons, or other objects and materials. Homemade playdough has large amounts of salt, which can be a problem if much is eaten. Use only unscented, water-based markers approved by the Art and Creative Materials Institute (ACMI), as some children are attracted to fruit-scented markers and may try to eat them.

Follow appropriate procedures when using manipulative art or sensory materials (see Figure 3.1). Do not allow children to eat or drink while using art materials, and be mindful of proper handwashing after art and craft activities. Children transfer the germs from their hands to manipulative materials, and their hands become heavily contaminated by whatever germs are in the materials. Whenever possible, provide each child with a separate portion. Hand hygiene, supervision of children, and discarding contaminated material are important hygienic practices when using these materials.

Special precautions are required to prevent children who have allergies to gluten, latex, or other substances from coming into contact with materials that could contain these allergens. These substances can be mixed into a material by contact with a tool or container that was previously used for play or to contain a different product. Before transferring art materials from their original containers or packaging, first clip or photocopy and then transfer the valuable safety information from the original package to the new container.

The Labeling of Hazardous Art Materials Act (LHAMA), established in 1988, requires that all art materials be reviewed to determine their potential for causing a chronic hazard and that appropriate warning labels be put on those found by ASTM standards to pose such chronic hazards. Under LHAMA, schools cannot provide art supplies with a chronic-hazard warning label to children in sixth grade and below. LHAMA gives the CPSC the authority to bring legal action against schools that do not comply.

Since 1940, ACMI has sponsored a certification program for children's art materials. The ACMI AP (Approved Product) label identifies art materials that are safe for children, meet voluntary standards of quality and performance, and have been certified in a toxicological evaluation by a medical expert; this label replaces the previous nontoxic seals of CP (Certified Product) and HL (Health Label). Families and others buying art materials (e.g., crayons, chalk, paint sets, clay, and pencils) for the program should be reminded to purchase only products that are accompanied by the statement "Conforms to ASTM D4236" or similar indication by the ACMI. Additional tips on purchasing art supplies are

> **Figure 3.1.**
>
> ## Using Playdough and Other Manipulative Art or Sensory Materials
>
> The child care program should have the following procedures on the use and life span of manipulative art or sensory materials such as clay, play dough, etc:
>
> a. If handmade, these materials should be made fresh each week, labeled, dated, and stored in airtight containers.
>
> b. If purchased, these products should be stored in their original packaging.
>
> c. Products that are labeled as toxic are prohibited.
>
> d. The surface upon which they are used and the tools used with these materials should be cleaned and sanitized before and after use.
>
> e. Children should practice hand hygiene before and after each use.
>
> f. Material should be discarded if it is sneezed upon, put into a child's mouth, or in any other way possibly contaminated.
>
> g. Children with latex or gluten allergies should be given their own portion of the material, and that individual portion should be stored separately if for repeat use.
>
> h. Children with cuts, sores, scratches, and colds with sneezing and runny noses should be given their own portion of the material, and that individual portion should be stored separately if for repeat use.
>
> Source: Standard 5.2.9.8, *Caring for Our Children*. Reprinted with permission.

given in Figure 3.2. If you have any questions, contact ACMI (**www.acminet.org**) or the CPSC (**www.cpsc.gov**).

For more details about the safety of art supplies, go to **www.acminet.org/Safety.htm**. If in doubt about whether a product is toxic, or if someone has contact with or ingests a possibly toxic substance, call the national line that connects to your regional poison control center: 1-800-222-1222.

Plants

Plants are a leading cause of poisoning in young children. If eaten, some plants can cause a skin rash or stomach upset; others can even cause death. *Many common household plants are poisonous.* Assume that a plant is poisonous unless you specifically know it to be nontoxic.

Nontoxic plants do not contain potentially dangerous chemicals. However, they may present a risk for choking or stomach upset, particularly for young children. To identify plants in your play area, check library books, garden and floral shops, or arboretums, or ask your local cooperative extension service. Then check with your regional poison control center to find out if any parts of the plant are poisonous. If in doubt, take it out.

Supervise young children closely around plants. Eating too much of any plant may make a child sick. Label plants in every area accessible to children, including around the perimeter of the building and in the play yard, so that if ingestion occurs, accurate information can be given to the poison control center. It is best to locate all plants out of children's reach if they are not being used in a specific activity. Teach children not to put plants, fruits, or berries in their mouth without first asking a grown-up.

The website of the Poison Control Center at the Children's Hospital of Philadelphia (**www.chop.edu/service/poison-control-center/**) offers tips and a list of nontoxic plants. At the time of this writing, this site lists the following plants as nontoxic:

African Violet	Honeysuckle
Aster	Hosta
Baby's Breath	Hoya
Baby's Tears	Jade Plant
Begonia	Kalanchoe
Boston Fern	Lilac
Christmas Cactus	Lilies: Day, Easter, Tiger
Crab Apple	Magnolia
Dracaena	Peperomia
Easter Cactus	Petunia
Echeveria (Hens-and-Chickens)	Prayer Plant
	Spider Plant
Gardenia	Swedish Ivy
Hibiscus	Violets

Batteries

The small button batteries used in some toys, cameras, and calculators present a choking hazard and can cause severe injury in just a few hours if swallowed. When replacing a button battery, be sure that you discard the old one immediately, away from children's areas. Keep remote control devices, cell phones, and other electronic gadgets away from infants, toddlers, and older children who might mouth a battery if the gadget is dropped or opens and releases the battery.

Hazards in the diaper-changing area

During diaper changing, use laminated pictures or other easily washed toys, mirrors, or interesting objects hanging out of reach to foster interaction and talking with the child at this special one-on-one time. Do not distract the child with something that may be hazardous, such as a pen or small or electronic objects. Only the supplies that will be used up in the course of a diaper change should be brought to the changing table and should be kept above the child's head or otherwise out of the child's reach so they do not become contaminated or used as toys during the changing procedure. If brought to the diaper-changing surface, containers of lotion, cream, wipes, or any other materials used in diaper changing will become contaminated, and these contaminated objects can spread the contamination to hands and objects that touch them. Powder can be dangerous if swallowed or inhaled. Talcum powder should not be used at all because some gets into the air and can be inhaled and damage the lungs. Lotions and creams can be toxic; a child mouthing a container might ingest some of the contents. Also, keep the disinfecting solution well out of reach of children. The recommended dilution of bleach and water is not toxic, but it can be irritating if sprayed into the eyes or mouth. Many commercial disinfectants are toxic.

Safety beyond the classroom

Playgrounds

A well-designed and well-managed play environment provides a wide range of opportunities for children's development, including motor development, decision making, social development, and learning experiences enhanced by seeing the world from new perspectives. Playgrounds provide the space in which children can challenge themselves physically. While it is important for children to take risks and experiment, they can get seriously hurt. Most injuries are preventable. Injuries are usually the result of unsafe equipment and/or poor supervision. While supervision cannot make hazardous equipment safe, children should be supervised on all equipment to be sure they use it safely. Some common playground equipment is not appropriate for younger children; in fact, some have design flaws that make them unsafe and even deadly.

To check the safety of your active play areas, use Figure A.5 the Safety Checklist for Active Play Areas in Appendix A and the information in the playground safety publications from the CPSC at **www.cpsc.gov**. For a quick look at the 12 most significant playground hazards, use the "Dirty Dozen" list available through the National Recreation and Park Association (NRPA). Search for "Dirty Dozen" at **www.nrpa.org**. To find and arrange for a Certified Playground Safety Inspector (CPSI) to evaluate your outdoor active play area, search for "CPSI" on the NRPA website, then select Registry. NRPA provides in-person and online training for people who want to be CPSIs. An NRPA-registered CPSI must successfully complete an examination every three years to provide evidence of competence. The issues involved in playground safety are fairly technical. Special testing devices are used to check for head entrapment and protrusion. The cost of an inspection by a CPSI is usually reasonable, and the results are very helpful.

Outdoor and indoor play areas must include equipment that is age-appropriate and developmentally appropriate for the specific children who will be using it. Recognize the range of developmental differences in children when planning the type, size, accessibility, and layout of equipment. If your program offers climbing opportunities indoors, then equipment, spacing of landing zones, and cushioning surfaces must meet the same safety standards specified for climbers outdoors. Play areas designed for school-age children are not safe for preschool-age children; those designed for preschool-

---

Figure 3.2.

How to Choose Art Supplies

AVOID powdered clay, which contains silica that is easily inhaled and harmful to the lungs.
USE wet clay that cannot be inhaled.

AVOID glazes, paints, or finishes that contain lead.
USE poster paints/water-based products.

AVOID materials with fumes and paints that require using solvents (such as turpentine) to clean brushes.
USE water-based paints, glues, etc.

AVOID cold-water or commercial dyes that contain chemical additives.
USE natural dyes such as vegetables or onion skins.

AVOID permanent markers that may contain toxic solvents.
USE water-based markers.

AVOID instant papier-mâché that may contain lead or asbestos, and **AVOID** use of color-print newspaper or magazines with water.
USE newspaper (printed with black ink only) and library paste or liquid starch for papier-mâché.

AVOID epoxy, instant glues, or other solvent-based glues.
USE water-based white glue or library paste.

AVOID aerosol sprays.
USE water-based materials/pump sprays.

AVOID powdered tempera paints.
USE liquid tempera paint or any nontoxic paint.

For additional information, visit the Art and Creative Materials Institute (ACMI) at **www.acminet.org**.

age children are not suitable for toddlers. For applicable requirements for play areas and playgrounds, see *Caring for Our Children* Standards 6.1.0.1 through 6.4.2.3. The National Program for Playground Safety (**www.playgroundsafety.org**) recommends that schools and child care centers have risk management policies regarding playgrounds. Minimally, these include a system for reporting playground injuries and playground maintenance/repair problems, and a detailed supervision plan.

Whether your play area is indoors, on the outside grounds of your property, or down the street, you can reduce the chance that a child will be injured. Teach children the basic safety rules shown in Figure 3.3. Many injuries occur due to misuse of equipment. The safest equipment is designed to prevent misuse. Perform regular maintenance checks of the active play areas, as factors such as children's play, weather, and aging materials create hazards that were not present when the area was first set up. No matter how well the play areas are designed, good supervision is essential. Follow these tips to maintain safe play environments:

- Supervise children closely at all times to prevent significant injury, such as climbing where it is not safe, swinging too high, running close to moving swings, or playing with equipment that is too advanced. Position extra staff members in areas of high risk.

- Check play equipment daily and the whole active play area before use. Programs should develop a plan for systematic inspection and maintenance. A Suggested General Maintenance Checklist is included as an appendix in the *Public Playground Safety Handbook* available from the CPSC at **www.cpsc.gov**.

- Because most injuries that occur in early care and education programs are due to falls, the most important safety feature for play areas is an impact-absorbent surface that is in accordance with ASTM standards. The standards specify the size of the area under and around equipment (the fall zone) that should be covered with the recommended amount of specific types of impact-absorbing material. The CPSC has conducted tests on the shock-absorbing properties of commonly used loose-fill surfacing materials to develop recommendations for appropriate depths for specific fall heights. (See Figure 3.4.)
  - Commonly used loose-fill materials include wood chips, shredded bark mulch, sand, pea gravel, and shredded rubber tires. All of these loose-fill materials scatter during

Figure 3.3.

Basic Playground Safety Rules

SWINGS
- Sit in the center of the swing. Never stand or kneel.
- Hold on with *both* hands.
- *Stop* the swing before getting off.
- Stay *far away* from moving swings.
- Be sure only *one* person is on a swing at a time.
- Use empty swings or exercise rings on swing sets only for swinging people, not for swinging or twisting while empty.
- Keep head and feet out of the exercise rings.

SLIDES
- Wait your turn. Give the person ahead lots of room.
- Use the ladder to climb up, and use the slide to come down.
- One person on the slide ladder at a time.
- Hold on with *both* hands climbing up.
- Before sliding down, make sure no one is in front.
- Slide down feet first, sitting up, one at a time unless the slide is double or triple width.
- After sliding down, *get away* from the front of the slide.
- Check whether metal slides that have been in the sun are too hot to use.

CLIMBING APPARATUS
- Only ____ people at a time (fill in your limit, depending on the manufacturer's instructions).
- Use *both* hands, and use the lock grip (fingers and thumbs).
- Stay away from other children who are climbing.
- Use climbers only when they are dry and cool to the touch.

HORIZONTAL LADDERS AND BARS
- Only ____ people at a time (fill in your limit, depending on the manufacturer's instructions).
- Everybody starts at the same end and goes in the same direction.
- Use the lock grip (fingers and thumbs).
- Keep a *big space* between you and the person in front.
- Use ladders and bars only when they are dry.
- Drop down with knees bent. Try to land on both feet.

OTHER
- Stay away from active play equipment when digging and doing other play activities.
- Do not play on seesaws because using them is not safe.

Source: Adapted and updated from U.S. Consumer Products Safety Commission, *Little Big Kids*, Washington, DC: U.S. Government Printing Office, 1980. Online: www.cpsc.gov/cpscpub/pubs/kids.pdf.

use and must be raked to maintain or exceed the required depth to accommodate the displacement that occurs while children play. In cold climates, loose-fill materials can get wet and then freeze, making the surface too hard to be safe. Each type of loose-fill material has drawbacks that must be addressed. Wood and bark chips compress, harbor insects, and usually deteriorate in less than a year. Uncovered sand attracts insect nests and animal feces. Pea gravel has pieces small enough to fit into noses and ears. Shredded rubber may contain toxic substances and will burn if a lit match is dropped onto it.

- Commercially manufactured playground surfacing materials (often described as unitary materials), such as poured-in-place composites and linking rubber squares, are a good option. These materials may be expensive to install, but doing so will save money in three or four years because they require less maintenance and less frequent replacement. If a manufactured surface is used, it should be one that the manufacturer warrants to meet ASTM standards.
- Cement, asphalt, grass, and hard-packed or frozen sand/soil are dangerous surfaces underneath or around equipment such as swings, climbers, and slides, even when children are supervised.

■ Teach children how to play safely. Involve them in making rules for playground behavior, and enforce these rules consistently. Compliment children when they use the playground appropriately.

■ If children are not playing safely, use developmentally appropriate behavior management techniques, such as redirecting them to safe activities, modeling safe behavior, or offering a positive direction or choice. If these measures do not change the unsafe behavior, remove them from play for a short time to reconsider how they can play safely, explaining how their actions could hurt someone.

■ Protect all play areas from streets, traffic, and access by people with inappropriate intentions. Locate play areas and install physical barriers such as a combination of fences, trees, bushes, and bollards (thick traffic control posts) to minimize the chance of a child darting into the street, vehicles crashing into the play area, or intruders interacting with the children.

■ If water is nearby (e.g., a stream, pond, drainage ditch), be sure there is adequate fencing to keep children from reaching the water and possibly drowning.

■ Check the outdoor environment for poisonous plants and remove them.

■ Avoid poisonous wood preservatives. Instead, use pressure-treated wood that is certified free of toxic substances such as creosote or arsenic. For all types of treated wood, use a double coat of nontoxic, nonslippery wood sealer every two years.

Riding toys

Have several sizes of tricycles or other riding toys available for older toddlers and preschoolers. A riding toy that is too large for a child is unstable and may be difficult to control properly.

■ Be sure that children who ride wheeled vehicles with wheels greater than 20 inches in diameter—even those with training wheels—wear properly sized bicycle helmets and that they remove the helmets when they get off the vehicle. (See additional tips about how to use helmets under Toys, earlier in this chapter.)

■ Use low-slung riding toys with seats close to the ground and a wide wheelbase; they are more stable.

■ Avoid vehicles with sharp edges, particularly fenders.

■ Look for pedals and handgrips with nonskid surfaces to prevent hands and feet from slipping.

■ Teach children safe riding habits and monitor their performance frequently.

Figure 3.4.

Minimum Compressed Loose-Fill Surfacing Depths

Inches	of	(Loose-fill material)	Protects to	Fall height (feet)
6*		shredded/recycled rubber		10
9		sand		4
9		pea gravel		5
9		wood mulch (non-CCA)		7
9		wood chips		10

*Shredded/recycled rubber loose-fill surfacing does not compress in the same manner as other loose-fill materials. However, care should be taken to maintain a constant depth as displacement may still occur.

Source: U.S. Consumer Product Safety Commission, *Public Playground Safety Handbook*, Bethesda, MD: Author, 2010. Online: www.cpsc.gov/cpscpub/pubs/325.pdf.

- Do not allow wheeled vehicles on sidewalks near streets. Low toys cannot be seen by cars or trucks.
- Do not allow children to ride double. Carrying a passenger makes the vehicle unstable unless the vehicle is designed for two.
- Teach children that riding down a hill is dangerous. A wheeled toy can pick up so much speed that it may be almost impossible to stop.
- Teach children to avoid sharp turns, to take all turns at a low speed, and not to ride down steps or over curbs.
- Advise children to keep hands and feet away from moving spokes.
- Keep the vehicles in good condition. Check regularly for missing or damaged pedals and handgrips, loose handlebars and seats, broken parts, and other defects.
- Cover any sharp edges and protrusions with heavy waterproof tape.
- Don't leave riding toys outdoors overnight; moisture can cause rust and weaken metal parts.

Pedestrian safety

Children learn by imitation and experience. Walks to a nearby playground offer teachable moments that can be used to introduce and practice safe pedestrian behavior. Both children and adults should cross the streets only at crosswalks. Most pedestrian/motor vehicle injuries happen when children dart out in the middle of the block. Basic rules of preschool pedestrian safety should be practiced. Teach the first five of the following rules to toddlers and preschool-age children; all eight rules should be taught to school-age children.

1. Sidewalks are for people—streets are for cars, trucks, and buses.
2. Cars and trucks are bigger than you are and can hurt you.
    - To be safe, you must be seen.
    - Walk with a grown-up wherever cars go—driveways, streets, parking lots—until you're at least 8. When you're old enough and big enough to go where cars and trucks ride, you must be responsible for observing all the safety rules yourself.
3. Stop at the curb or the edge of the road. Never go into the street or across a driveway without an adult.
4. Keep away from cars in driveways. Do not play in driveways.
5. When crossing a street or driveway, look left, right, then left again to be sure it is safe to cross. Scan for cars; use your eyes like a flashlight. Stop, look, listen. Practice this method at every street and every driveway.
6. Cross only at crosswalks or corners, not between cars or in the middle of a block.
7. Use a flashlight and wear clothing that reflects light if you go out when it is dim.
8. If there is no sidewalk, walk so the drivers on your side of the road can see your face.

Use a travel rope or have the children hold hands to keep younger children together. Children can hold onto spaced knots in a rope. Make the walk fun, not confining, by playing Follow the Leader or singing songs. Explain safety rules for crossing the street and enforce the rules consistently, even with adults. By talking about safety often, you encourage children to think and talk about the reason behind the actions in the rules. During walks, ask children to point out traffic warning signs (stoplights, signs, and crosswalks) and to explain how they help pedestrians and traffic. Older children may be able to stay with a "walking buddy," taking care of each other.

Young children have difficulty looking for oncoming traffic because they are too short to see around and over parked cars, bushes, and other barriers. Often they cannot tell from what direction a sound, such as that from a car motor or an emergency siren, is coming. Nor can they judge the speed and distance of vehicles coming toward them. They have difficulty waiting for an adult or a crossing signal to indicate that it is safe to cross a street. Worse, they imitate the inappropriate behavior of adults who take chances, such as crossing where there is no crosswalk when one is close enough to use, crossing when the signal says it is not safe to do so, or running across the street. Be sure to hold the child's hand, and select a safe place to cross. Model and verbally reinforce scanning for traffic—looking left, right, and then left again. (The vehicle closest to hitting you would come from your left.) When walking, children should learn to stop at a driveway as if it is a street to check for an oncoming vehicle. They need to learn to watch for turning vehicles at intersections. Just because they can see a car does not mean that the driver sees them.

Field trips

Pay extra attention to safety during field trips. Children tend to get excited about new and unfamiliar surroundings and may take risks that lead to injury. Increase children's safety during field trips by taking these steps:

- Recruit family members, volunteers from senior citizen centers, or students from early childhood courses to help supervise.
- Obtain a signed permission slip from parents/legal guardians for *each* excursion. This should include notifying them at the time of enrollment about

neighborhood walks that are part of the routine curriculum and getting special permission for those that differ from routes and destinations that the parents have been told are part of the usual curriculum. Knowing about the excursion routes ahead of time allows parents to raise any safety concerns that may otherwise be overlooked.

- Involve children in making and enforcing rules for field trips. Make sure children understand the rules *before* you leave.
- Identify children with a label that states the program's name and telephone number. Do *not* put the child's name on the label.
- Prepare for an emergency by bringing a small first aid kit with you. Bring a mobile phone and a list of emergency telephone numbers, a folder with copies of emergency forms, and signed permission slips. You may need to verify your authorization to be responsible for a child's care if an emergency occurs.
- If you are traveling by car, be sure in advance that there are enough vehicles so that each child and adult has a size- and age-appropriate seat restraint.
- Be a positive role model: Wear seat restraints when riding in vehicles, and cross traffic areas correctly when walking.
- Make sure that all safety seats and/or safety belts are properly used. (See Chapter 10 for more on motor vehicle transportation safety.)
- If possible, check out the field trip site in advance so that staff members are familiar with locations; hazards; mobile phone signal usability; emergency procedures; restroom facilities; and water for drinking, handwashing, and first aid.

Sun safety

Exposure to the sun even on cloudy days, in all seasons, presents additional areas of concern for outdoor play. Children can be sunburned easily or get skin burns from contact with hot surfaces such as sand, asphalt, and playground equipment. Dehydration and heat-related illness can also occur. Make sure children have access to drinking water before and after vigorous play. Purposely offer water to drink at least every two hours during the day. If the National Weather Service says the heat index is above 90° F, it is too hot to play safely outside. Find a cooler environment for children to engage in gross motor activity.

The risk of skin cancer from sun exposure is significantly increased by time spent in the sun in childhood. If there is no natural shade on your playground, create some with tents or canopies. (These add lots of new fun and adventure, too.) When the hot midday sun shines, during the hours of 10 a.m. to 2 p.m., limit the amount of time children and staff members spend outdoors without protective clothing and properly applied sunscreen in any area that lacks shade.

Skin must be protected against ultraviolet (UV) radiation in the UVA and UVB spectrum. Ask families

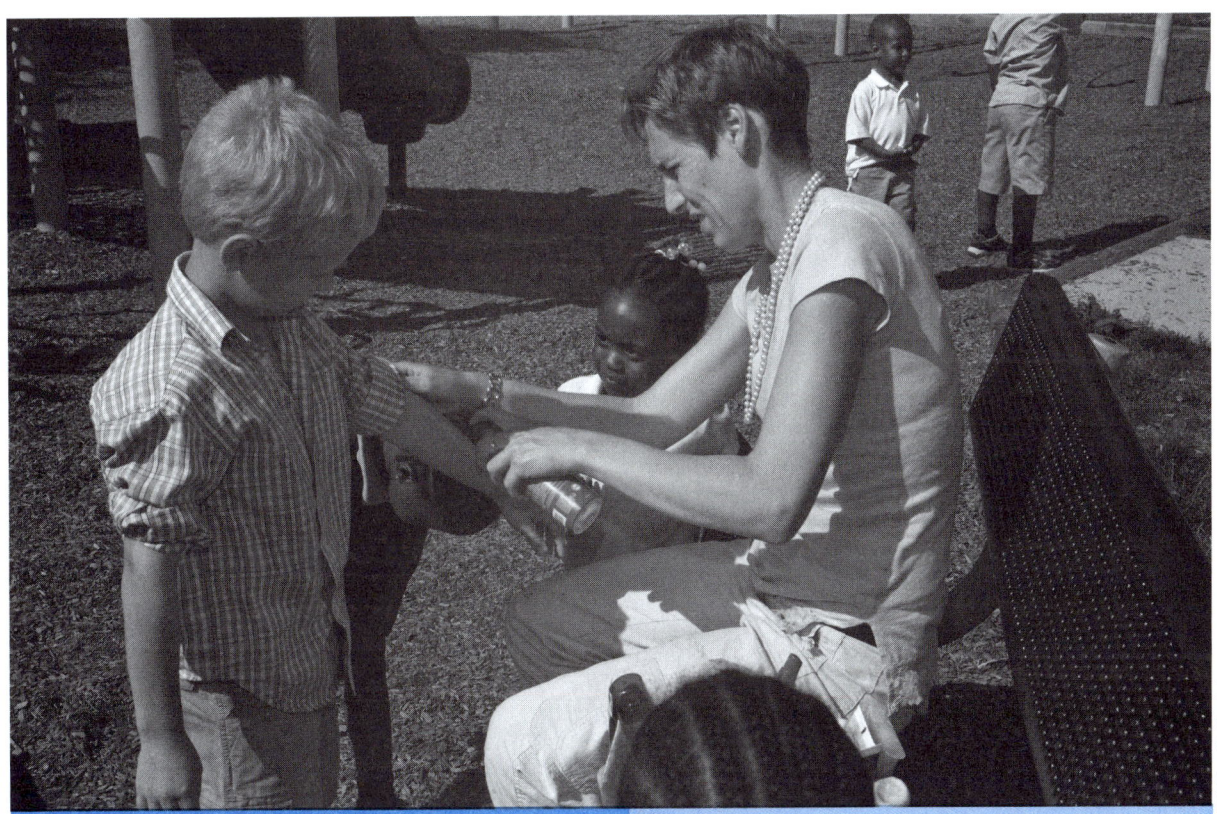

to authorize the use of sunscreen and to dress their children in protective clothing (or send protective clothing with their children to the program), such as long-sleeve, loose shirts and hats or visors. You should need a parent's consent only, not an order from a health professional, to apply sunscreen. However, some state regulations do require a health professional's note since the state may consider these products over-the-counter medications.

Use a broad spectrum (UVA and UVB) product that is labeled with a sun protection factor (SPF) of at least SPF 15. SPF means the multiple of the time the user would expect to get sunburned without using the product. So SPF 15 means that if the skin would start to show injury after 20 minutes of exposure, the product extends this time to 300 minutes, or five hours. Products with an SPF of 50 or more do not offer greater protection than those with a lower SPF.

Apply the sun protection product 15–30 minutes before exposure to the sun to allow time for the sunscreen to bind to the skin. Then, because children perspire when running around, reapply it at least every two hours whenever the children are outside, even if it is cloudy or cool. No sunscreen is waterproof. They all become less effective when wet. After June 2012, Federal Drug Administration (FDA) regulations require that sunscreen products that protect against both UVA- and UVB-induced skin damage will be labeled "Broad Spectrum" and "SPF 15" (or higher). The label on these products will also say that these products reduce the risk of cancer and early skin aging when combined with other sun protection measures as directed on the label. Other products that do not qualify for the Broad Spectrum label must say: "Skin Cancer/Skin Aging Alert: Spending time in the sun increases your risk of skin cancer and early skin aging. This product has been shown only to help prevent sunburn, not skin cancer or early skin aging."

Manufacturers can no longer use the terms "sunblock," "waterproof," or "sweat-proof" on their labels. Water-resistance claims must be based on testing that shows how much time a user can expect to get the declared SPF level of protection while swimming or sweating. Two times will be permitted on labels: 40 minutes or 80 minutes. No product can claim instant protection. To learn more about sunscreen labeling, go to **www.fda.gov/sunscreen**.

Each afternoon, the Environmental Protection Agency (EPA) and the National Weather Service post the predicted UV Index for the next day. The UV Index is a measure of the risk from sun exposure, from 1 (low) to 11+ (extremely high). For the UV Index for your ZIP code, go to **www.epa.gov/sunwise/uvindex.html**.

Swimming/wading safety

Drowning is still one of the leading causes of death among young children. Children can drown in less than an inch of water. Most drowning incidents occur in backyard pools, and the young drowning victim is generally missing for only a few minutes before the drowning occurs. States with warm climates have more drowning incidents than average. Make sure that entrances to pools have secure locks and latches that are child resistant. Fencing needs to surround the pool on all four sides (that is, a building cannot serve as part of the enclosure). Whenever children are near water (including swimming pools, wading pools, ponds, streams, or salt marshes), there must be constant, active adult supervision, with the supervising adult within an arm's length to provide touch supervision. At least one adult present must be certified in water safety and infant/child CPR. Be sure to assign one adult as a designated water watcher, whose only job is to watch for problems. This person can wear a tag to identify the responsibility and must hand off the tag to another adult if her attention must be elsewhere.

Buckets filled with water or other liquids—especially the large five-gallon size—present a drowning hazard to young children. Never leave a bucket unattended when small children are around. Even a partly filled bucket can be a drowning hazard to curious young children learning to walk, who pull themselves up using the bucket and then topple into it.

Teach children these basic water safety rules right from the start:

- Go through a gate or approach a swimming pool only when you are with an adult.
- Swim or play in the water only when an adult agrees to watch you.
- Wear a life jacket (authentic personal flotation device, not water wings, noodles, or inner tubes) when you are near or in the water until you have learned to swim well.
- Do not run, push, or dunk in or around water.
- Keep glass out of any swimming area.
- Do not swim with something in your mouth.
- Yell for help only when you need it.

Teach all adults how to manage a blocked airway and give rescue breathing. When possible, teach CPR to school-age children, too. For water safety videos from the CPSC, tips, and a water watcher tag, go to **www.safekids.org**. Also visit **www.cdc.gov** and search for "swimming" and "drowning."

Insect bites and stings

Bugs like summer, too. Stinging insects often swarm around sugary containers, trash cans, and ripe fruits. Although most insects will not sting unless provoked, they seem to be more easily irritated during late summer and early fall. To prevent stings, adults and children should learn to avoid getting excited and moving around rapidly when they see stinging insects. Such activity is more likely to result in a sting. Keep trash cans away from outside play areas. During picnics, avoid sweet foods such as fruits and fruit juices unless water is available to rinse off sticky areas after eating. Because perspiration and overheated skin seem to attract stinging insects, sponge off, sprinkle, or spray children with water to keep them fresh and cool. (Refer to Chapter 2 for information on insect repellent.)

Obtain and use the first aid instructions from the AAP (**www.aap.org**). These include details on how to handle insect bites and stings. Staff members should know if any child is allergic to insect stings and should be prepared to treat them as recommended by the child's family and physician.

Winter outdoor play

Children of all ages enjoy and benefit from playing outdoors in all except the most extreme weather. Although "extreme" weather varies according to what people are accustomed to, *Caring for Our Children* permits outdoor child care activities as long as the windchill is above -15° F, as determined by the National Weather Service. In winter, be sure children dress warmly but are not overdressed. If they are overdressed and play actively, they will get sweaty and then chilled. Go outside, however briefly, if the weather conditions are above the windchill limit and it is not raining or snowing too hard to stay dry with appropriate clothing. Going outside in snow and rain provides opportunities to learn about these natural events. Splashing in puddles or making tracks in the snow can be a lot of fun. Staff members and children alike feel refreshed when fresh air is part of the daily routine.

Snow safety

Encourage children to play in and with snow. Take advantage of this wonderful natural resource for daily winter play activities. Remember these snow safety precautions:

- *Snowballs can be dangerous,* especially when the snow is packed hard or when children put rocks or other items in them. Being hit in the face or head with this type of snowball can cause serious injury.
- Be sure that children do not throw snowballs into parking lots, into streets, or at moving cars.
- Encourage children to play in and with the snow, but don't let them eat it. Although eating snow is fun, it is *not* healthy, particularly in cities, where it can contain dirt or toxic atmospheric substances.
- Be sure scarves and hoods do not have strings or parts that can get caught on playground equipment. These can cause strangulation and other serious injuries.
- Keep children dry. Wet clothing allows for rapid cooling and frostbite.

Special safety tips for infants and toddlers

Never assume that a child's motor abilities will remain the same from day to day. One day an infant cannot possibly turn over and fall off a changing table; the very next day he can give a successful push and end up on the floor. In a safe environment, an infant's or toddler's natural curiosity can be encouraged if you give special consideration to indoor and outdoor equipment.

Equipment and toys

Keep safety in mind when you buy and use furniture and equipment for children younger than 3 years of age. Injuries involving cribs, baby walkers, and high chairs are fairly common yet usually preventable. Reduce the possibility of injury by selecting appropriate equipment that meets CPSC guidelines (go to **www.cpsc.gov** to view CPSC publications by product type), properly maintaining it, and supervising its use. Walkers that infants can move across the floor should not be used because many children fall over, pull objects down on them, or go down steps while in them. Stationary walkers that allow children to stand and turn around do not help teach children to stand and walk any earlier and may actually delay motor development. However, using a stationary walker for typically developing children who cannot yet hold themselves upright is acceptable if children spend very little time in them. Using a prescribed walker for children with disabilities is an appropriate accommodation.

The Juvenile Products Manufacturers Association (JPMA) has a testing and certification program for high chairs, play yards, carriages, strollers, walkers, gates, and expandable enclosures. When purchasing such equipment, look for labeling that certifies that these products meet the standards. ASTM also maintains a website at **www.astm.org** with the latest standards on high chair specifications. The label should indicate the weight limit and other restrictions for using the equipment.

For all equipment intended to be used by children of any age, contact the manufacturer of any equipment for which you do not have the original label and instructions to ask for them, and to be sure the equipment has not been recalled. The CPSC maintains a recall list that you can use to check for recalls of all the equipment in a facility. It's a good idea to check the recall list at least once a year for products that are in the facility.

Changing surfaces

Even though the floor may seem to be the safest place to change diapers, disposable training pants (such as Pull-Ups), or soiled underwear, it is not a good changing surface in child care. It is hard to prevent extensive contamination of the floor and other nearby objects. Standing older children on the floor to change them puts the teacher in an ergonomically difficult position and makes it hard to clean the child's soiled skin adequately. Each group of children should have at least one changing table that is not used by any other group. The table should have a changing surface that is at least three feet above the floor to prevent adult back strain.

Always keep at least one hand on the child. Do not use safety straps; they are neither sanitary nor safe. Never leave the child, even for a moment. Whenever possible, use a table with guardrails or a recessed top; these offer some additional protection against falls. Keep areas for changing, food preparation, and play separate.

Indoor play areas

Programs with infants and toddlers should make sure that enough free floor space is available for crawling and toddling children. These floors should be clean, free of splinters and cracks, and not highly polished. The amount of space per child affects the risk of injury as well as the risk of spread of infectious disease. Standard 5.1.2.1 in *Caring for Our Children* defines the space required as a minimum of 42 square feet of usable floor space, with 50 square feet preferred. Usable floor space does not include any areas covered by furnishings or used as walkways, toilet or changing areas, or staff member work space or administrative areas.

Separate infant and toddler play areas from the general play area for older children. This encourages the younger children to explore without the danger of being knocked down by older children. These areas should be furnished with developmentally appropriate surfaces and materials. For example, the surface should not be a particulate, loose-fill material such as pea gravel that could pose a choking hazard for infants and toddlers. Tunnels to crawl through should be at ground or floor level for infants and toddlers. Such equipment for older children may be elevated. Provide an easily washed area for quiet activities and gross motor movement. If an area is covered by a textured surface such as a rug, be sure it can be picked up and laundered. Bolt down top-heavy furniture such as shelving or cubbies to avoid toppling by children pulling up on furniture.

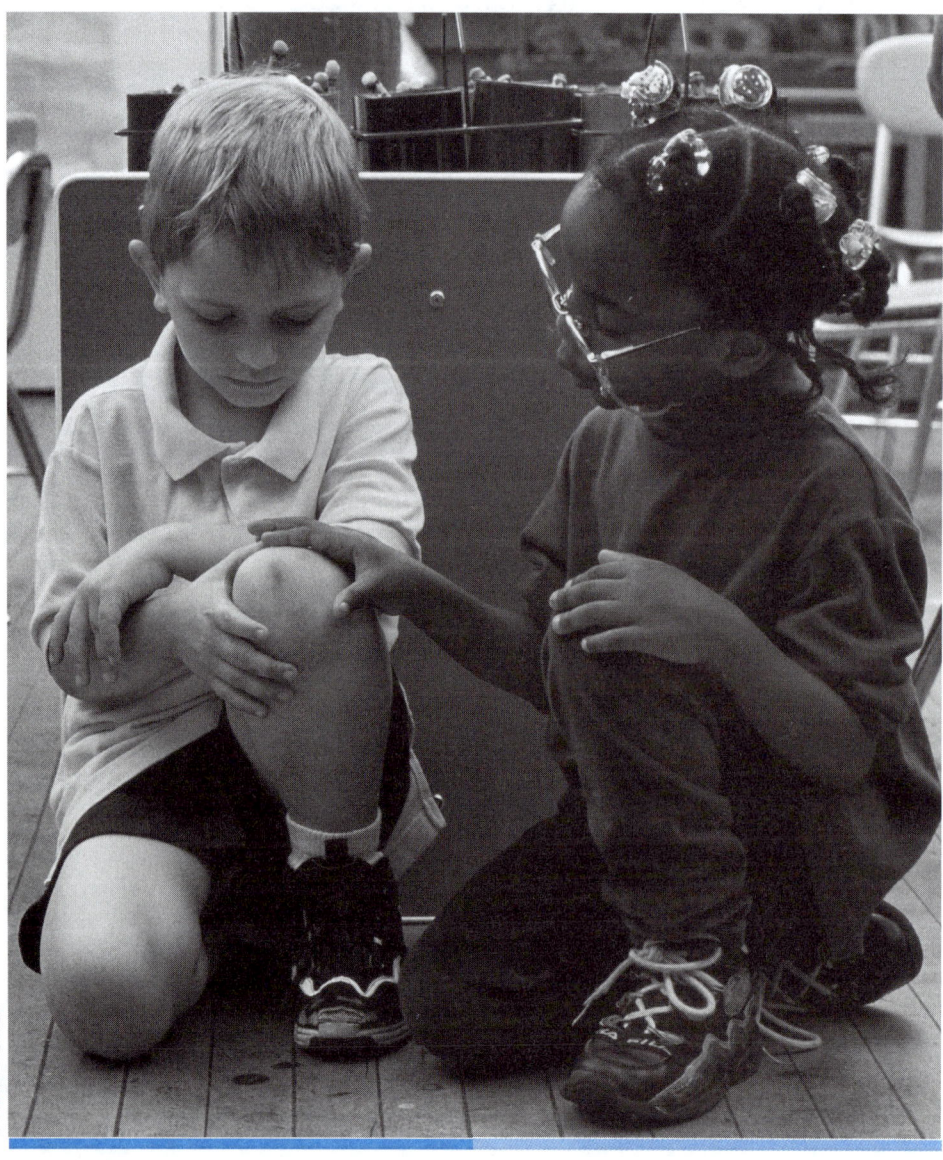
© Ellen B. Senisi

Figure 3.5.

Safe Sleeping for Infants

Facilities should develop a written policy that describes the practices to be used to promote safe sleep when infants are napping or sleeping. The policy should explain that these practices aim to reduce the risk of sudden infant death syndrome (SIDS) or suffocation death and other infant deaths that could occur when an infant is in a crib or asleep.

All staff, parents/guardians, volunteers, and others approved to enter rooms where infants are cared for should receive a copy of the Safe Sleep Policy and additional educational information and training on the importance of consistent use of safe sleep policies and practices before they are allowed to care for infants (i.e., first day of employment/volunteering/subbing). Documentation that training has occurred and that these individuals have received and reviewed the written policy should be kept on file.

All staff, parents/guardians, volunteers, and others who care for infants in the child care setting should follow these required safe sleep practices as recommended by the American Academy of Pediatrics (AAP):

a. Infants up to twelve months of age should be placed for sleep in a supine position (wholly on their back) for every nap or sleep time unless the infant's primary care provider has completed a signed waiver indicating that the child requires an alternate sleep position.

b. Infants should be placed for sleep in safe sleep environments, which includes: a firm crib mattress covered by a tight-fitting sheet in a safety-approved crib (the crib should meet the standards and guidelines reviewed/approved by the U.S. Consumer Product Safety Commission [CPSC] and ASTM International [ASTM]), no monitors or positioning devices should be used unless required by the child's primary care provider, and no other items should be in a crib occupied by an infant except for a pacifier.

c. Infants should not nap or sleep in a car safety seat, bean bag chair, bouncy seat, infant seat, swing, jumping chair, play pen or play yard, highchair, chair, futon, or any other type of furniture/equipment that is not a safety-approved crib (that is in compliance with the CPSC and ASTM safety standards).

d. If an infant arrives at the facility asleep in a car safety seat, the parent/guardian or caregiver/teacher should immediately remove the sleeping infant from this seat and place them in the supine position in a safe sleep environment (i.e., the infant's assigned crib).

e. If an infant falls asleep in any place that is not a safe sleep environment, staff should immediately move the infant and place them in the supine position in their crib.

f. Only one infant should be placed in each crib (stackable cribs are not recommended).

g. Soft or loose bedding should be kept away from sleeping infants and out of safe sleep environments. These include, but are not limited to: bumper pads, pillows, quilts, comforters, sleep positioning devices, sheepskins, blankets, flat sheets, cloth diapers, bibs, etc. Also, blankets/items should not be hung on the sides of cribs. Swaddling infants when they are in a crib is not necessary or recommended, but rather one-piece sleepers should be used (see Standard 3.1.4.2 for more detailed information on swaddling).

h. Toys, including mobiles and other types of play equipment that are designed to be attached to any part of the crib, should be kept away from sleeping infants and out of safe sleep environments.

i. When caregivers/teachers place infants in their crib for sleep, they should check to ensure that the temperature in the room is comfortable for a lightly clothed adult, check the infants to ensure that they are comfortably clothed (not overheated or sweaty), and that bibs, necklaces, and garments with ties or hoods are removed (clothing sacks or other clothing designed for sleep can be used in lieu of blankets).

j. Infants should be directly observed by sight and sound at all times, including when they are going to sleep, are sleeping, or are in the process of waking up.

k. Bedding should be changed between children, and if mats are used, they should be cleaned between uses.

The lighting in the room must allow the caregiver/teacher to see each infant's face, to view the color of the infant's skin, and to check on the infant's breathing and placement of the pacifier (if used).

A caregiver/teacher trained in safe sleep practices and approved to care for infants should be present in each room at all times where there is an infant. This caregiver/teacher should remain alert and should actively supervise sleeping infants in an ongoing manner. Also, the caregiver/teacher should check to ensure that the infant's head remains uncovered and re-adjust clothing as needed.

Source: Standard 3.1.4.1, *Caring for Our Children*. Reprinted with permission.

Toddlers must be well supervised, especially near water tables and in bathrooms near toilets and deep sinks. These are naturally of great interest to young children and, with the unsteady gait of toddlers, present a potential drowning hazard. They also pose a significant sanitation challenge that requires one-on-one supervision.

Sleeping arrangements

Placement of cots and cribs is an important safety issue.

- Leave a clear aisle between cribs. Separations for infectious disease control require three feet between children who are using sleeping or rest equipment. However sleep/rest equipment is arranged, staff members must have quick access to each child in an emergency.
- Place cribs away from open windows, window blinds, and shade cords. Do not use stacking cribs or bunk beds.
- Be sure all cribs comply with the most recent CPSC requirements for crib safety. Malfunction of cribs made before July 2011 has resulted in infant deaths. For more information, see **www.cpsc.gov/info/cribs/index.html**.
- Follow the guidelines for safe sleeping that are detailed in Figure 3.5. These will help prevent sudden infant death syndrome (SIDS), described below.

Sudden infant death syndrome

Sudden infant death syndrome (SIDS) is the death of a seemingly healthy infant from no apparent cause. The death of a child is always a tragedy, and a SIDS death is one of the most frightening types. Until the roles of sleep positioning and sleep environment were discovered, SIDS, also known as crib death, was the major cause of death in infants after the first month of life (up to 2 deaths per 1,000 live births). Researchers do not yet fully understand all the causes of SIDS, but a 40 percent reduction in SIDS deaths has been associated with putting infants down on their backs to sleep. More recently, researchers have identified other contributing factors: soft bedding and objects, co-sleeping, overheating, exposure to secondhand smoke, and unsafe cribs. Other cases of presumed SIDS have been found to involve child abuse, and some still have no known cause. Many SIDS deaths can be prevented by using a snug-fitting mattress; removing soft objects such as toys, bumpers, and blankets (use clothing for warmth instead) from the crib; avoiding overheating; and putting infants down to sleep on their backs in a crib that meets current CPSC safety standards.

Studies show that infants are more likely to be positioned on their sides or stomachs by child care workers than by parents as a group. Also, data suggest that hour-for-hour of time spent in each setting, infants are more likely to die of SIDS in child care settings than in their own homes. Always put infants down to sleep on their backs, unless there are specific medical conditions for which a physician prescribes prone (stomach) sleeping with the medical reason for this request. These conditions are very rare. If a child is placed on her back and subsequently rolls over, there is no need to return the child to the back-sleep position. It could be argued that failing to put an infant down to sleep supine is a form of maltreatment.

Studies by the CPSC have associated soft bedding with infant deaths. Families and caregivers should put infants on a firm, flat sleeping surface and never on top of soft, fluffy items such as pillows, couches, comforters, and sheepskins. Infants should also never sleep with an adult in the adult's bed. In child care, blankets should never be used for warmth, as comfort objects in the crib, or for swaddling. Use clothing that allows free movement of the infant's legs and unrestricted expansion of the chest for breathing.

Be aware that if an apparent SIDS death occurs in a child care program, an autopsy can verify that there was no identifiable cause of death (e.g., disease or suffocation). If a potential SIDS death occurs, contact your state public health department and state chapter of the national SIDS program for help for the family, staff members, and other families in the program, who will understandably be very upset.

Shaken baby syndrome

Shaken baby syndrome, also called abusive head trauma, is a type of traumatic brain injury of infants and young children. The term refers to the consequences of a young child's head whipping back and forth during shaking or another activity that causes rapid movement of the child's head, such as throwing the child up in the air. The average age of shaken baby syndrome victims is 3–6 months, but the condition may be seen in children up to 5 years of age. Injuries from shaking a young child's head are the result of the brain slamming back and forth inside the skull cavity. Swelling and bleeding inside the brain can occur, but even without swelling or bleeding—and without ever hitting the head—the force of acceleration and deceleration can injure brain cells. Shaken baby syndrome can result in blindness, deafness, seizures, learning difficulties, cerebral palsy, speech impairment, and death. It is the leading cause of death and long-term disability from child maltreatment. Staff members and families should be reminded not to engage in activities that cause rapid movement of a young child's head and consequent brain injury.

Supervision

Caring for children in a group setting is different from caring for your own children in your own home. More children of the same age usually are in a group program. In group care children also participate in a relatively high level of activity during waking hours and share an environment with other children whose usual rules of behavior differ from their own. Teachers must be vigilant about supervising children in ways appropriate for their age and must know where every child is at all times. To be sure of the whereabouts and activity of each child, assign a specific teacher to supervise certain children, and have that teacher routinely conduct name-to-face checks of each child at preset intervals and before and after each transition (e.g., from the classroom to the playground or from the restroom to the classroom).

Several methods are used for assigning accountability to a specific teacher for individual children. One way is to use a token for each child marked with that child's name (and any other key information). The teacher carries, wears, or posts the token visibly. Timed intervals between checking for all the children assigned to the teacher should not be longer than 15 minutes. A signal-giving wristwatch, vibrating pocket alarm, or some other not-too-intrusive reminder helps ensure that the teacher does not become distracted and fail to do a name-to-face check at short intervals. Teachers need to be able to see and hear all children assigned to their care at all times, as appropriate for the child's age and developmental stage. Knowing individual children well and analyzing the layout of specific program sites may alert teachers to other steps they can take to prevent a child from slipping out of sight or becoming involved in something that could cause injury.

Use of high-risk equipment requires even closer supervision. Stationing adults within an arm's reach of children engaged in potentially injurious activities allows prompt intervention when a challenge becomes an unacceptable risk. For example, a teacher should be at the slide to monitor and ensure safe use of the steps and sliding bed or chute. Swings need close monitoring to be sure children do not stray into the path of the swing, twist, stand up on the seats, or otherwise improperly use the swings. Children and adults need to have clear rules about what is allowed and have those rules restated often. Posting key rules as "dos" rather than "don'ts" reminds staff members to tell the children in a positive way about what they may do. (See Figure 3.3.)

Safety education and hazard checks

Injuries are the result of unsafe conditions in the environment, a mismatch between a child's abilities and activities, and/or a lack of adult supervision. Sometimes there are hidden dangers seen only after a child or staff member is injured. Injuries can often be prevented by:

- Being aware of potential hazards
- Taking action to eliminate or reduce these hazards
- Knowing what to do in an emergency
- Teaching children about safety

Provide children with the skills to prevent injuries and to help care for themselves and others in case of emergency. Keep in mind that your own attitudes and behaviors toward safety are as important as the physical setup of the facility. Use the following ways to give safety messages to children and staff members:

- Be a positive role model.
- Give clear statements when explaining the correct, safe way to do something.
- Compliment children for doing things safely.
- Involve the children in making and enforcing rules to increase their safety awareness and help them feel involved. As soon as children understand words, involve them in making safety checks. Even the youngest toddler can be asked to look for toys on the floor to put away after play.
- Teach children what to do in an emergency and where to get help.
- Use teachable moments to discuss safety (e.g., when a child gets a minor bump or bruise, talk to all the children about ways to prevent similar injuries).

A Special Note on Federal Standards for Infant Sleep Equipment and Recalled Products

Do not buy or use old infant cribs or other infant sleep equipment without first checking that they meet CPSC standards. Many cribs manufactured before the effective date of the crib safety standards (June 28, 2011) do not meet the requirements, especially cribs with drop sides. Inventory all cribs and other equipment so you can check with the CPSC at least annually for product recalls on all equipment used in the child care facility. Recalls of toys and children's products are posted online at **www.cpsc.gov**. Consider subscribing to the CPSC list to automatically receive recall notices as they are issued, and share this information with families.

Many recalled articles are still in use and cause injury because users do not know the product has been recalled. If a product has been recalled, disassemble and discard it. Do not sell, donate, or store it where it may be used at a later time by someone who does not know it was recalled.

Planned lessons on safety are most effective when integrated with other curricular activities. Classroom routines, math, science, language arts, creative drama, social studies, art, and music can all be taught along with safety messages. Safety can be a part of a game with a serious motivation. Children love to be hazard-hunters. Have each child or a team of children search for a specific type of hazard or inspect a part of the building, then notify an adult about any hazards found.

In addition to your own ideas, you may wish to use safety curricula from a variety of resources. Risk Watch® is one excellent curriculum designed with input from the nation's leading safety and early childhood education organizations to teach children how to keep themselves safe. Available from the National Fire Protection Association, the curriculum addresses the eight most common causes of injury to children. Go to **www.nfpa.org** and search for "Risk Watch." You'll find many tools on this site, including lesson plans, workshop support materials, letters for parents, handouts, worksheets, and much more.

Community-based Safe Kids coalitions (go to **www.safekids.org** to find a coalition in your area) and other safety promotion programs often have educational materials and people who will come to do special programs. Local fire, police, and disaster preparedness personnel may be willing to come teach children about safety and their role as community helpers. Instructors who teach pedestrian, passenger, bike, and school bus safety may be funded by your state's Department of Transportation. Regional poison control centers usually have community outreach and education programs.

Select the age-appropriate safety curriculum that best fits your program's needs and philosophy. Whatever you choose, remember that safety education is more than just a one-time activity. The following list offers examples of ways to integrate safety concepts into all of your activities:

- Use storytelling, story reading, and classroom role play with chairs and seat belts to review passenger safety rules and other safety lessons.
- Include poison prevention in nutrition education conversations at the table, at circle time, during cooking experiences, when doing routine cleanup, and when taking walks outside.
- With the children, make a dollhouse from cardboard boxes or hollow blocks, then use dolls or paper figures to act out home hazards (e.g., hot surfaces, poisonous products, and toys left on stairs).
- Weave messages about clothing into discussions on weather and appropriate dress (e.g., wearing light colors and reflective clothing at night or on dark, rainy days; wearing dark colors on bright, snowy days).

Suggested activities

- With a partner, conduct a safety check of a child care center or family child care home. Look for hazards independently, and then compare observations. What hazards did you find? Are the observations of your colleague the same? When you and your colleague differed in your observations, did either of you overlook a hazard or disagree about what is hazardous? How could hazards be corrected? How can families, staff members, and children be involved to make safety checks more effective?

- Contact the local licensing agency. Accompany a licensing inspector, a building/fire inspector, and a sanitarian to a child care site. See how hazard checks are done, whether they overlap, and whether the findings conflict with or support one another. What is done when a problem is identified? How do staff members in early care and education view official inspectors?

- Discuss how to correct safety problems in child care when expense is involved. Discuss the role of staff members, families, public authorities, and children in identifying and participating in correcting safety problems.

- Discuss how routine safety checks should be done in an early childhood program. Who should do them? How often should they be done? How can follow-up on problems be ensured?

- Think about activities that could be used to teach safety to toddlers, preschoolers, school-age children, families, or more than one of these groups at the same time. What would you need to do this activity? Try to find an early care and education program where you could try out an activity.

- Go to the Safe Kids website, **www.safekids.org**. Look for topics and tips that you can use to make attractive, informative parent and staff education posters. Make at least one poster, and then give it to a child care program.

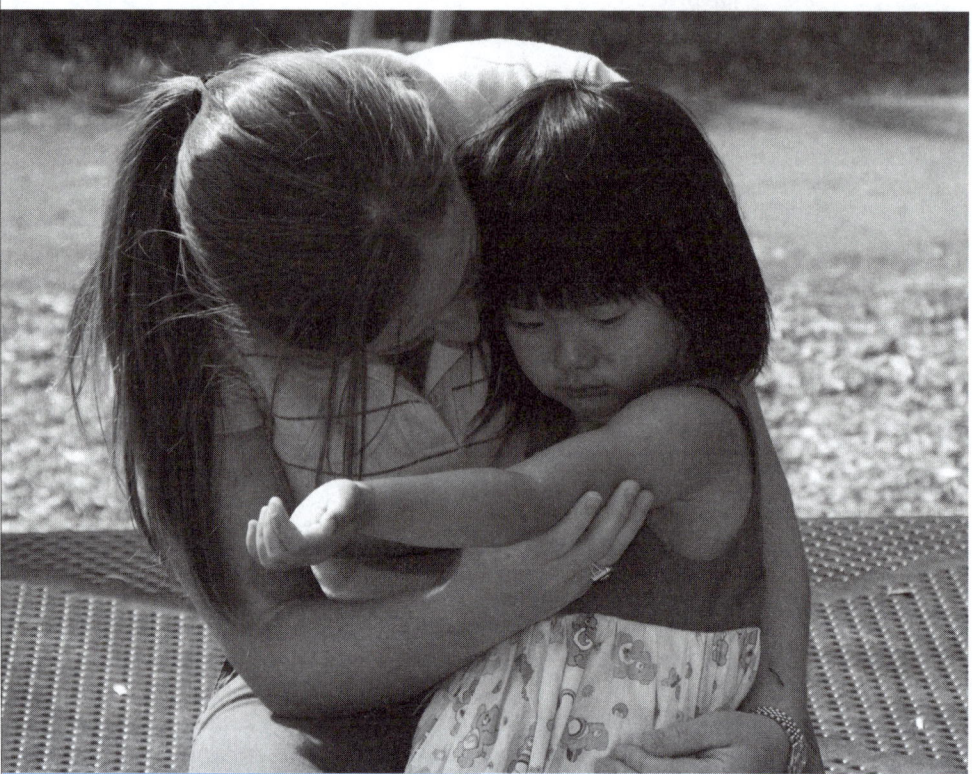

Ready for Emergencies and Injuries

MAJOR CONCEPTS

- Advance planning for emergencies leads to sound decisions in a crisis.
- An emergency arouses fears that must be put aside temporarily so that the emergency can be managed appropriately.
- When an injury or a sudden illness occurs, all adults who are responsible for the care of children should be prepared to provide first aid and an emergency response appropriate to the group care setting.
- Practicing emergency procedures involving role-playing is key to responding appropriately in a time of stress.
- Staff members, parents, children, and community emergency personnel must coordinate their response to an emergency.

A child falls from a playground climber. A child chokes while eating a snack. A parent acts in a threatening fashion. Electrical power is lost during a storm. You smell gas in the kitchen. A tragic event occurs in the community that involves some families in your program. What would you do?

No matter how careful or safety conscious you are, emergencies will occur. If a facility has a comprehensive, written emergency policy, known and practiced by everyone, the result will be better handling of such situations. Use *Model Child Care Health Policies* and *Caring for Our Children* Standards 9.2.4.1 through 9.2.4.10 to be sure your facility has planned for all potential emergencies and has appropriate practices in place. Some elements to cover include the following:

- Handling specific incidents and notifying a parent or guardian: What is the plan for each of the following?
    - A lost or missing child
    - Suspected maltreatment of a child or abuse of an adult (staff member, family member, or visitor) while on the child care premises
    - Injuries requiring medical or dental care, emergency treatment, or hospitalization: Who will give first aid? Who will call 911? Who will provide medical care personnel with health information about the child, an authorization form signed by the parent for emergency medical care, and informed consent to share the child's health records with other service providers?
    - Mental health emergencies
    - Death of a child or an adult who is known to those in the program
    - Presence of a threatening individual who attempts to gain or succeeds in gaining entrance to the facility or to outdoor play areas
    - No authorized person arrives to pick up a child
- If the building and grounds need to be evacuated, or if it is necessary to shelter-in-place, who will be responsible for the daily roster of children and adults who are at the facility, and for family notification information?
- Where will everyone go if you must shelter-in-place, if you cannot go back into the building after an evacuation, or if you must evacuate some distance from the building? How will this situation affect the facility's emergency procedures?
- What is the plan for emergency transport to a local emergency facility? Who will respond when you call 911? Will an ambulance come, or will the police come first to assess the situation? What will they do when they come? Where will they take a child who needs hospital care? Will they allow the child's teacher to accompany the child until the parent can assume responsibility for the child? What, if anything, will be done differently if it is an adult who has a medical emergency?
- Do all children with known medical conditions that might require emergency or urgent care have a care plan created by the child's health care provider that addresses such situations? (See Appendix O of *Caring for Our Children* for sample forms from New Jersey and California.)
- Is there a plan in place to handle a disease outbreak, such as seasonal and pandemic influenza?
- Who is responsible for keeping the first aid kits supplied in serviceable condition, including immediate restocking when the kit is used and a monthly check that the contents are as specified in *Caring for Our Children* Standard 5.6.0.1?
- Who is responsible for maintaining an unexpired 72-hour supply of food and water for each child and adult in the facility to use in the event of a natural disaster or other community-wide situation that requires sheltering-in-place?
- Who will take charge and implement plans to respond quickly to electrical, plumbing, gas, heating, or natural disaster emergencies?
- How often will staff members be required to demonstrate their ability to locate and operate fire extinguishers to fight a small fire or clear an escape path and to determine quickly when a fire is too large to fight with a fire extinguisher?
- What developmentally appropriate lessons about emergency preparedness are teachers expected to provide to children? How will staff members coordinate this teaching with supportive messages for families?
- What is the plan for emergency drills/exercises for the following events that pose relevant risks to the facility? (Include shelter-in-place, evacuation to nearby location, and out-of-the community drills at different times of the day, including naptime.)
    - Fire—monthly
    - Tornadoes—monthly in tornado season
    - Floods—before the flood season
    - Earthquakes—every six months
    - Hurricanes—annually
    - Threatening person outside or inside the facility—at least every six months (more often if the facility is located near a prison)
    - Rabid or aggressive animal
    - Toxic chemical spill
    - Nuclear event

Figure 4.1 outlines procedures to follow for a medical emergency situation. These procedures can be adapted to fit your program's size and location and the children's ages. A program policy should clearly state the roles and responsibilities of the children and each staff member in such an emergency. Families also need to be informed about the emergency medical procedures and their roles in them.

Prepare for emergencies

Be sure that each staff member and family reads the facility's written emergency policies and procedures, signs to indicate understanding, and then subsequently refers to them. Whenever an emergency occurs, use the occasion to review how well the policy or procedure worked, and update the written document with improvements you identify. Even when handled well, an emergency offers a teachable moment. Encourage everyone to take another look at the written policies and procedures they signed to be sure to be ready for another incident, perhaps one that will be of a different type. Ask the public education division of local police and fire departments to arrange on-site visits to help staff members make appropriate emergency plans.

Make sure first aid and emergency supplies are available wherever the children go—including on neighborhood walks and trips and near all high-risk areas, such as the kitchen and playground. These supplies need to be stocked with the proper contents, restocked after each use, and checked monthly to be sure the contents are all there and do not need to be replaced. Ensure that the first aid and emergency supplies are sufficient to follow the current pediatric first aid instructions and deal with possible emergencies. Supplies are sold at drugstores, supermarkets, and discount stores, and over the Internet. Use Figure 4.2 as an inventory of the contents for first aid and emergency supplies. Keep a record of inspections of the supplies.

Store the supplies in a labeled, closed container (box, cabinet, or drawer) or in a backpack or closed tote bag that is large enough to hold all the necessary supplies for first aid or emergencies in the facility or on trips. Arrange the contents so you can reach items easily without emptying the kit. Be sure that the contents are wrapped tightly and are sanitary. The location of these supplies should be known and accessible to all staff members, but not accessible to children.

Keep emergency information for children and staff members up to date. Appoint a specific person responsible for having this information on hand in emergencies, on trips, and in the event of evacuation. Ask parents to update emergency contact information every six months, and verify information periodically by testing it with a telephone call to be sure that parents or emergency contacts can be reached quickly. An easy way to implement this is to call a few emergency contacts each day until everyone's contact numbers have been tested, then start from the beginning of the list to do it again.

Be sure all directors, teachers, and other staff members involved in providing direct care have documentation of satisfactory completion of training in pediatric first aid and pediatric CPR skills. The documentation should be current according to the requirement for renewal of the training and skills assessment. The course should include all the topics listed in *Caring for Our Children* Standard 1.4.3.2 (topics to be covered for everyone) and Standard 1.4.3.3 (for swimming and water play). Teaching pediatric CPR skills should involve demonstration, practice to acquire the skills, and then return demonstration by the learners to show the instructor that they can perform the skills competently. First aid for children in the early education setting requires a more child-specific approach than standard adult-oriented first aid offers. Several national organizations provide curriculum and training of instructors, but not all include the full list of topics that should be

Figure 4.1.

Emergency Medical Procedures

1. Remain calm. Reassure the victim and others at the scene.
2. Stay at the scene and give help at least until the person assigned to handle emergencies arrives.
3. Send word to the person who handles emergencies for your program. This person will take charge of the emergency, assess the situation, and give any further help as needed.
4. Do not move a severely injured or ill person except to save a life.
5. If necessary, telephone for help. Give all the important information slowly and clearly. To make sure that you have given all the necessary information, *wait for the other party to hang up first*. Arrange for transportation of the injured person, if necessary by ambulance or other vehicle. Do not drive unless accompanied by another adult. Bring your child care emergency information with you.
6. Do not give any medication unless authorized by your local poison control center (for poisonings) or physician (for other illnesses).
7. Notify parent(s) of the emergency and agree on a course of action.
8. If the parent(s) cannot be reached, notify the emergency contact person specified by the parent(s).
9. Be sure that a responsible individual from the program stays with the injured child until parent(s) take charge.
10. Fill out an injury/incident report within 24 hours. (See Figure A.6 in Appendix A.) File in the child's folder. Give the family a copy, preferably that day. Put a copy in the central injury log.

Figure 4.2.

Inventory for First Aid Kits and Emergency Supplies

First aid and emergency supplies should be kept wherever the program is caring for children. Include the following items in first aid and emergency supplies:

a) Disposable nonporous, latex-free or non-powdered latex gloves (latex-free recommended)
b) Scissors
c) Tweezers
d) Non-glass, non-mercury thermometer to measure a child's temperature
e) Bandage tape
f) Sterile gauze pads
g) Flexible roller gauze
h) Triangular bandages
i) Safety pins
j) Eye patch or dressing
k) Pen/pencil and note pad
l) Cold pack
m) Current American Academy of Pediatrics (AAP) standard first aid chart or equivalent first aid guide such as the *AAP Pediatric First Aid For Caregivers and Teachers (PedFACTS) Manual*
n) Coins for use in a pay phone and cell phone
o) Water (two liters of sterile water for cleaning wounds or eyes)
p) Liquid soap to wash injury and hand sanitizer, used with supervision, if hands are not visibly soiled or if no water is present
q) Tissues
r) Wipes
s) Individually wrapped sanitary pads to contain bleeding of injuries
t) Adhesive strip bandages, plastic bags for cloths, gauze, and other materials used in handling blood
u) Flashlight
v) Whistle
w) Battery-powered radio

When children walk or are transported to another location, the transportable first aid kit should include ALL items listed above AND the following emergency information/items:

a) List of children in attendance (organized by caregiver/teacher they are assigned to) and their emergency contact information (i.e., parents/guardian/emergency contact home, work, and cell phone numbers)
b) Special care plans for children who have them
c) Emergency medications or supplies as specified in the special care plans
d) List of emergency contacts (i.e., location information and phone numbers for the Poison Center, nearby hospitals or other emergency care clinics, and other community resource agencies)
e) Maps
f) Written transportation policy and contingency plans

Source: Standard 5.6.0.1, *Caring for Our Children*. Reprinted with permission.

---

covered. (See Chapter 3 for additional discussion of pediatric first aid and CPR training.)

Have these important forms on hand for emergencies:

- *Parental permission forms.* Hospitals and emergency rooms have the right to refuse to give emergency treatment to any minor child, except in a life-threatening situation, without parental informed consent at the time of treatment. Remind parents that they must be reachable *at all times* to give consent for medical care. Ask parents to complete emergency permission forms before enrollment, and keep these on file. Take a copy of all permission forms with you on field trips. (See Appendix KK in *Caring for Our Children* for a sample form.)
- *Injury/Incident report forms.* Every program should use a standardized form for reporting all injuries or illnesses that require first aid or additional care (Figure A.6 in Appendix A is a sample form from *Model Child Care Health Policies*). Give one copy of the report to the child's parents and keep another copy in the child's folder. Find out which incidents or injuries must be reported to state or local authorities. Maintain one central file of copies of all injury/incident reports so patterns of injury or other incidents can be monitored to improve program safety.

Getting help

Teachers should carry a mobile phone to parks, playgrounds, and other places they visit with the children. Since mobile phones do not always have a reliable signal, know the locations of nearby places where you can use a telephone or fire alarm box, or places to go for help. Make sure that everyone in the building has ready access to a telephone to call for help.

Usually you can reach emergency assistance by dialing 911 everywhere in the United States. Verify this by checking the local phone directory. Near the phone in your facility, post your program's address, description of the building, and directions to it from a major road, since these may be hard to remember in a crisis. (See Figure A.7 in Appendix A for a sample emergency number form.) Be sure your facility is well marked, with signs visible from the street, so rescue workers can find it easily. Contact the local police to find answers to the following questions about your emergency and medical services:

- Who answers the emergency telephone—police, fire, ambulance, dispatcher?
- What steps does the dispatcher have to take before sending the ambulance? Call another dispatcher? Call emergency medical technicians?
- Who provides the ambulance service—police, fire, volunteer, private company, a facility in another town?
- How far do the emergency service providers have to travel to get to your program? Where is the nearest point where they wait for a call?
- How long will it take them to get to your program?
- Where is the nearest emergency department that is capable of providing competent pediatric care? Some emergency departments do not provide pediatric care or provide only life-saving stabilizing care to transfer a child to another hospital set up to care for children.

Try to visit your local helpers *before* you need them in a crisis. Most ambulance services are happy to show groups of visitors their equipment, and some will even visit your facility if you ask. Emergency departments are harder to tour, but you can at least visit the waiting area and become familiar with check-in procedures. These visits also will help reassure children and their families.

Emergency evacuation

Saving lives is the first priority in any emergency. Saving property should be considered *only* when everybody is safe.

Planning, preparation, and practice are the essential ingredients of a successful evacuation plan. Have a written, well-rehearsed plan for handling any conceivable disaster or emergency that might require evacuating from the portions of the facility generally used. This plan should include specifics such as routes, assignments for all staff members, and how to alert emergency service personnel about the situation. For example, post the key words to say when you need help right away from the local fire department, police, ambulance, or emergency management agency. Often, if you say a child is involved, the priority for an immediate response increases.

To plan for an evacuation:

- Make sure everyone knows where to go if the building has to be evacuated. Be sure that the arrangements are reconfirmed periodically for a more remote location as a second backup in case the nearby refuge is involved in the problem that required evacuation of the child care facility. Families must know where to look for their children. Stock the emergency shelters where you will take the children and inform parents by letter about these locations.

- Be sure that the daily roster records everyone who is on the facility premises: children, staff members, volunteers, and guests. Designate appropriate staff members to carry the list to the evacuation location so that it can be used to make sure the evacuation is complete.

- Post emergency telephone numbers and a copy of emergency procedures beside every telephone. All adults using the building should be familiar with these numbers and the procedures to be used in an emergency. On field trips, take a copy of the list and a list of each child's emergency contact numbers.

- Plan two exit routes from every area of the building. Post emergency evacuation exit instructions in every room where they can be seen easily.

- Stage unannounced evacuation drills at least once a month. Practice using the alternate as well as the usual exit routes. Vary the time of day to cover all activities (including naptime) and times when the fewest adults are with the children. Naptime drills will be least disruptive but still effective by carrying them out unannounced and close to the usual wake-up time for the children. A week or so before a drill will occur, staff members and children should talk about what to do when there is a drill.

- Maintain logs of evacuation drills for on-site inspection and review by the building inspector. For most buildings, evacuation in less than two minutes is possible. In large buildings, fire-resistant exit routes are usually required.

Maintain Self-Control in an Emergency

In the event of an emergency, remember three important things:

- *Keep calm*—if you panic, the children are likely to panic too.
- Follow your emergency policy and procedures.
- Act quickly.

Fire preparedness procedures

- During a fire, get out of the building, and then call 911 to alert the fire department.
- Post a diagram showing the main shutoff switches for electricity, gas, and water.
- Test fire and smoke alarms at least once each month.
- Post diagrams of exits and escape routes in each room. Mark exits clearly, and do not block them with furniture or other objects.
- Teach children who can follow these instructions to stop, drop, and roll if their clothing is on fire and to crawl under smoke to get out of a smoke-filled building. Teach younger children to come to a grown-up when they spot something hot, or something scary happens. Practice these actions with children.
- Practice leaving the building with the children at least once a month so that they recognize the sound of the alarm and know where to go.
- Include fire and burn prevention in the children's curriculum. The website **www.firesafety.gov/kids** has activities and online hazard recognition practice for older preschool and school-age children. The National Fire Protection Association, at **www.nfpa.org**, has materials and lesson plans to teach fire safety to preschool and school-age children. Be sure to choose developmentally appropriate materials and activities that promote children's learning. For example, some of these websites have pictures to color. Coloring a picture does not teach a concept unless the teacher uses the picture to teach the concept.
- Have fire extinguishers inspected annually. Place them where they can be reached easily. Know when and when not to use a fire extinguisher. Use an extinguisher only if:
  - You are nearby when a fire starts or the fire is small (confined to its origin—in a wastepaper basket, cushion, or small appliance) and discovered in its early stages
  - Other staff members get all children out of the building and call the fire department
  - You can fight it with your back to an exit and you can get out fast if your efforts fail
  - The extinguisher is in working order and you know how to use it (see box)

Using a Fire Extinguisher

1. Stand back about 8 feet.
2. Aim at the base of the fire, not the flames or smoke.
3. Squeeze or press the lever while sweeping from the sides to the middle of the fire.

If the fire spreads beyond the spot where it started or if it could block your exit, don't try to fight it. If you have the slightest doubt about whether to fight or not to fight—then don't. Get out and call the fire department.

Helping children during emergency or evacuation procedures

To calm a group of panicked children, remove them from the scene and reassure them. Explain simply and carefully what has happened and what will happen. Answer their questions truthfully. Then redirect their attention with a game or quiet activity. Most important: STAY CALM. If you panic, the children will too. If you need to evacuate the building and children are frightened, have them hold each other's hands. Human touch is very reassuring in scary situations.

To evacuate nonambulatory children, carry two or three infants or use a large wagon or evacuation crib to transport infants, toddlers, or children who are severely disabled outdoors (if your building has ramps) or at least to the door where someone else can take them.

To remove a child who is too scared to leave the building, use your legs to press gently on the back of the child's knees to push him forward, or hold his hands with one of your arms across his back.

Closings due to power failure or natural catastrophe

Some power failures are short and require no action, but they can pose a serious health hazard when heat or air conditioning is lost. Nearly every part of the country has some risk of weather-related or other natural catastrophe (snow, heavy storm, flood, tornadoes, hurricanes, earthquakes, and so on). Some of these events can be predicted before the facility opens, but others may occur during the child care day.

Every facility needs a plan to alert families about situations that require unexpected closings. When a need for closing occurs, families may not be able to get to the facility quickly, so alternative care plans must be made for children. Sometimes staff members will have to take children to an alternate shelter until parents can arrive. An emergency supply of food, water, clothing, blankets, flashlights, diapers, and other necessary supplies should be kept ready, either to support care at the facility or at an alternative facility to which the children must be evacuated until families can arrive to assume their care.

Security and handling persons who pose security risks

Unfortunately, security breaches at child care facilities have occurred. Both strangers and relatives who have mental health or substance abuse issues have taken threatening and even fatal actions involving children and staff members in child care facilities. Noncustodial parents have used pickup time as an opportunity to abduct their children.

Every child care facility needs a plan for maintaining security to prevent entry of any individual into child care areas until that person is screened by a member of the staff in direct interpersonal interaction, including visual contact through windows or a reception area. To control access to the facility, use buzz-in gates, cameras with an intercom system, or a person who closely monitors entrances. All programs should also require people to sign a visitor's log upon entry and exit, declaring the purpose of the visit. These precautions provide a psychological deterrent for individuals who may have an impulse to walk into a facility when they don't belong there.

If an individual can enter the premises without first going through a locked door that separates the office or lobby area from the child care area, or if a person can have direct access to the children upon entering your site, both children and staff members are at risk. All staff members should be taught how to properly identify people before allowing them to enter the site. They should always obtain a reason for the person's presence in the building. Anyone who works in the program should be prepared to challenge any person who is unfamiliar or a familiar person who is acting strangely, asking courteously if they need help.

If the stranger or strangely acting familiar person does not accept escort, or acts nervous or evasive, the facility needs a method to alert someone to call the police and someone to activate a lock-out procedure that prevents access to the children by the potentially dangerous person. A false alert is better than an adverse event. Ideally, the routine entrance process will shield the program from entry by undesired visitors, but there should be a back-up process in case someone does get through the entrance, either by slipping in with someone who is permitted to enter or by coming in before anyone realizes that the person's presence poses a problem.

A safe area to go to if there is a threatening individual in the facility should be designated for all staff members and children. All staff members should know the layout of the facility and be familiar with the name or label for all its areas. Make sure every staff member knows where the safe area is, but do not post or announce it beforehand to anyone who does not work in the program.

Once an emergency arises, staff members need to have a mechanism of communicating room to room and calling emergency personnel. Emergency preparedness experts recommend that staff members use codes to

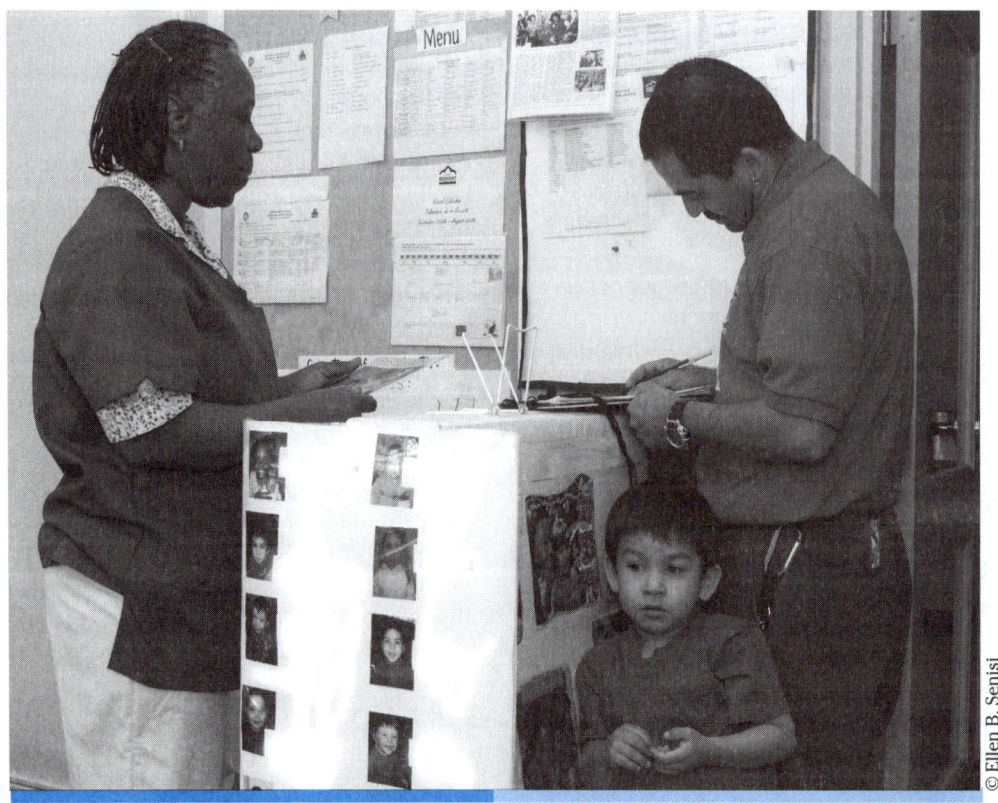

alert others to the presence of an intruder. Staff members at one center, for example, use a specific sentence when there is an intruder or threatening situation, using their telephone intercom to say something like "Sheri left her red earring in the front classroom [or whatever area has been compromised]." This signals other staff members to stay away from a particular area and to get the children to safety.

Security measures at entrances must be carefully planned so that they do not present barriers to emergency personnel. Local police may have some ideas for reasonable ways to improve security at child care facilities.

Play areas located next to a street are more hazardous than those in a more interior and less visible location. These sites are vulnerable to accidental or intentional stranger and vehicle penetration. The importance of providing protection of play areas is highlighted by a real-life tragic breach of security. A man drove around a child care playground, smiling at the children and staff members in a play area that was located near the street and protected only by a chain-link fence. He then deliberately drove his vehicle into the group, killing two children and wounding other children and a staff member.

Experts suggest placing play areas at the farthest side from the street to remove children from both auto exhaust and stranger intrusion. If the play area must be close to the street, install bollards (steel-reinforced posts) that are at least four feet tall and secured 24–36 inches into the ground to reinforce an existing fence. When placed at four-foot intervals, bollards can stop an out-of-control car from breaking through a fence, thus saving children's lives. Although a block wall looks like a sturdy barrier, it may not stop a car without the addition of the steel-reinforced posts at four-foot intervals. Trees make excellent natural bollards if they line the fence.

A chain-link fence does little to protect children. It is not a sufficient barrier to stop impact, and it can be easily climbed—by intruders and by children. Both chain-link and wrought iron fences provide visual and potential conversation contact with strangers from the outside. There is value in having children able to see outside the child care property, but weigh this against the risk. If your program uses barriers that block an outsider's view of the children, make sure teachers and directors still have the ability to see the surrounding property from the inside out. Natural buffers such as bushes and trees provide excellent visual and physical barriers if the foliage is kept trimmed to prevent someone from hiding in them.

While opening windows for fresh air dilutes germs and removes indoor odors, the window openings should have guards that prevent exit by children and entry by intruders. The guards should be able to be opened by staff members or emergency personnel if the window must be used to evacuate. Hinged window bars are inexpensive and easy to install on the interior frames. Alternately, windows can usually be adjusted with a window stop on the inside, such as a block of wood, or a guard that extends above the window opening.

Lighting is another often overlooked but very important aspect of security. Darkness hides those who wish to enter the premises uninvited. As the length of day shortens during the fall and winter, reevaluate outside lighting, turning it on earlier in the afternoon and perhaps using it also in the early hours of the morning. If your site is equipped with security cameras, make sure there is enough lighting to create a clear recording, particularly during dusk and darkness.

Security concerns include not only the possibility of an intruder coming onto the property and entering the building but also the possibility of children leaving the premises on their own. Sometimes children run out of a gate simply because it is open. Sometimes gates open into a busy street or parking lot. Use self-locking gates, the kind sold for swimming pool enclosures, so that the gate automatically closes and locks when nobody holds it open. A double gate with one gate separated from the other by a small corral-like area is another good safeguard. Even if a child can open the gate latch, the double-gated "corral" space will at least slow the child's departure and increase the chance that a supervising adult will be able to reach the child in time.

Families, children, teachers, and directors must have a safe procedure for picking up and dropping off children that is understood and practiced by all concerned. Failure to observe the procedure should be grounds for disciplinary action for families or staff members. Parents or guardians should sign in and sign out verbally and in writing in view of the teacher who cares for the child, not just in a notebook or with a receptionist at the entrance.

Make sure children do not cross streets or any traffic unescorted when entering or exiting the building. Do not open any gates or doors only to stand and talk; an open door may permit a child to run out or could allow someone who shouldn't enter to run in. Open doors and gates only when you are ready to use them.

Many child care programs suffer high rates of staff turnover and hire substitutes or other temporary workers who are less familiar with parents. Staff members should ensure that an adult picking up a child is authorized to do so. For anyone the staff members do not know by sight, they should identify the person by, for example, requiring photo identification or matching the adult's signature with a signature on file. Telephone authorization of a family member who is not authorized or known to the facility should not be accepted because it is too easy for someone to pose as parent or to coerce a parent to make such a request. While thinking about such possibilities is unpleasant, it is critical to the safety of the children and their families.

Suggested activities

- Ask a local child care director to tell you about a time when an emergency involved an individual child or was a threat to the whole facility. Discuss with the director what happened and how such an emergency had been planned for or might have been planned for.
- Research media coverage of emergencies that have occurred in child care facilities. What happened when there was a fire? What happened when someone unstable came into a child care facility with a gun? What happened when a child care program was in a building that was targeted by terrorists?
- Obtain the inexpensive chart of pediatric first aid instructions from the AAP bookstore at **www.aap.org** (or call the AAP publications department, 847-434-4000). Review each instruction to see which ones differ from what you might have thought was the correct thing to do.
- Where did you learn first aid procedures? Did the training include CPR? Where in your community might you find current and appropriate pediatric first aid training? What does such training cost per person?

5

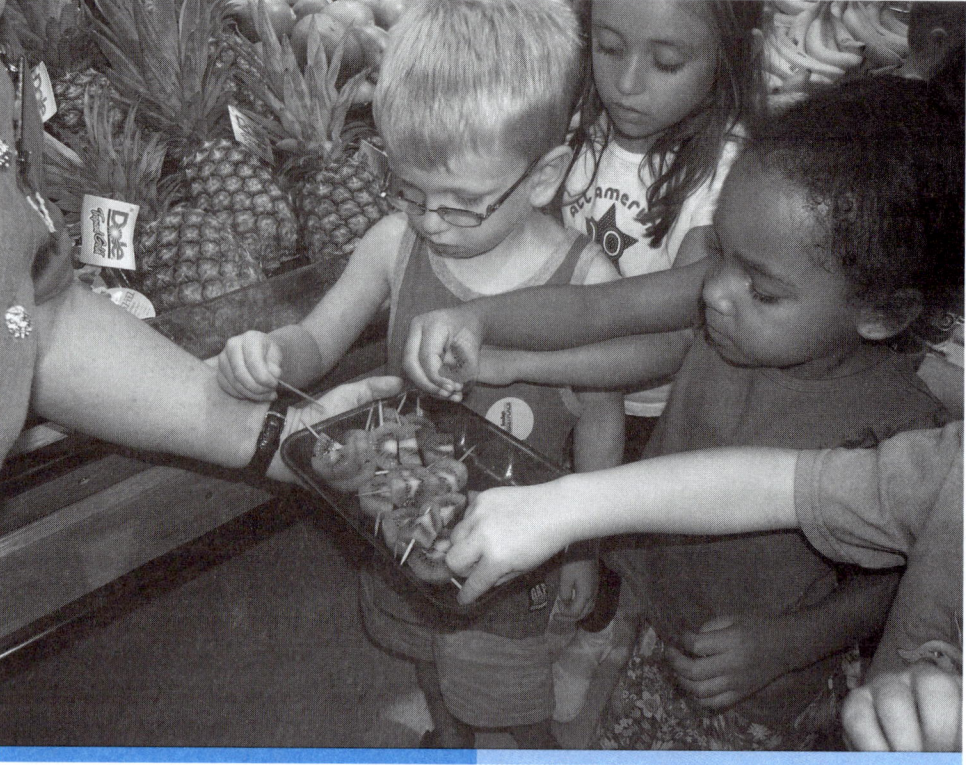

Promoting Health with Good Nutrition

MAJOR CONCEPTS

- Child care programs should ensure that children are offered a variety of foods each day.
- The food offered to children must be developmentally appropriate for a child's ability to chew, swallow, and digest. It must contain the nutrients required for growth in portions that promote healthy weight.
- Children need regular times for meals and snacks.
- Nourishing snacks between meals round out a well-balanced diet. Snacks should provide important nutrients because a child may prefer them to foods at a regular meal.
- National recommendations and standards for nutrition define best practices for promoting young children's health, including much needed measures to prevent overweight and obesity. (See also Chapter 6: Promoting Health with Physical Activity.)
- Nutrition experiences in child care teach children lifetime food habits.
- Following food safety practices while obtaining, storing, preparing, and serving food is essential whether food is prepared in the child care facility or brought from home.
- Significant health benefits are associated with meeting the national recommendations for nutrition for children in group care.
- Early educators can use updated evidence-based resources prepared by experts in food and nutrition science to support implementation of healthful nutrition in their programs.

Good nutrition is an essential ingredient of quality child care. Providing recommended types and amounts of food and beverages in a healthful way as discussed in this chapter is essential to children's growth and brain function. Alarming increases in overweight and obesity rates are occurring in the United States, even among preschoolers. Since being overweight or obese is associated with significant adverse social-emotional and physical health consequences, this national issue deserves everyone's attention. It requires intervention even in the earliest years.

Tasty, colorful, nutritious foods and a pleasant, relaxed eating environment contribute to a child's sense of well-being. A child develops lifelong eating habits through early eating experiences. Teachers need to know children's nutritional requirements and how to provide a nutritious diet. Equally important is creating a positive social atmosphere during meals and snacks.

The nutrition consultant

Every program, even one that mostly serves food the children bring from home, needs input from a qualified nutrition consultant, preferably a registered dietitian (RD). Many RDs have earned an undergraduate degree focused on nutrition or dietetics. The American Dietetic Association (ADA) recognizes courses that RDs must take to acquire nutrition and food knowledge, competency, and skills. Those seeking the RD certification must complete a recognized internship program of 1,200 to 1,500 hours. After the internship, the RD candidate must pass the national examination of the Commission on Dietetic Registration. Thereafter, the RD must complete continuing education to maintain the RD status. Many RDs specialize in a particular area, such as pediatrics or care for people with specific diseases.

In contrast, the qualifications of "nutritionists" vary greatly. Some have no professional qualifications at all. Some states license nutritionists, but many do not. Whoever performs this role for the early childhood program should have the appropriate training and background. Appendix C: Nutrition Specialist, Registered Dietitian, Licensed Nutritionist, Consultant, and Food Service Staff Qualifications in *Caring for Our Children* provides a helpful table showing titles, level of professional responsibility, education, and experience for individuals involved in nutrition consultation and food service work. If an RD with experience in early childhood programs is not available, look for someone with a bachelor's degree in foods, nutrition, or dietetics and at least two years of experience in community programs serving young children. Places to look for an appropriate nutritionist include: public health departments; agencies that work with children with special health needs; children's hospitals; college nutrition departments; the Special Supplemental Nutrition Program for Women, Infants, and Children (WIC); state cooperative extension services; school food services; state administrators of the Child and Adult Care Food Program; and nutritionists who are members of the American Dietetic Association, the American Public Health Association, and/or other recognized national organizations to which health professionals belong.

Every early childhood education program should develop a written nutrition, feeding, and food service plan, and then have the nutrition consultant review it. The plan needs to address the following key topics:

- Layout, equipment, and maintenance of food preparation areas
- Food budget
- Tasks involved with food procurement, storage, preparation, and serving
- Staffing for each food task, including mealtime activities
- Feeding practices and policies for each age group in the program
- Adult modeling of healthful eating
- Menu planning and nutritionist review of menus for meals and snacks
- Meal-service practices, such as holding perishable food at safe temperatures until ready to be eaten, letting children serve themselves, availability of second helpings, discarding leftovers that have been handled after leaving the kitchen or (if perishable) have been out of the safe temperature zone for two hours
- Eating as part of social development, learning about cultural and ethnic differences, and promoting a positive social atmosphere during mealtimes
- Preparing foods at home and for special events
- Assessing the adequacy of nutrition for individual children
- Addressing children with special dietary needs that require written plans from a child's health care provider (e.g., food intolerance, food allergies, and special diets)
- Written infant/toddler feeding practices and plans
- Coordination of feeding in the program and at home to meet and not exceed children's needs
- Nutrition education as a part of the curriculum
- Use of community nutrition resources

Obesity

Health professionals identify children who are overweight and obese using the body mass index, or BMI. BMI is calculated by dividing weight (in kilograms) by height squared (in meters). BMI helps to determine whether and to what extent a person is over- or underweight. Tools to obtain the BMI using weight and height are available from the National Heart, Lung, and Blood Institute at **www.nhlbisupport.com/bmi/**. Those with a BMI less than 18.5 are considered underweight. Those with a BMI between 18.5 and 24.9 are at normal weight. However, those with a BMI between 25 and 29.9 are between the 85th and 95th percentile of BMI by sex and age and are overweight. Those with a BMI of 30 or above are above the 95th percentile and are obese. The 2007–2008 United States National Health and Nutrition Survey (NHANES) found that 17 percent of the nation's children were obese. Among children 2–5 years of age, 10.4 percent were obese. Among children 6–11 years of age, 19.6 percent were obese.

If overweight begins before 8 years of age, obesity in adulthood is likely to be more severe. (See **www.cdc.gov/obesity/childhood/** for more on this issue.) National data released in 2011 indicate that the significantly increased risk of obesity for young children begins very early. In fact, researchers found that at 9 months of age, 31.9 percent of U.S. children were either at risk (overweight) or obese. This percentage increased to 34.3 percent by age 2 (Moss & Yeaton 2011).

Being overweight is linked to health problems in adulthood such as high blood pressure, Type 2 diabetes, and increased risk for coronary heart disease. When people take in more calories than they need, their bodies use the imbalance between calories consumed and calories used to store fat. The imbalance occurs because of a combination of genetic, behavioral, and environmental factors. Obesity is a major health challenge in the United States. Early educators have a key role to play in reducing overweight and obesity. The necessary approaches discussed in this chapter include interventions for both nutrition and physical activity. (See Chapter 6 for more information on physical activity.)

National standards and recommendations for nutrition in early care and education programs

The Child and Adult Care Food Program (CACFP) of the United States Department of Agriculture (USDA) feeds more than 3.3 million children who are enrolled in participating child care and emergency shelter programs each year. The CACFP sets the standards for meal patterns and specific foods for children in group care. Complying with this standard is best practice, even if the early education program does not receive reimbursement from the CACFP.

In 2010, the Institute of Medicine (IOM) recommended updates to the Child and Adult Care Food Program. The IOM report *Child and Adult Care Food Program: Aligning Dietary Guidance for All* (2010) offers general recommendations and specific meal pattern tables to address not only daily feedings but also variations in daily feedings across the week. (The recommendations that are most pertinent to early care and education programs are found in Chapter 7 of the IOM report.) Excerpts from this report (pp. 114–135) are paraphrased here:

For infants (birth to 1 year of age)

- Provide only breast milk or iron-fortified infant formula for children less than 6 months of age without other supplemental foods. Encourage breastfeeding.

- Gradually introduce meats, cereals, fruits, and vegetables of a type selected and prepared for infant feeding beginning at 6 months of age. When solids are introduced at 6 months, make meat the first solid food introduced to help ensure a sufficient source of iron. The small amount of iron in breast milk is maximally absorbed as long as the infant is not receiving any other food. When the exclusively breastfed infant receives solids at 6 months of age, meat is a better source of iron for the infant than cereal and seems to be as well digested. Feeding infants meat as their first solid food instead of cereal changes long-standing traditions for the sequence of introduction of solid foods. However, recent studies have shown many children have an insufficiency of iron that affects their brain functions and sleep behaviors, even when their iron levels are not low enough to cause lowering of the number or size of their red blood cells, resulting in measurable anemia.

- Give no fruit juice of any type before 1 year of age.

For all children age 1 year and older

Plan meals and snacks to increase the variety of fruits and vegetables, increase the proportion of whole grains, and decrease solid fats, added sugars, trans fats, and sodium. Specific recommendations for menu planning include the following:

- Serve one fruit and two vegetables at each lunch/supper meal. Over the course of a five-day week, serve different types of vegetables at each lunch and supper (tailoring serving sizes to meet the nutritional needs of the child's age group), as follows:
  - Dark green vegetables at least twice per week
  - Orange vegetables at least twice per week
  - Legumes at least once a week
  - Starchy vegetables no more than twice per week
  - Other vegetables at least three times per week

- Serve fruit rather than fruit juice at most meals; unsweetened 100 percent juice is allowed only once per day in a serving size specified for the child's age. *Caring for Our Children* Standard 4.2.0.7 limits the volume of juice to 4–6 ounces per day, including the juice a child drinks at home. Programs that serve juice need to discuss with parents how much juice children get at home to adhere to this standard. It might be easier not to serve juice in the program.

- Over the course of the week and day, at least half of the grain/breads served in meals and snacks should be those labeled as containing 100 percent whole grains. Whole grains contain more nutrients than refined grains, which have had parts of the grain removed. Other grain/bread must be enriched. Gradually increase the proportion of grain foods that are whole-grain rich to well above half of the grain foods, and include 100 percent whole grain foods often.

- For each morning and afternoon snack, provide two different food components in a serving size tailored to the needs of the child's age group. Over the course of a five-day week, ensure that each child receives the following:
  - Two servings of fruit
  - One serving of an orange vegetable
  - One serving of a non-starchy vegetable
  - Two servings of grain/bread
  - Two servings of lean meat or meat alternate
  - Two servings of low-fat or nonfat milk

- To limit the amount of solid fats, added sugars, trans fats, and sodium in all meals and snacks, follow these guidelines:
  - Choose milk and yogurt that is low-fat or nonfat for those age 2 years or older (whole milk for 1-year-old children).
  - Meats must be lean.
  - Fruits and juices must be free of added sugars.
  - Foods with nutritional labels should be labeled as containing zero grams of trans fat.
  - Foods high in added sugars and/or sodium should be served infrequently, if at all.

Specific daily meal and snack patterns with sample menus are shown in Figures A.8 and A.9. (These are drawn from Tables 7-1 through 7-5, 7-8, and 7-9 in the IOM report available on the website of The National Academies Press at **www.nap.edu/catalog/12959.html**. A link to this publication is also on the website of the Food and Nutrition Service of the United States Department of Agriculture, the administrator of the CACFP, at **www.fns.usda.gov/ORA/menu/Published/CNP/FILES/cacfpiom.pdf**.) For categories of foods children should be offered, see Figure 5.1.

Since 1980, the Departments of Agriculture and Health and Human Services have been required by law to issue an updated set of national standards every five years called "Dietary Guidelines for Americans." The federal government uses the Dietary Guidelines for Americans as the basis for food assistance programs, nutrition education initiatives, and decisions about national health objectives. The 2010 Dietary Guidelines recognize that two-thirds of the United States population is overweight or obese. The report emphasizes a health-promoting, total diet that addresses the intake of food, calories, and nutrients, and it recommends eating patterns that help people implement the guidelines in their everyday lives. (For more information about these guidelines, go to **www.health.gov/dietaryguidelines/**.)

General approaches to eating

A pleasant, relaxed eating environment helps children and adults develop positive attitudes about food and eating. Establish regular times for meals and snacks. Prior to a meal, encourage some physical activity so that children will be hungry and ready to sit calmly during the meal. To help them settle down before eating, use a calming transition activity such as singing a song or reading a story. If children have not done something that involves moving their bodies, or they have come directly from vigorous physical activity to a meal or snack, they may not feel like eating.

Make sure everyone sits at a comfortable height in relation to the table top. The table surface should be as close as possible to midway between the waist and armpit to make it easy to use arms and hands properly for self-feeding. Feet should touch the floor or a foot rest, as it is harder to adjust body position for comfortable eating without a firm surface to push the feet against.

Unless specifically prohibited by state regulations, food should be served in family-style food containers. Provide age-appropriate portions in the serving dishes; for children, provide a dish that is sized for the child's appropriate portion size. Adults may use a dish that accommodates their proper portion. When children are just learning how to serve themselves, the serving dishes can hold a few individual portions put in the serving dish to make it easy for each child to take a portion without handling food that others will eat. For example, put quarters of a sandwich on a plate separated from one another; put soft foods in a wide-bottomed bowl with a portion-sized scoop so children can easily take a portion with a serving utensil. This helps teach children about portions. As children become more skilled at serving themselves, serving plates may contain bulk soft foods. Put only enough for a few children in the serving dish, keeping the rest of the food and a few clean bowls and utensils in reserve. That way, if the food is contaminated when a child serves it, you can replace the contaminated food with a clean serving bowl, utensil, and a few untouched portions for the next child. The adults should model these actions for children and encourage them to help themselves to all the food components for the meal.

Figure 5.1.

Categories of Food Offered

Children in care should be offered items of food from the following categories:

Making Healthy Food Choices*

Food Groups	USDA †	CFOC Guidelines for Young Children
Fruits	All fresh, frozen, canned, dried fruits, and fruit juices	• Eat a variety, especially whole fruits • Whole fruit, mashed or pureed, for infants seven months up to one year of age • No juice before twelve months of age • 4 to 6 oz juice/day for one- to six-year-olds • 8 to 12 oz juice/day for seven- to twelve-year-olds
Vegetables	Dark green, red, and orange; beans and peas (legumes); starchy vegetables; other vegetables	• Dark green, red, orange, deep yellow vegetables • Other vegetables, including starchy ones like potatoes • Other root vegetables, such as viandas • Dried peas and beans (legumes)
Grains	Whole grains and enriched grains	• Whole and enriched grains, breads, cereals, crackers, pasta, and rice
Protein Foods	Seafood, meat, poultry, eggs, nuts, seeds, and soy products	• Fish, chicken, lean meat, eggs • Nuts and seeds (if appropriate) • Avoid fried fish, meat, and chicken
Dairy	Milk	• Human milk, infant formula for infants at least up to one year of age • Whole milk for children ages on up to two years of age or reduced fat (2%) milk for those at risk for obesity or hypercholesterolemia • 1% or skim milk for children two years of age and older • Other milks such as soy when recommended • Other milk equivalent products such as yogurt and cottage cheese (low-fat for children two years of age and older)
Oils	Oils, soft margarines, includes vegetable, nut, and fish oils and soft vegetable oil table spreads that have no trans fats	• Choose monounsaturated and polyunsaturated fats (olive oil, safflower oil) • Soft margarines
Solid Fats and Added Sugar	Limit calories (% of calories) of these food groups	• Avoid concentrated sweets such as candy, sodas, sweetened drinks, fruit nectars, and flavored milk • Limit salty foods such as chips and pretzels

*All foods are assumed to be in nutrient-dense forms, lean or low-fat, and prepared without added fats, sugars, or salt. Solid fats and added sugars may be included up to the daily maximum limit identified in the Dietary Guidelines for Americans, 2010.

†Recommends: Find your balance between food and physical activity.

Source: Standard 4.2.0.4, *Caring for Our Children*. Reprinted with permission.

Children can be finicky about the appearance of their food and may prefer to have different foods not touch each other on the plate. Encourage children to taste new foods, and occasionally praise them when they eat a variety of foods (e.g., "I see that you ate foods of different colors"). Don't praise children for eating large quantities, because this interferes with self-regulation. Suggest (once or twice, but do not badger) that a child who is reluctant to try a new food might taste just one bite. Special accommodations should be made for children who cannot have certain foods or who need monitoring to limit their portions. For all children, eating should require sitting down without other distractions. They should not eat while standing, walking, running, playing, participating in video or computer screen activities, or riding in vehicles. Children should be allowed to be done eating when they are full. If an infant starts to fall asleep while eating, the feeding should stop.

Except when feeding infants or older children who need feeding assistance, teachers should sit at the table and eat with the children. This promotes socialization while eating and helps prevent undesirable behavior. The goal is to foster positive attitudes about eating and social interaction while eating. Model for children how to serve foods, how to pick up food with a fork or spoon, and how to eat different foods. Eat items that meet the nutrition standards. Ask politely for a particular food to be passed. Children will learn language and manners from listening to and watching adults. As children approach school age, help them fine-tune their table manners by giving direct instruction about appropriate table etiquette. As with all instruction, whenever possible, explain what is expected rather than telling children what *not* to do.

Involve children in food-related experiences beyond simply eating. Have them participate in mealtime activities such as setting and clearing the table. At mealtime, talk about the color, shape, size, quantity, and temperature of the food; where it grew; different ways to prepare it; the events of the day; the weather; or any other topic of interest. Offer opportunities for them to see how food grows and how it is sold in stores. The experiences can include touching, smelling, and exploring food they will be served and food that is from different cultures than their own. Young children are more likely to eat food that they have learned about in such activities.

Feeding infants

During the first year of life, infants experience more changes in diet than at any other time in life. They grow rapidly and develop motor skills and progress from eating only liquids to feeding themselves table foods. Although children develop feeding in a predictable sequence, the pace of progress varies considerably from one child to another. During this period, interaction with adults has a strong influence on the infant's development of self-feeding skills and acceptance of a variety of foods.

Infants should be fed on cue unless the child's health care provider and the parent give written instructions otherwise. An infant expresses hunger with an open mouth, making suckling sounds, and moving hands. It should not be necessary for an infant to cry to be fed, nor is it appropriate to feed an infant who is alert and seeking interaction but is not showing signs of hunger. Hungry infants should receive food, not a pacifier. Limit pacifier use to soothing when a child is falling asleep in a crib. Feeding should stop when the infant seems full, even if more food remains in the bottle or dish. Infants may show they have had enough to eat by turning away from the nipple, closing their mouth, or paying more attention to what is around them. For infants, feeding is an essential one-on-one activity that builds trust, a sense of security, and appropriate eating patterns for life. It should be a time for a consistent caregiver to build a warm, positive relationship with the child.

Breast milk is best

Human milk is the most important recommended food for at least the first year of life. It is uniquely suited to support infant growth and brain development, and it

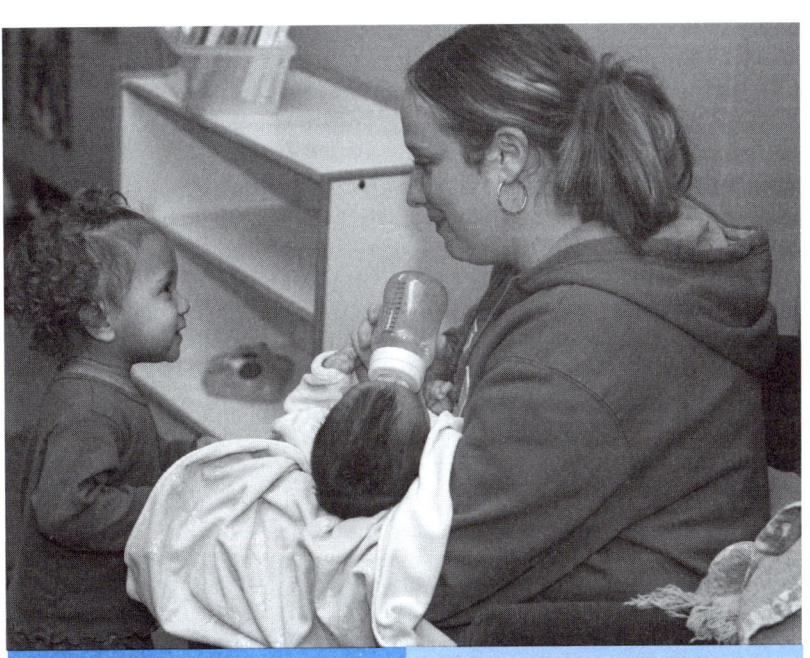

protects infants against infection and even some diseases that appear later in life. These include decreases in the incidence of diarrhea, respiratory disease, middle ear disease, bacterial infection of the blood, bacterial meningitis, botulism, urinary tract infections, necrotizing enterocolitis, SIDS, diabetes, lymphoma, allergic diseases, ulcerative colitis, other chronic digestive diseases, and childhood obesity. Mothers benefit from breastfeeding their infants, too, with lowered risk of diabetes, breast cancer, and heart disease.

The advantages to infants are greatest with exclusive use of human milk for the first 6 months of life and no other type of milk until after 12 months of age. Any amount of breastfeeding, however, provides some benefit to the infant, even if the infant receives some formula during the day. Concerns about the need to supplement breastfed infants with vitamin D and iron should be addressed by the infant's health care provider. Some will need supplements, while others will not. Some may need introduction of solid foods as early as 4 months of age, but most will not. Each infant in group care should be fed as specified by that child's health care provider.

Many factors determine how eager mothers are to continue breastfeeding. Since feeding human milk offsets the increased risk of infection from group care for infants, staff members should do all they can to support families to maximize their infant's use of this very special food. When infants cannot be fed human milk, they should receive iron-fortified formula of a type recommended by the child's health care provider.

The following guidelines for early education programs will help promote breastfeeding and support nursing mothers:

- Encourage the mother to breastfeed her infant on arrival, before departure, or during her work breaks.
- Provide a quiet, private place with a comfortable chair and stepstool, and a place for the mother to wash her hands. Have water available for the mother to drink so she has enough fluid for herself and her milk. These arrangements will help the mother to relax and secrete the hormone that allows her milk to flow (letdown).
- Encourage mothers to use effective breast pumps that empty their breasts without making them sore in 15 to 20 minutes. The more expensive but more effective hospital-type electric breast pumps can be rented. Include a place at the facility with an outlet where mothers can use an electric breast pump after nursing the infant to encourage milk production as much as possible. Mothers should pump at least every four hours while they are away from their infants. Feeding the infant at the breast as often as possible will help maintain milk supply. A healthy, mature infant's suckling is a better stimulus to milk production than any pump. When infants and mothers are together, the infant should feed at the breast. If the mother and infant are together, it's not helpful to bottle-feed to maintain the workday schedule.
- Before the infant needs bottle-feedings in the program, ask the mother to have someone other than her give the infant a bottle of breast milk at least several times to teach the infant how to feed from a bottle when the mother will be unable to breastfeed. It is easier for the infant to learn to bottle-feed if it is attempted when the infant is hungry and the mother is not in the same room. With the mother, plan a bottle-feeding schedule at the program that ensures that the infant is eager to nurse when the mother arrives. Make the last feeding time at least two hours before the mother's expected arrival. Ask the mother to call if she will miss or be late for a feeding.
- Follow the guidelines for preparing, feeding, and safely storing expressed human milk (milk removed from the breast by some method other than suckling) in *Caring for Our Children* Standard 4.3.1.3. Keep a backup supply of small amounts of frozen or refrigerated expressed breast milk to supplement feedings when the infant seems to want more than the usual volume.
- Be informed about the basics of breastfeeding and support mothers in this endeavor. With adequate rest, nutrition, and fluids, most mothers are able to maintain their milk supply when they bottle-feed part time. Most women do not need to use formula if they express their milk at least once every four hours while away from their infants and breastfeed full time while with the infant. Some women prefer to feed some formula. Their decision may make it more difficult for them to maintain their breastfeeding, but the decision should be respected.
- Breastfeeding may continue into the second year of life if the infant and mother are comfortable and want to nurse.

Preparing and handling human (breast) milk and infant formula sent from home

Follow the guidelines for preparing, feeding, and safely storing expressed human milk in *Caring for Our Children* Standard 4.3.1.3. Figure 5.2 shows the guidelines for storing human milk from this standard. Arrange to have a backup supply of frozen or refrigerated expressed human milk on site.

Staff members should thoroughly wash their hands prior to preparation of all infant feedings. Only cleaned and sanitized bottles and nipples, or equivalent factory-prepared nursing bottle bags, should be used. Only human milk and formula in factory-sealed containers can be brought into the facility. Transport time and uncertainties about preparation and holding temperatures until the formula arrives make it hazardous to use for-

Figure 5.2.

Guidelines for Storing Human Milk

Human Milk That Was Never Frozen

Location	Temperature	Duration	Comments
Countertop or table	Room temperature (up to 77° F or 25° C)	6–8 hours	Containers should be covered and kept as cool as possible; covering the container with a cool towel may keep milk cooler.
Insulated cooler bag	5° F–39° F or -15° C–4 °C	24 hours	Keep ice packs in contact with milk containers at all times; limit opening cooler bag.
Refrigerator	39° F or 4° C	5 days	Store milk in the back of the main body of the refrigerator.

Frozen Human Milk

Location	Temperature	Duration	Comments
Refrigerator's freezer section	5° F or -15° C	2 weeks	Store milk toward the back of the freezer, where temperature is most constant. Milk stored for longer durations in the ranges listed is safe, but some of the lipids (fats) in the milk undergo degradation, resulting in lower quality.
Separate freezer compartment of refrigerator with separate door	0° F or -18° C	3–6 months	
Chest or upright deep freezer	-4° F or -20° C	6–12 months	

Source: Adapted from Standard 4.3.1.3, *Caring for Our Children*. Reprinted with permission.

---

mula prepared at home. While some parents may object to providing factory-sealed containers of formula, the program can point out that transporting formula made up at home has been found to be a cause of illness and that it is safer to make fresh bottles of formula when the infant needs a feeding.

Human milk. The mother's expressed milk should be fed only to her own infant. If human milk is inadvertently fed to another mother's child, it is possible that the infant fed this milk may have been exposed to hepatitis B, hepatitis C, or HIV in this body fluid. Staff members should follow a procedure that includes informing the mother who expressed the milk about the mistake and when the bottle switch happened. The mother should be asked about how the milk was handled before it was brought to the facility, whether she has been tested for hepatitis B, hepatitis C, and HIV, and if so, when and whether she is willing to share the results of such tests with the parents of the child mistakenly fed her milk. If she doesn't know whether she has been tested, ask if she would be willing to check about it with her health care provider and then have a blood test and share the results if she hasn't been tested. The parents of the child mistakenly given another mother's milk need to be informed of the mistake, told that the risk is very low of exposure to infection, encouraged to notify the infant's health care provider of the exposure, and given the information available about the milk and the blood test results of the mother whose milk was given. If there is a possibility of exposure to hepatitis B, the child who received the feeding by mistake may need blood testing and special attention to prevent this infection with prompt use of vaccine. Safeguards should be in place to prevent mix-ups in feeding human milk. Any occurrence should be assessed to determine how to prevent it in the future.

Chilled or frozen human milk may be transported from home to the child care facility in a cooler bag (at a temperature of 40° F or lower) as long as the air temperature is below 86° F and the out-of-refrigerator time is less than two hours. Human milk should come to the facility in a clean and sanitary bottle with the nipple fitted tightly to prevent spilling. All containers of human milk should be of the ready-to-feed type and bear the date of collection and the child's full name. Labels should be resistant to loss of the name and date when washing and handling, as confusion may occur if there are several bottles from different mothers being thawed and warmed at the same time in the same place.

Infant formula. Formula should be the same brand that the child is fed at home. If it is not of the ready-to-feed type, it should be a liquid concentrate or powdered infant formula product to be diluted with water according to the manufacturer's instructions on the label. It is safest to use water that is boiled for one minute in an automatic kettle or in a pan and then cooled for no more than 30 minutes to prepare a fresh bottle as it is needed. The freshly boiled water should be from a source approved by the health department. Adding formula to boiled water that is still warm (but not hot enough to burn) makes it unnecessary to heat the milk before giving it to the child. Room temperature tap water may be used to make formula if the water is approved by the health department for this approach. Guidelines for preparing formula are available in many languages at **http://who.int/foodsafety/publications/micro/pif2007/en/index.html**.

No matter what type of milk is used, discard any remaining in the bottle after a child has fed from it. For formula, discard any fluid milk in a factory-sealed container that has been open for 48 hours. Human milk containers that have more than an ounce and have not been used for feeding may be returned to the mother at the end of the day. (Bottled milk that has been fed will have been contaminated with saliva and bacteria.)

Warming formula bottles and infant foods

Teachers may warm infant foods and infant bottles of human milk or formula if infants do not accept them at the refrigerated or room temperature at which they were stored. (Many infants are quite happy with cold bottles and room temperature infant foods.) When human milk, formula, or food is warmed, use running warm tap water or a container of water no warmer than 120° F. Don't leave bottles in water to warm for more than five minutes. When bottles of milk or infant foods are warmed at room temperature or in warm water for an extended time, they provide an ideal growth medium for bacteria. Do NOT use a microwave oven to warm anything fed to an infant. Microwave ovens heat foods unevenly and the microwave energy continues to heat up food after it is removed from the microwave oven. This can result in burns to the infant.

After warming, mix bottles gently. Do not shake human milk as this breaks some of the cellular components that help protect the infant from infection. Test the temperature of the milk before feeding. Stir infant foods to distribute the heat evenly. When preparing food and testing food temperature, use two hands to do so safely. Mishaps can easily occur while holding a child and working with food, hot water, or hot surfaces. It is also harder to perform proper hand hygiene, prepare food, and keep food and utensils off unsanitary surfaces when you are juggling a child and food at the same time. A smooth transition to feeding requires that teachers respond to the infant's earliest hunger cues, use simple preparation methods, and then pick up and interact with the infant if a little more time is needed for the food to warm.

If a device such as a slow cooker is used for warming infant formula, human milk, or infant food, the device and its cord should be out of children's reach. The water inside should not exceed 120° F. Some infants have received burns from water dripping from a bottle removed from a slow cooker or when they pulled on a dangling cord and the slow cooker came down on them. Keep a thermometer in the slow cooker to check the temperature when food is put into it. Empty, sanitize, and refill the device with fresh water daily.

Bottle-feeding technique and weaning from bottle-feeding

Bottle-feeding should simulate breastfeeding. It should occur when the infant's cues indicate hunger rather than be used to pacify a child who needs comforting. For example, rooting (eager turning of the face) and sucking movements are hunger cues. While feeding, the caregiver should interact with the infant, stimulating socialization with eye contact and conversation. Infants should always be held in the caregiver's arms or sitting on the caregiver's lap for bottle-feeding. Only one infant should be fed at a time. When the infant seems to want

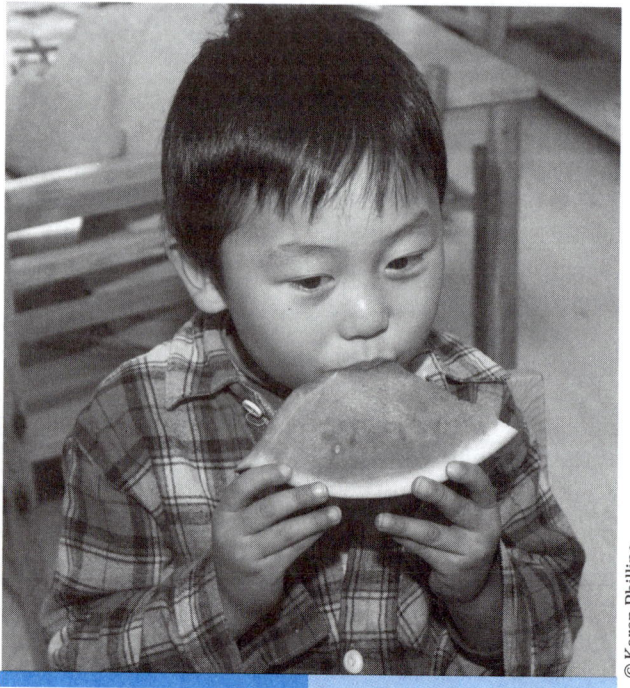

to stop the feeding, gently rubbing the infant's back while upright may help the infant burp swallowed air. Gentle rubbing stimulates a reflex that makes babies stretch their backs a little. This helps air bubbles move upward from the stomach toward the infant's mouth. If after a burp the infant does not seem to want to eat more, this is a cue that the feeding should stop.

The bottle nipple should have a wide base and be of a size and shape that allows the nipple to lie against the roof of the infant's mouth with the lips closed over the base of the nipple. Do not use bottle propping at any time. It is associated with choking, ear infections, and oral health problems. It also misses a key opportunity for the caregiver to foster a warm relationship and sense of emotional security for the infant during feeding.

Weaning from bottles to a small cup with two to three ounces of fluid in it at a time should occur when the infant seems ready. Many infants are ready to drink from a cup held by the adult as early as 6 months of age. The American Academy of Pediatric Dentistry recommends completing weaning from a bottle by no later than the child's first birthday.

Avoiding baby bottle tooth decay and other issues related to feeding from bottles and sippy cups

Do not allow infants or toddlers to drink from a bottle while lying down, to go to bed with a bottle, or to walk around with a bottle or sippy cup. Falling on the bottle or cup and drinking over a prolonged period are risks for oral injury and tooth decay. Formula, milk, juice, and sweetened drinks contain sugars that feed bacteria that often infect the mouth. The bacteria release chemicals that can decay existing or erupting teeth, creating a condition known as nursing-bottle mouth. In this condition the lower teeth are somewhat protected by the tongue, and the upper teeth are more affected. This may lead to early loss of teeth, particularly the front upper teeth. As a result, the child may not be able to chew food properly. The decayed teeth may damage the teeth still growing in the gums. Loss of these primary baby teeth may reduce jaw growth, leading to crowding when the adult teeth erupt. In addition, as mentioned above as a reason not to allow bottle propping, children who drink their bottles lying down also are prone to ear infections and choking. If parents want an infant to take a bottle to bed, explain that it is not safe to follow this practice. Instead, offer the infant a drink before putting him to bed.

While many infants like fruit juices, drinking beverages other than breast milk or formula makes them drink less of the more nutritious liquids that help them grow. Children should not drink fruit juices before 1 year of age. On very hot days, breastfed infants should be offered more breast milk; formula-fed infants should be offered small amounts of plain water.

Introducing solid foods

Experts recommend starting solid food when infants are between 4 and 6 months old, preferably closer to 6 months. Earlier introduction of solid foods interferes with the infant's intake of breast milk or iron-fortified formula that contains the balance of nutrients needed for growth in early infancy. Early introduction of solid foods may be associated with allergy and digestive problems. Also, many infants do not develop the neuromuscular skills needed for eating solid foods until 6 months of age. Around 6 months, breastfed infants may require vitamin drops with iron that should be given by the family at home.

Eating solid foods does not help children sleep through the night; development of the brain determines when children can sleep for longer periods. Infants show readiness for solids when they can hold their heads steady by themselves, open their mouths and lean forward in anticipation of food being offered, close their lips around a spoon, move the food from the front of their mouths to the back, and then swallow it.

Giving a child solid foods should proceed according to a written plan made in consultation with the child's parents and health care provider.

Commercially packaged baby food should be fed with a spoon from a dish, not from the factory-sealed container. The container and lid should be washed off with detergent and water and then rinsed in fresh tap water before opening. Carefully examine the food removed from the commercial packaging to be sure it is free of foreign material and fragments of glass and for any signs that it is not wholesome. Solid foods should not be mixed with breast milk or formula in a bottle or in an infant feeder unless the child's health care provider recommends it. Infant feeders are devices that look like large syringes and are used to push solid food into an infant's mouth. Teachers may use infant foods brought from home if the foods were prepared, transported, and stored in a sanitary manner and are clearly labeled for feeding to one specific child. Any food left in the dish from which the infant was fed should be thrown away. Food should be fed to only one infant from the same dish and spoon.

To avoid problems with food intolerance, serve a child only foods that have already been introduced without a problem at home. Food intolerance is far more common than food allergy. Symptoms from a particular food may be the result of an immature digestive system or lack of particular elements of digestion required for that food. Infants who were born full-term have enough blood cells to give them the iron reserves to last for four to six months. They use iron as they grow to make new blood cells to fill their larger bodies and supply the many places in the body that need iron, including brain cells. Infants need zinc for healthy growth and immune function. The first solid food should provide needed iron and zinc, such as meat or a semisolid form of an iron-fortified infant cereal. Meat is recommended for the first solid food for breastfed infants because it has more accessible iron than infant cereal. For infants who have been fed iron-fortified formula, meat is a good first food too. Between 6 and 8 months of age, vegetables and fruits can be added to the diet. At about 8 or 9 months, offer table food. Choose table food the infant can easily gum/chew, mash, or swallow whole. By the end of the first year, the infant should be eating most table foods.

Use these guidelines to feed solid foods:

- Allow time for the infant to get used to the feel and taste of solid foods. Use the infant's cues to tell you when it is time to offer another spoonful. If the infant looks at the spoon with an open mouth, that is a strong positive signal. If the infant turns away and seems interested in something else, wait until the infant's attention returns to the food on the spoon and talk about it to encourage tasting. Never push the food into the infant's mouth when the infant does not seem to want it. If the infant seems overeager for one bite after another, try talking and playfully interacting with the child to slow the feeding to a reasonable pace. This will help the child learn a healthful eating behavior.

- As indicated above, families should introduce new foods at home before they are tried in the child care setting. Be sure families wait two to three days to see if the new food is well tolerated before trying another new food.

- At around 8 to 10 months of age, or when infants seem interested in bringing food to their own mouths, they can begin to have some food put on their tray to feed to themselves with their fingers—with vigilant adults watching for choking.
  - All food should be cut into pieces no larger than 1/4 inch. Chop or cut cooked turkey, chicken, lean hamburger, or fish into small pieces to make chewing easier. Soft foods should be offered in similar-sized portions.
  - To infants interested in self-feeding, offer pieces of meat and cheese that are small enough to be swallowed whole, cooked or soft vegetable strips, and fruit pieces.
  - Serve cooked and mashed dried beans or peas for additional protein.
  - Offer eggs—scrambled until dry-cooked, hard-boiled, or in other foods—when the child's health care provider suggests the infant is ready for this nutrient-rich food.

- An adult should always sit with children while they are eating. The adult should be with only one infant at a time and, when working with children who can feed themselves with adult assistance, should be seated with no more than three children and within arm's reach of all three. This encourages social interaction and allows the adult to be alert for children who are showing signs of choking, squirreling away several pieces of food in their mouth at one time, or failing to chew food.

Beginning whole, low-fat, or skim cow's milk

Provide breast milk or iron-fortified formula to infants until they reach at least 12 months of age. Breast milk and infant formulas may be continued for as long as parents want to feed their children these milks and their health care providers recommend it. For children at risk for obesity or high cholesterol, health care providers may recommend reduced-fat (2 percent) milk. Between 1 and 2 years of age, children who do not have a plan to receive breast milk, formula, or reduced-fat milks should receive whole cow's milk. Milk contains the nutrients toddlers need for brain and nerve development. Unless the child's health care provider recommends it, do not serve reduced-fat, low-fat, or skim milk until 2 years of age. Children who are 2 years of age or older should be served skim or 1 percent pasteurized milk.

Feeding toddlers and preschool-age children

A toddler's growth rate slows down between 18 months and 3 years. As a result, a toddler eats less. In the preschool years, children grow at a steady, but slower, pace. Toddlers are demanding and energetic by nature. As they explore and gain control over themselves and their environment, they experience success and become more independent. They begin to take more responsibility for what and how much they eat. For example, they may go on food jags, eating only a few foods or going through periods when they seem to eat almost nothing at all.

Teachers and families are responsible for what children are offered to eat, as well as where, when, and how food is offered. However, children determine whether they eat what is offered. Adults should work to help the child establish positive attitudes toward eating and to ensure that a nutritionally adequate diet is offered. Most toddlers and preschool-age children will be well-nourished if a variety of nutritious foods are available.

- Help toddlers become independent by allowing them to select from a variety of acceptable foods placed in age-appropriate, small-sized portions in serving dishes. The food should be divided so that a few child-sized portions are in a serving dish with the rest held in reserve in case a child accidentally dumps the food on the floor or contaminates the servings intended for others. If necessary, a spare serving dish can be refilled from the reserved food and a clean utensil provided for children to continue to serve themselves. The serving dishes should include the right number of appropriately sized portions for the adults who are eating with the children to serve to themselves also. The adults may serve themselves first to show the children how to do it.

- Age-appropriate portions are specified in the CACFP guidelines at **www.fns.usda.gov/cnd/care/Program Basics/Meals/Meal_Patterns.htm**.
- Food should be served in plates, bowls, and cups that are appropriately sized to accommodate a portion for the child or adult, and not larger. Research shows that larger plates, bowls, and cups promote overeating. If a child wants more food, offer additional servings of foods that are low in fat, sugar, and sodium to meet the caloric needs of the individual child.
- For toddlers, provide child-sized tableware (e.g., a short-handled spoon with a broad bowl; a blunt-tined, short fork; and a small cup) to let them learn how to use these utensils along with their fingers for self-feeding. By preschool age, most children will be able to use ordinary spoons and forks. If provided, knives should not be sharp. Preschool-age children may use blunt knives to apply a spread to foods such as vegetables, bread, and crackers.

Feeding school-age children

Follow the CACFP guidelines (found at **www.fns.usda.gov/cnd/care/ProgramBasics/Meals/Meal_Patterns.htm**) to plan meals and snacks for children who are in kindergarten and higher grades. Children in an early care and education facility or in school should have breakfast either at home or in the program, and those who are in the facility for two or more hours need at least one snack. A snack should be offered around two hours after a meal. Plan to have at least two hours between the end of a snack and the beginning of another meal to give children time to empty their stomachs from the previous feeding. Plan at least three hours between the end of one meal and the beginning of the next meal.

Basic nutrition facts

Snacks

Snacks are an important part of a well-balanced diet. They are especially important for preschoolers because their stomachs are small and they may not be able to eat what they need in three meals to meet their energy needs or satisfy their appetites. Within two or three hours after a meal, most young children will be hungry. Snack time must provide nutrients missing from the rest of the day's food. The challenge is to help children eat nutritious snacks at appropriate times during the day. Good snacks are those that provide essential nutrients.

They may have to substitute for a meal that the child decides to skip. If children are hungry, snack time can be a good opportunity for them to try new foods.

Serve nutritious snacks that meet the CACFP guidelines mentioned in the previous sections. The CACFP guidelines are expected to be updated based on the IOM recommendations to require more variety among nutrient sources for snack foods over the course of a week. A list of nutritious snack ideas is provided in Figure 5.3. Avoid snack foods such as commercial chips, sweet cakes, candies, fruit juices, and fruit drinks; these have limited nutritional value for the calories they contain. For sweets, serve whole fruits cut into appropriate-sized pieces. Unsalted pretzels are acceptable as a bread substitute for children older than 4 years of age. Avoid salted snacks/foods of any type. Cook with olive or canola oil. Select whole grains when grain-containing foods are served for snacks and meals.

Appetite

After infancy, children's appetites decrease. Many preschoolers have unstable eating habits. Children may be less hungry because they are in a slow growth stage or are practicing newly discovered independence. A small appetite may be a signal that a child is tired, excited, ill, or in strange surroundings. Be aware of any change in a child's appetite that lasts longer than a few days, and discuss the change with the child's family.

Variety is essential

Because no single food contains all the nutrients our bodies need, teachers should serve children a variety of available fruits, colorful vegetables, lean proteins, and whole grains. Preschoolers generally enjoy eating the same foods that they see adults around them eat.

Adults also can help children develop good food habits by offering (and eating for themselves) both new foods and the same foods prepared in different ways (e.g., cooked carrots and carrot salad). Gradually introduce foods to increase food acceptance. Pay attention to what foods children eat and encourage them to eat foods from different food groups.

Food habits are learned: Nutrition education

Food habits and the ability to eat wisely are *learned*. The early education facility's written curriculum should integrate teaching about food characteristics, food choices, and food handling, while also including separate food-related curricular activities. These activities can teach about how and where foods grow, the food parts we eat, how food is sold, and how to choose healthful foods. Involve a nutrition consultant, teach-

Figure 5.3.

Ideas for Nutritious Snacks

Fruits and vegetables

- **Apple sandwich**—Slice an apple, thinly spread peanut butter on the slices, and make a sandwich. Or put a piece of cheese between apple slices.
- **Yogurt sundae**—Let children make their own; just supply bowls, plain yogurt, and toppings of fresh fruit pieces, wheat germ or dry cereal, and for children over 4 years of age, chopped nuts.
- **Kabobs**—Use a straw pinched at one end to make a skewer. Prepare these or other combinations to place on the skewers:
- **Fruit and cheese**—Place fresh fruit and low-fat cheese cubes, pitted dates, or prunes on long straws. Serve kabobs with a dip made with plain, low-fat yogurt sprinkled with cinnamon or a few drops of vanilla flavoring.
- **Veggies**—Skewer cut-up fresh vegetables such as halves of cherry tomatoes, zucchini, steamed carrot rounds, cucumbers, green peppers, mushrooms, and low-fat pieces of cheese. Serve with salad dressing or a dip made with mashed beans, yogurt, or cottage cheese and seasoned with herbs.
- **Toss a salad**—Invite children to a homemade salad bar. Set out dishes of cut-up veggies for children to create their own salads.
- **Celery stuff-its**—Fill celery with part-skim ricotta cheese mixed with unsweetened crushed pineapple. Or, fill celery with a thin layer of peanut butter and add a few raisins (this is called "Ants on a Log").
- **Lettuce roll**—Spread tuna or chicken salad, a thin layer of peanut butter, or low-fat ricotta cheese on a lettuce leaf, roll it up, and eat.

Freezer delights

- **Frozen Dixies**—Freeze unsweetened applesauce or crushed unsweetened pineapple in a paper cup with a Popsicle stick.
- **Frozen strawberry yogurt pops**—Blend 1 cup of frozen strawberries or other fruit until smooth. Mix the blended fruit with 1 cup of plain, low-fat yogurt. Pour into paper cups with a Popsicle stick in the center and freeze 1–2 hours until firm. Remove cup from frozen yogurt and serve. Makes seven pops.
- **Banana pops**—Mix 2 cups of low-fat, plain yogurt with 1 cup of mashed banana and 1 teaspoon of vanilla. Pour into six 4-oz. paper cups, insert Popsicle sticks in the center, and freeze until firm. Remove cup from frozen pop and serve.
- **Banana rockets**—Coat peeled, ripe bananas with orange juice or orange juice concentrate (to prevent discoloration), wrap in foil or plastic wrap, and freeze. Or, roll chilled, juice-coated bananas in finely chopped nuts or granola, press firmly to coat, and freeze until firm.

Homemade convenience snacks
(for kindergarten-age or older children)

- **Trail mix**—Combine dried fruits and dry cereal together, and divide into plastic bags or paper cups.
- **Cheese popcorn**—Make air-popped popcorn and sprinkle with grated Parmesan cheese.
- **Going crackers**—Serve *low-salt* crackers and cheese or a cottage cheese and herb dip. Be sure to choose your crackers carefully. Crackers that are lower in fat or sodium include low-salt wheat crackers available in many brands, unsalted matzo, plain low-salt breadsticks, and graham crackers.
- **Yummo wrap-ups**—Have children make their own wrap-ups using flour tortillas spread with a thin layer of peanut butter, dried fruit, and raisins—ideal for hikes. Or, for fresh-from-the-refrigerator snacks, wrap up part-skim ricotta cheese and cinnamon or fresh fruit.
- **Nachos**—Cut low-salt corn tortillas into six triangles and top with grated mozzarella cheese. Place in the oven (or toaster oven) at 350° F to crisp the tortillas and melt cheese. Serve with salsa.

Blender snacks

- **Blender basics**—For a shake, blend 1 cup of plain yogurt, 1 cup of chopped fruit (e.g., strawberries, bananas), and ½ cup of milk. The shakes will be thicker if made with frozen fruit. (Optional: Add ¼ to ½ teaspoon of vanilla.)
- **Melon cooler**—In blender, mix 1½ cups of ice cubes; 1½ cups of cubed watermelon, honeydew, or cantaloupe; and ½ teaspoon of lemon juice until smooth. Serve immediately. Makes 2½ cups.
- **Ambrosia shake**—In blender, mix four sliced, ripe bananas; ½ teaspoon of lemon juice; ¼ teaspoon of vanilla; and 5 cups of low-fat, skim, or reconstituted nonfat, dry milk. Makes six servings.
- **Fruit soup**—In blender, combine 1 banana; 1 peeled and cored apple; ½ to 1 cup of strawberries; 1 tablespoon of orange juice; 1 cup of plain, low-fat yogurt; a dash of cinnamon; and a dash of dried mint. Chill before serving. Makes six ½-cup servings.
- **Mango delight**—In a blender, mix 1 cup ice cubes, 1 cup frozen mangos, 1 cup fresh or frozen pineapple, 1 banana, fresh mint, and ½ teaspoon lime juice until smooth. Makes 4 cups.
- **Strawberry smoothie**—In a blender, mix 1 cup ice cubes, 1 cup frozen strawberries, 1 banana, and 1 cup soy milk until smooth. Serve immediately. Makes 3½ cups.

ers, and any food service personnel in developing the concepts and learning activities for nutrition education for children and families.

For children, nutrition education promotes acquisition of knowledge and skills that are key components of child development. When they plan, prepare, serve, and then eat tasty and healthful snack foods, children can be creative, learn how to choose foods that are both tasty and good for their bodies, and build their self-esteem. Food preparation helps children practice their fine and gross motor skills and teaches safety and sanitation, as well as cultural similarities and differences. Visits to farms, farmers' markets, neighborhood food stores, and home gardens make good field trips if they are well planned and include related educational activities before and after the visit. Search the website of the USDA Food and Nutrition Service at **www.fns.usda.gov/fns/** for preschool materials on nutrition education. For example, the organization has a curriculum suitable for children ages 3–5 called *Grow It, Try It, Like It! Preschool Fun with Fruits and Vegetables.* This curriculum includes detailed instructions and downloadable materials. See Figure 5.4 for suggested sources of advice about nutrition activities for children.

Family involvement is essential so that health-promoting messages are reinforced at home. Here are some ideas for ways to include families:

- Ask family members to help plan menus. For those who are interested, schedule an educational meeting on the principles of good nutrition involved in menu planning for young children.
- Ask families to share creative meal and snack ideas. Have a contest for the favorite idea.
- Include nutrition articles in the program's newsletter, classroom posts, or email announcements about nutrition education activities. Ask families to suggest topics for future family education programs so that nutrition education is responsive to their interests.
- Invite family members to participate in classroom nutrition education activities.
- Send printed menus home with children to show what meals and snacks are planned, and post the menu where families can see any last-minute changes.
- Ask families to share their ideas for interesting and safe foods that are appropriate for their child's nutritional needs and developmental feeding abilities that families can send with their children or the program can provide.
- Invite families to attend a potluck dinner and bring a special food from a favorite family recipe or something that is unique to their culture. Be sure to give families instructions for safely preparing and transporting foods to be shared. Ask them to list all the ingredients in their dishes, and then post this information where the food is served.
- Talk with families about any eating or nutritional issues you notice in children. As appropriate, refer them to community nutrition programs and health professionals. Provide families with regular progress reports on their children's eating in the program.
- Sponsor educational programs on nutrition and food consumer issues. Use the print materials, videos, and graphics available at **www.choosemyplate.gov** as a starting point. For example, the website offers a series of tip sheets, each of which includes 10 tips for implementing a specific nutrition recommendation, such as how to add more vegetables or how to feel satisfied with smaller portions. Each tip sheet is provided in English and Spanish. These tip sheets make for good additions to newsletters, bulletin boards, and email messages to families to post on their refrigerators at home.
- Talk with families about how they can foster positive eating habits at home, such as the following:
  - Encourage good eating behaviors, such as always sitting down for snacks and meals.
  - Involve the child in food-related activities (e.g., letting the child help prepare food with age-appropriate, safe kitchen tasks; sharing in cleanup activities; and talking about nutritious food in a positive way).
- Make available a list of community food and nutrition services, including school nutrition programs, food stamps, WIC, Commodity Supplemental Food Program (CSFP), and emergency feeding agencies.

Food as reward, punishment, and celebration

Children are more likely to learn unhealthful eating behaviors when adults use food as a reward, pacifier, or punishment. You have probably heard many times, "No dessert until you finish the food on your plate." This statement encourages the child to continue to eat all of the food served instead of stopping when feeling full, and implies that dessert is a better part of the meal. Children need positive encouragement, but using food as a reward places undue emphasis on the desirability of eating certain foods, which may lead to eating too much of them. Similarly, focusing celebrations on food rather than on games and other activities emphasizes external signals for eating rather than children's awareness of hunger and satiety. Desserts for meals should be nutritious and not withheld, even if they are the only food the child eats at a meal. Plan desserts so that if children eat only the dessert, they will have received the nutrients they need. Use praise, smiles, or hugs, but not food, as rewards for desired behavior. Choose healthful foods for parties.

> **Figure 5.4.**
>
> ### Sources for Nutrition Education
>
> Local resources for nutrition education include:
>
> a. Local and state nutritionists/RDs in health departments, in maternal and child health programs, and divisions of children with special health care needs
> b. Nutritionists/RDs at hospitals
> c. The Women, Infants, and Children (WIC) Supplemental Food Program and cooperative extension nutritionists/RDs
> d. School food service personnel
> e. State administrators of the Child and Adult Care Food Program
> f. National School Food Service Management Institute
> g. Healthy Meals Resource System of the Food and Nutrition Information System (National Agricultural Library, U.S. Department of Agriculture)
> h. Nutrition consultants with local affiliates of the following organizations:
>   1. American Dietetic Association
>   2. American Public Health Association
>   3. Society for Nutrition Education
>   4. American Association of Family and Consumer Sciences
>   5. Dairy Council
>   6. American Heart Association
>   7. American Cancer Society
>   8. American Diabetes Association
>   9. Professional home economists like teachers and those with consumer organizations
>   10. Nutrition departments of local colleges and universities
>
> Source: Standard 4.7.0.1, *Caring for Our Children*. Reprinted with permission.

Food safety

A public focus on ecologically safe and sustainable food has led to an array of choices in markets, which offer both healthful foods and marketing hoaxes. Local food may or may not be fresher than food transported long distances. Local produce is not available year-round in many places. Foods that are marked "certified organic" by the United States Department of Agriculture or an independent third-party certifier are supposed to be grown without pesticides, herbicides, hormones, or antibiotics. However, as is true of other foods, they can still be contaminated by naturally occurring toxins or illness-causing germs. Certified organic foods cannot be assumed to be safe, nor are those that are not certified organic necessarily harmful.

Concerns about animal rights have led to labeling food that is allegedly produced in more natural ways—for example, "grass-fed" or "free-range." However, such production methods may not necessarily be better for animals or the environment, and they do not always result in better-quality food.

Small traces of pesticides may be found in many foods. While minimizing exposure to pesticides is desirable, rejecting foods that have levels of pesticides that have not been found to be harmful makes little sense. To minimize exposure to pesticides and select healthful foods, thoroughly wash all vegetables and fruits.

Drink water from a tested public health water source whenever possible. Bottled waters are not regulated. Much of bottled water comes from the same municipal water systems that provide tap water. When tested, some brands of bottled water have been found to be contaminated with chemicals and bacteria. When you need portable water, use water from a safe source to fill reusable water containers, preferably those made of stainless steel. If plastics are used, choose products labeled as BPA and phthalate free.

Food brought from home

When facilities allow food to be brought from home, they must have written guidelines for families about what is acceptable. Food brought from home should be nourishing and safe, complying with the CACFP guidelines. However, unless the food is a commercially prepared food in the original, sealed container, the quality of preparation and the content of the food cannot be assured. Therefore, food brought from home must be carefully inspected to try to determine whether it is safe to give to the child. If in doubt, throw it out. Food must be available to supplement inadequate or inappropriate food brought from home. Teachers are responsible for seeing that children eat in a way that supports their growth and health, and they must follow best practice even if families want their children fed otherwise.

Foods brought from home should be clearly labeled with the child's name, the date, and the type of food. Meals and snacks prepared at and brought from home for one child should not be shared with another child. Inadvertent sharing will occur, but it should be discouraged to minimize the risk to other children. Perishable foods should be checked to be sure they are at a safe temperature when they arrive, and then refrigerated until served. Food-borne illness is very common. The Centers for Disease Control and Prevention (CDC) estimates that every year about one in six people in the United States gets sick from food.

Use the following list of specific food-related risks for children to check that program policies and procedures address the issues involved.

- See Chapter 3 for precautions to take to prevent choking from foods and to prevent improper use of food service articles (e.g., using feeding bottles and cups when children are not seated on a lap or in a chair).

- Do not feed honey to children younger than 1 year of age. Honey can cause botulism in infancy. Check food and formula labels to be sure that honey has not been used as a sweetener.

- Be sure all staff members are aware of children's food allergies and of the emergency steps to take if an allergic child consumes a problem food. Be especially alert at occasions when foods are brought into the facility by family members or staff members that are not foods planned for and provided by the facility. For the safety of some highly allergic children, the offending food may need to be banned from any room the child uses. Recent research suggests that washing off surfaces that have been in contact with peanut products may be sufficient to protect children allergic to peanuts. It is rarely necessary to ban a food from the entire facility (see Food allergies and intolerances later in this chapter).

- Be sure foods brought from home are prepared, transported, stored, and served following food safety guidelines.

Activity and physical exercise affect appetite

Activity has a lot to do with appetite and nutritional status. Active children need more calories than inactive ones; this means that they have a better chance of getting all required nutrients. Adequate physical exercise year-round, preferably on a daily basis, is important to a child's nutrition (as well as development) because it stimulates a healthy appetite, uses calories, and maintains muscle tissue. (See Chapter 6 for more about how physical activity affects health.)

Common nutritional concerns

Preventing overweight and obesity

Obesity is a complex problem with multiple causes that is now epidemic in the United States. Some combination of overeating, poor food choices, inactivity, social or emotional factors, and genetics is responsible for obesity. Helping children learn healthy eating and exercise habits and limiting screen time (e.g., TV, videos/DVDs, and computers) are the keys to preventing obesity. Although overweight children will not always become overweight adults, many children who are overweight become obese and will remain so throughout life. Obesity can significantly affect a child psychologically and emotionally and can result in low self-esteem. People who are overweight suffer many health problems. These problems both shorten their lives and increase their pain and suffering even when they are still quite young.

The goal of weight management for children who are of normal weight is to teach them healthful habits that will prevent excess weight gain. The goal of weight management for overweight or obese children is to limit further weight gain. Then these children will grow slimmer as they grow into their weight. Actual weight loss may not be recommended, as children need adequate nutrients and calories for growth. Nutritious meals and snacks are essential to good weight management for all children.

Early childhood programs can manage and prevent obesity in young children by taking the following measures:

- Encourage children to be physically active, as discussed in Chapter 6.

- Have designated mealtimes and designated eating places, and focus on social interaction during the meal.

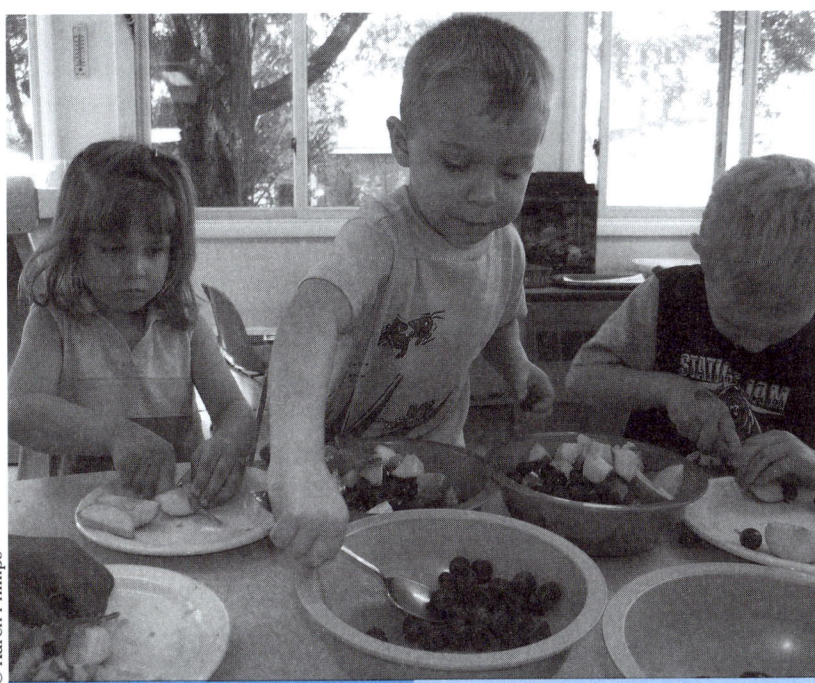
© Karen Phillips

- Prohibit screen time (TV, videos/DVDs, computers, and other electronic screen devices) for children younger than 2 years of age. For older children, limit screen time to no more than 30 minutes once a week in the early education facility. Such use should be for educational or physical activity only. Limit computer use to no more than 15 minutes at a time except for school-age children using the computer to do their homework. Make sure all screen time is free of advertising and brand placement. Remember, do not let children eat while watching television or doing other activities.
- The majority of children watch TV every day at home. Early care and education programs must severely limit screen time so the child does not exceed the AAP recommendation to limit screen time to a total of less than two hours a day. Remind all adults who watch TV programs on any electronic device when children are present not to watch programs that are not intended for children. The content of many programs, including news, talk shows, and reality and drama programs, expose children to inappropriate language, frightening images, and dangerous risk-taking behaviors.
- Limit high-calorie foods (high in fat, sugar, or both).
- Limit juice intake to no more than four to six ounces per day, including drinks consumed in the program and at home. Avoid sweetened beverages such as fruit drinks, powdered or syrup-based drink mixes, and chocolate-flavored milk, which add extra calories. Commercial chocolate milk often is made with skim milk, but it has extra calories from the fat in the added chocolate. Chocolate is a stimulant like caffeine. Frequent use of chocolate teaches children to look for it as a regular part of their diets. Most of the time, a child's thirst should be satisfied with water after the proper amount of milk is consumed.
- Use low-fat or skim milk with children older than 2.
- Put food on small plates.
- Provide high-fiber, filling, crunchy foods.
- Limit eating to appropriate portion-controlled meals at designated eating times (three meals plus two snacks, preplanned for portion control and nutrient balance).
- Provide lots of nonfood rewards. Instead of high-calorie foods, plan activities as the centerpiece for birthday parties, holidays, and other celebrations, and serve fresh fruit and vegetables as the party foods.
- Help children learn to deal with emotions or stress without turning to food.
- Remember, the behaviors of teachers and family members influence children's attitudes and behaviors. Be a good role model.

Fats

Fats play a significant role as a cause of heart disease. Polyunsaturated and saturated fats are important nutrients to include in the proper ratio. *Polyunsaturated fats* are usually found in liquid vegetable oils that contain essential fatty acids the body cannot manufacture. *Saturated fats,* the solid fats found in beef, pork, lamb, chicken, and dairy products, are the ones to be limited. Some fat from both sources, however, is necessary to maintain the proper balance of fatty acids in the body. Hydrogenated or partially hydrogenated vegetable oils have been treated to convert some of the polyunsaturated fats to saturated fats, so watch out for foods with labels that indicate that, although they contain healthful oils, these oils have been hydrogenated. Foods such as hot dogs, luncheon meats, and potato chips are high in saturated fat and salt and should be limited in a child's diet.

Sugar

Many factors determine how foods affect children's teeth. The more often children snack on foods containing sugars and starches, the greater the chance for tooth decay. Serve foods with little or no added sugar. The only reason to sweeten food is for taste, and much of the sweetening of food is not necessary. In nature, few foods have the concentration of sugar people commonly put in prepared foods. Highly concentrated sugar loads put a heavy demand on the body to process this quick source of energy, and the excess is often stored as fat.

Avoid foods or drinks with added sugars on the ingredient list, such as sucrose, glucose, high-fructose corn syrup, corn syrup, maple syrup, and fructose. Honey, molasses, raw sugar, and refined sugar all contain the same number of calories. Avoid adding natural or artificial sweeteners to vegetables, fruits, fruit juice, or cereal. Limit foods such as candy, sweetened beverages, and sweetened baked goods that provide many calories and low levels of essential nutrients.

Salt

Preference for salty foods is learned. Teachers should not teach this unhealthy salt-craving lesson. Diets high in salt may cause high blood pressure in people with a susceptibility to this problem. Reduce salt intake by not salting food at the table, decreasing the amount of salt used in cooking, and limiting salty foods (e.g., pickles, canned soups, chips, some crackers, and salted nuts). Foods may be flavored with spices or herbs instead of salt for taste. Be aware of hidden salt commonly found in hot dogs, bacon, sausages, condiments, and many canned and some frozen foods.

Vegetarian diets

Vegetarian and vegan cuisine excludes some or all animal products. Vegetarian diets, often high in fiber and low in cholesterol and saturated fat, can have positive health benefits. A well-planned vegetarian diet can provide all the nutrients a child needs for growth and activity. However, a professional who understands children's growth and nutritional needs and the nutrient content of the foods in these diets must carefully check the child's intake to be sure it provides sufficient amounts of what the child needs. Meeting with an RD to plan menus for a child who eats a vegetarian diet may be necessary to ensure that the child receives enough calories and nutrients.

Vegetarian diets vary. Vegetarian diets that include dairy products and eggs readily provide all needed nutrients for young children. Vegan or total vegetarian diets that omit all animal protein may not provide enough protein, calcium, iron, zinc, vitamin D, and vitamin B12. Very strict vegetarian diets also may be low in calories due to their high bulk and low fat content. Children eating strict vegetarian diets should be assessed for health issues such as short stature, low weight, and rickets.

Legumes, seeds, or nuts, when combined with grains, provide a good protein source. To get enough protein, children on vegan or strict vegetarian diets need to eat more than children who eat meat, fish, poultry, and cheese. The number of servings from each food group is different for a child eating a vegetarian diet, particularly a vegan diet. Families who wish to have their children follow a vegan diet should consult an RD and their child's health care provider to ensure that intake of nutrients and calories is adequate for growth.

Milk

If children who are also eating solid foods drink too much milk, they may not be hungry for solid foods and may develop iron-deficiency anemia. Offer water if a child is thirsty and has already had sufficient milk. A preschooler needs approximately 16–24 ounces (2–3 cups) of milk daily. If a child doesn't drink much milk, do not make an issue of it. Left alone, the child will probably go back to drinking milk. Other foods rich in calcium, such as hard cheese and yogurt, can be substituted for milk (see Figure 5.5).

Some children have lactose intolerance, a lack of intestinal enzymes to digest the milk sugar, lactose. This problem can be avoided with special milks, calcium supplements, or use of enzyme preparations before having a milk product.

Nutritional problems and special diets

Early childhood programs must follow the instructions of the family and the child's physician in preparing and feeding a special diet. Sometimes special diets are requested for cultural or religious reasons. Where possible, accommodate these requests as long as the child's nutritional needs are met and the preparation does not pose an undue burden for staff. For diets required due to health problems, the child care facility must address the special need just as it must accommodate any child with a disability. Consult an RD for assistance in menu planning and feeding adjustments to meet the child's needs.

Iron deficiency

Anemia occurs when too little blood is produced or too much blood is lost. Barring blood loss, the usual reason for anemia is an inadequate intake of iron. This problem occurs most commonly during periods of rapid growth, such as early infancy and adolescence. Recent studies

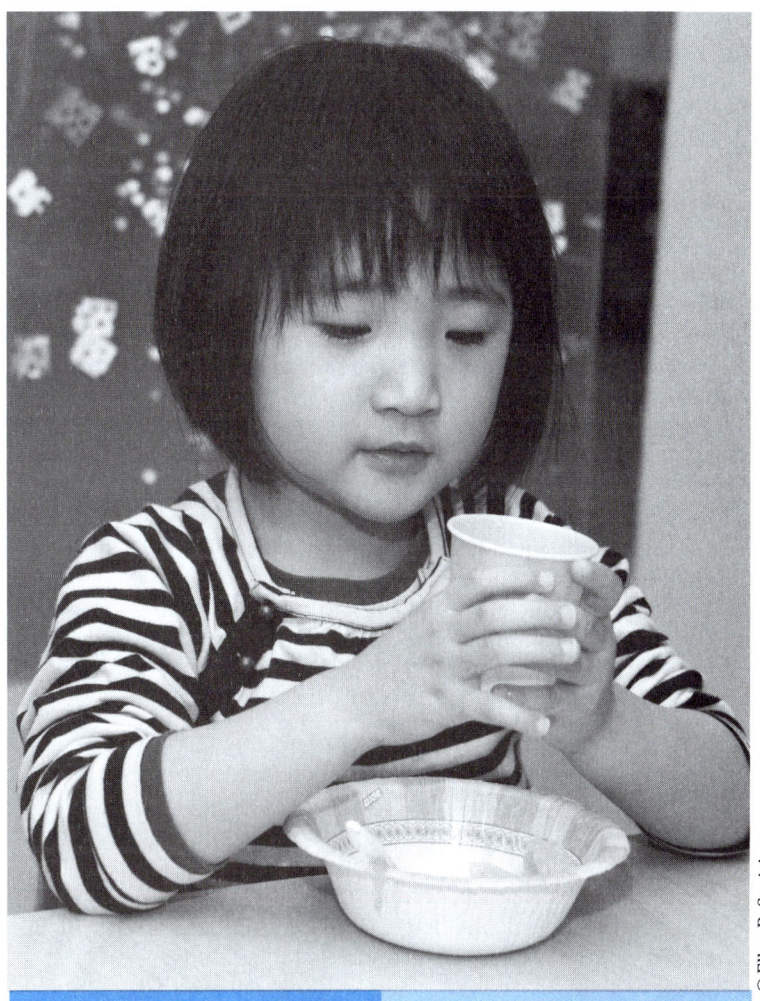

Figure 5.5.

Dietary Sources of Calcium

Excellent

Yogurt (low-fat or whole milk)
Skim milk
Low-fat milk (1 percent or 2 percent)
Buttermilk
Whole milk
Swiss cheese
Sardines (Pick the low-salt canned variety. Serve the fish mashed with its bones and then mixed with a little mayonnaise as a sandwich filling or spread.)

Good

Cheeses (cheddar, Muenster, mozzarella, blue)
American or Swiss pasteurized process cheese food
Parmesan cheese, grated
Tofu*
Dry skim milk, instant
Salmon, pink, canned with bones
Collard greens, cooked

Fair

Blackstrap molasses
Vanilla, soft-serve, frozen dairy products (check sugar content)
Figs, dried
Kale, cooked
Mustard greens, cooked
Ice cream, vanilla (note that ice cream is a high-calorie, high-fat food that doesn't have a lot of calcium)
Chickpeas, cooked
Broccoli, cooked
Cottage cheese, creamed

*Calcium content of tofu differs according to the processing method. Tofu contains calcium if it is processed with a calcium coagulant such as sulfate. Look on the nutrition label or in the ingredient list. Nigari is a popular tofu coagulant that does *not* contain calcium.

---

of the role of iron in the body found that before anemia develops, other body tissues suffer from iron deficiency. For example, brain cells may not function properly with inadequate levels of iron.

Iron fortification of bread, cereal, and pasta reduces the risk of anemia from nutritional deficiency. In addition to anemia screening, checking blood iron levels is recommended when iron deficiency is suspected. Here are some things teachers can do to prevent iron deficiency:

- Encourage children to consume a varied, well-balanced diet that includes iron-rich foods.

- Provide iron-rich foods at meals and snacks. Good sources of iron include dried beans and peas, lentils, beef, pork, lamb, whole wheat and enriched breads, and cereal products. Raisins and peanut butter also contain a small amount of iron. Iron from animal sources is absorbed better than iron from plant sources.

- Serve iron-rich foods with a source of vitamin C. Vitamin C increases the body's ability to use iron. The amount of iron absorbed from plant sources increases significantly when these foods are combined with food high in vitamin C. For example, with chili serve spinach, broccoli, or tomato slices; with split-pea soup serve half an orange, cantaloupe cubes, or strawberries. These fruits and vegetables also provide fiber.

- Limit milk consumption to 24 ounces per day and ensure adequate intake of other foods, particularly iron-containing foods.

Failure to thrive

Some children do not grow properly. Their height may be short for their age, or their weight may be low for their height. They may tire easily and be inattentive, disinterested in eating, and undernourished. This complex syndrome, known as failure to thrive, may be due to medical, nutritional, or psychosocial factors.

When a child is suspected to be failing to thrive, immediately refer the child for a complete medical, nutritional, and social evaluation. Assist the family with carrying out a recommended treatment plan. If a child has been diagnosed in the past as having failure to thrive, watch closely for signs of poor growth even when the crisis is past.

Sometimes failure to thrive can signal child abuse or neglect. In these cases, be alert to other possible signs of child abuse or neglect (see Chapter 13) that would require immediate reporting to child protective services.

Food allergies and intolerances

Infants and young children sometimes have food allergies or are intolerant of certain foods. An allergic reaction occurs when a child is sensitive to a particular food and the immune system produces increased amounts of antibodies. The allergic reaction can be avoided only by avoiding the food.

The most common food to cause allergic reactions is peanuts, but other common causes are tree nuts, eggs, cow's milk protein, wheat, fish, shellfish, citrus fruits, and berries. Some of these products are present in very small quantities in ordinary foods where you might not suspect them to be present. For example, peanut oil is used in some spaghetti sauces. When a child has a food allergy, scrutinize every food and carefully read every food label.

Food intolerance is much more common than food allergy. A food intolerance is present when a person has some metabolic factors (e.g., lack of an enzyme or chemical) that make it difficult or impossible to digest or use certain food. Sometimes foods can be modified so that the child can tolerate them. Intolerance to the sugar in cow's milk (lactose) is a common problem in infants and children. Soy formulas are an alternative to cow's milk or regular formula for children with milk allergies or lactose intolerance. Sometimes the intolerance is relative, affected by the amount of the food the child takes. Some children can have a small amount of the food to which they are intolerant without difficulty.

Most children who are allergic to food have symptoms such as a rash when they eat the offending food. A few allergic children cannot even touch a surface that has a small amount of a food to which they are sensitive. When they have even the smallest contact, they develop symptoms such as diarrhea, vomiting, abdominal pain, rash, irritability, breathing problems—sometimes even death. Reactions may be immediate or delayed, and symptoms may be mild to severe.

When a child has a food allergy or intolerance, follow these guidelines:

- Confirm the nature of the food problem with the child's health care provider and obtain a clear set of instructions to follow routinely and in the event of inadvertent exposure of the child to the problem food.
- With permission from the child's parents, post the child's food allergies prominently in the areas the child will use. The child could wear a label warning of the allergy so that substitute staff members and visitors do not inadvertently expose the child to the offending food.
- Read labels to identify hidden sources of the problem foods or substances.
- Work with families to find acceptable substitutes for problem foods.
- Carefully plan menus with an RD to ensure adequate nutrition, particularly if a child has multiple food allergies or is allergic to other major food groups.
- Plan with staff members and families as necessary to protect the allergic child from exposure to the problem food.
- Use training, guidelines, materials, and warning notices available from the Food Allergy and Anaphylaxis Network (FAAN) for teachers. The website for this organization is **www.foodallergy.org**.

Hyperactivity

Hyperactivity is not caused by food allergies or food intolerance. The common myth that sugar makes children hyperactive is a misinterpretation of what happens in the body after a high sugar feeding. Within an hour or so after eating a sugary food, the blood sugar goes up quickly. This rise in blood sugar may make the person sleepy—which commonly happens after a big meal. In response to a high blood sugar level, the body puts out a big amount of insulin. If the sugary food does not contain more slowly digested protein and fat, the insulin quickly pulls the sugar level in the blood down. A quick lowering of blood sugar levels often makes the person irritable. Many people think this irritability from a high sugar feeding is because the sugar made the child "hyper."

Additive-free diets have not been found to be of value in the treatment of hyperactivity. While eliminating artificial food colorings and salicylates (aspirin-like compounds) does not harm children and may improve a diet's nutritional value, it does not affect the hyperactivity itself. Any diet for a hyperactive child should be carefully planned along with appropriate medical and psychological treatment. Consult the child's health care provider to ensure nutritional adequacy.

Feeding children who have other special needs

Children with special needs have the same basic care and feeding needs as all children. Often these basic needs are overlooked in the concern for the disability. Children may have nutritional problems (e.g., poor food intake, inability to chew or swallow normally, inadequate weight gain, short stature, obesity, or iron-deficiency anemia) *and* behavioral concerns associated with eating, placing them at nutritional risk. Infants or children with special needs may require more patience, time, and understanding for feeding than typically developing children. Special adaptive equipment also may be necessary.

Healthful foods and dietary supplements play an important role in helping the child with chronic illness maintain weight, strength, and energy and fight infections. Some children with chronic illness or other special needs can follow a normal diet most of the time. During bouts with fever, diarrhea, nausea, or weight

Figure 5.6.

MyPlate Mini-Poster

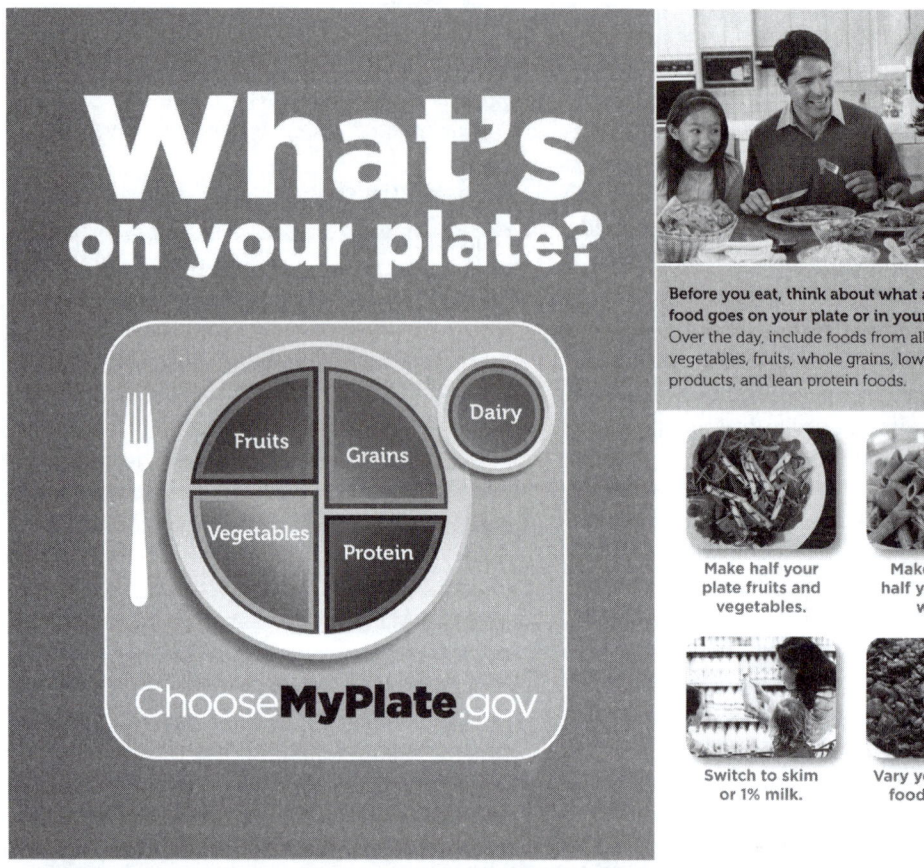

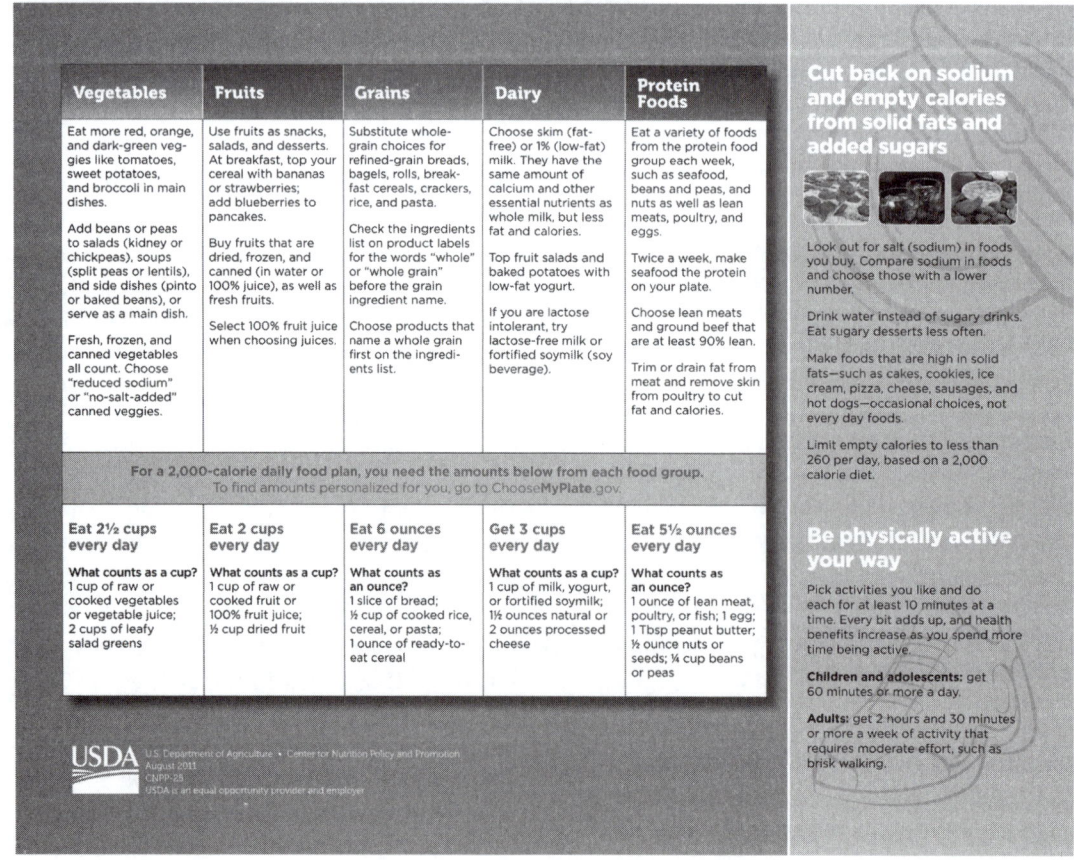

Source: United States Department of Agriculture, Center for Nutrition Policy and Promotion (CNPP).
Online: http://www.choosemyplate.gov/downloads/mini_poster_English_final.pdf.

loss, they may require a special diet and food supplements.

Whatever the disease, disorder, or disability, good nutrition always contributes to optimal growth and development and can decrease or prevent some debilitating effects. Use the services of a nutritionist or dietician to ensure that families and staff members have the knowledge, skills, and support to provide optimal nutrition for a child with special needs. Involving families in planning how to meet the special nutritional needs of a child with a disability is especially important. To help solve any complex problems, involve pediatricians, occupational and physical therapists, social workers, or other health professionals.

Dietary guidelines for young children

In support of the national standards mentioned earlier in this chapter, the USDA offers graphic images called MyPlate in separate versions for preschoolers, school-age children, and adults. These are available as a printable image and poster at **www.choosemyplate.gov** (see Figure 5.6).

Community nutrition resources

Familiarity with community nutrition programs, local nutritionists, and emergency food agencies will help you make appropriate referrals when necessary. Obtain information about locally helpful resources to share with families from the state agency that administers the CACFP. To learn about the CACFP and locate your CACFP agency, go to **www.fns.usda.gov/cnd/care/**. Search the CACFP website for links to other community programs, such as school nutrition programs, food stamps, and emergency feeding agencies. You can also search this site for information about WIC. These organizations and agencies may suggest other helpful resources available in your area. Ask about special grants or projects that target early care and education programs.

Running a food service

Operating a food service program for young children involves menu planning, food purchasing and preparation, food service, and a number of issues related to environmental health, sanitation, and infectious disease control. Even if all foods served are brought from home, the program is running a food service. Many issues must be addressed when food is brought from home:

- Selection and preparation
- Transportation of foods
- Labeling of foods and containers
- Safe storage in child care until foods are served
- How the food should be served to the child
- Sanitation in handling foods and food containers brought from home

For more details about how to run a food service, consult other resources such as those produced by the CACFP. For recipes, information on preparing nutritious meals, and tips on food safety, visit the Healthy Meals Resource System of the USDA, Team Nutrition, at **http://healthymeals.nal.usda.gov**. Also see Chapter 4 of *Caring for Our Children* and *Making Food Healthy and Safe*, 2nd edition, available on the website of the National Training Institute for Child Care Health Consultants at **http://nti.unc.edu**. This publication offers specific guidelines to implement the child care food service standards outlined in *Caring for Our Children*.

Menu planning

Plan your menus around young children's nutritional and developmental needs by using the meal pattern developed by the CACFP as a minimum standard. Incorporate the recommendations for revision of the CACFP from the IOM listed earlier in this chapter, under National Standards and Recommendations for Nutrition in Early Care and Education Programs. For sample menu planning worksheets and guidance, contact your state CACFP or state extension service. Prepare weekly written menus and post or distribute them to staff and families. Vary menus by season, and avoid repeating weekly menus more than once a month.

Centers should consider setting up a menu planning committee. This committee might consist of the program director, a teacher, a teacher assistant, a cook, parent(s), and a nutritionist. If you use cyclical menus, the committee may have to meet only once a month or every six weeks.

Food purchasing

- Be sure that food and beverage suppliers meet local, state, and federal codes.
- Be sure that the meats and poultry you purchase have been inspected and passed tests for wholesomeness by federal or state inspectors.
- Use only pasteurized milk and milk products. If you use dry milk for cooking, prepare it in a clean container and immediately refrigerate or use it.
- Do not use: foods canned at home; food from dented, rusted, bulging cans; or cans without labels. Fresh and frozen foods are preferable to canned foods, due to concerns about high salt content and potential BPA exposure in canned foods.
- Consider making arrangements with a local food

store to provide abundant fresh fruits and vegetables in the quantity the facility needs for a discounted price. Stores often run sales on overstocked items and may be willing to be proactive in selling the larger quantities that a child care facility requires.

Food storage

- Store all perishable foods at temperatures that will prevent spoilage (refrigerator temperature, 40° F or lower; freezer temperature, 0° or lower).
- Place thermometers in the warmest part of the refrigerator and freezer (near the door), and check them daily.
- Set up refrigerators to allow for air circulation around shelves and walls. This helps maintain proper food temperatures.
- Always examine food when it arrives to make sure it is not spoiled, dirty, or infested with insects.
- Store unrefrigerated foods in clean, rodent- and insect-proof, covered metal, glass, or hard plastic containers. (Check local bakeries for containers that they consider disposable, or get them from restaurant equipment suppliers.)
- Store food containers above the floor (about six inches) on racks or other clean slotted surfaces that permit air circulation.
- Keep storerooms dry and free from leaky plumbing or drainage problems. Repair all holes and cracks to prevent insect and rodent infestation.
- Keep storerooms cool (about 60° F) to increase the food's shelf life.
- Store all food items separately from nonfood items.
- Use an inventory system: *The first food stored is the first food used.* This ensures proper rotation. Inspect food daily for spoilage. Many food safety tools are available on the USDA website, including food storage guidelines and food service training tools. Go to **www.usda.gov** and search for "food storage" to find current materials available for free.

Preparing and handling table foods

The following guidelines apply to all foods, whether they are prepared at the facility, brought to the facility by a catering service, or brought from home.

- Wash all raw fruits and vegetables before use. Wash tops of cans before opening.
- Thaw frozen foods in the refrigerator or put quick-thaw foods in plastic bags under cold running water for immediate preparation. DO NOT thaw frozen foods by allowing them to stand at room temperature.
- Use a thermometer to check the internal temperatures of the following foods to be sure they have been cooked evenly and held at a safe temperature until they are served:
  - Poultry: Heat to a minimum of 165° F
  - Stuffing: Heat to a minimum of 165° F in a separate pan (do not cook inside poultry)
  - Pork and pork products: Heat to a minimum of 160° F
- Prepare potentially hazardous foods (e.g., meat salads, poultry salads, egg salads, seafood salads, potato salads, cream-filled pastries, and other prepared foods containing milk, meat, poultry, fish, and/or eggs) as quickly as possible from products that have been kept chilled. Serve immediately, and refrigerate leftovers immediately.
- Prevent bacterial growth by maintaining all potentially hazardous foods at temperatures lower than 40° F or higher than 140° F during transportation and while holding until the food is served. Bacteria multiply most rapidly between 40° F and 140° F.
- Cover or completely wrap foods during transportation.
- Never reuse a spoon that has been used even once for tasting.
- Make sure each serving bowl has a spoon or other serving utensil.
- Keep foods that might be needed for second servings refrigerated or heated in the kitchen (below 40° F or above 140° F). That way, if they are not eaten as second servings, they can safely be served as leftovers at another meal. Discard if the foods have not been held at these safe temperatures for two hours.
- Throw away leftover food from serving bowls on the table with these possible exceptions:
  - Whole, raw fruit and cut or raw vegetables that can be thoroughly washed
  - Packaged foods that have not been unwrapped and do not spoil
- If foods are to be stored after they are cooked and then served later, place them in shallow pans and refrigerate or freeze immediately to rapidly bring the temperature to 40° F or lower.
- After two days, discard prepared casseroles or leftovers that were not served, even if they were properly stored in the refrigerator. Do not send leftovers home with children or adults because of the hazards of bacterial growth during transport.
- Keep lunches brought from home in the refrigerator until lunchtime. Encourage parents to use cold packs to transport any perishable food at safe temperatures. (Spot-checking whether food was transported at safe temperatures is simple: Put a food thermometer in the perishable food just before putting the lunch box in the facility's refrigerator.) Remember, the outside of a lunch box is not sanitary; put the contents, not the lunch box itself, onto a sanitized table where children eat.

- Let children choose what to eat from the contents of the lunch boxes, but put out the most nutritious foods first.

Storing nonfood supplies

- Store all cleaning supplies (including cleaning agents) and other poisonous materials in *locked* compartments or in compartments well above the reach of children and separate from food, dishes, and utensils.
- Store poisonous and toxic materials (other than those needed for kitchen sanitation) in *locked* compartments *outside* the kitchen area.
- Store insect and rodent poisons in *locked* compartments in an area apart from cleaning materials to avoid contamination or mistaken usage.
- Make sure any bait put into food storage areas is boxed, labeled, and separated to prevent possible contamination of food supplies.
- Keep all poisonous materials in their original containers and use them only according to the manufacturer's instructions.

Cleaning and caring for equipment

- Throw away cracked or chipped dishes or utensils that may harbor bacteria. Avoid utensils with chipped or painted handles.
- Wash dishes using a method approved by the local department of health. (See also Chapter 10.)
- Set up a food service cleaning schedule according to the one shown in *Caring for Our Children*, Appendix W.
- Be sure there are sufficient garbage cans to hold all garbage. They should have tight-fitting lids and be leak-proof. Line the cans with plastic liners; empty and clean cans frequently. Keep the garbage area clean at all times.

Insect and rodent control in food areas

Programs should use Integrated Pest Management (IPM) to reduce the risk of pesticide exposure to children. IPM is the application of a combination of methods for managing pests such as insects, diseases, weeds, and rodents. It is an environmentally sensitive approach to pest management that includes pest prevention techniques, pest monitoring methods, biological controls, pest attractants and repellents, bio-pesticides, and pesticides. One excellent, child-care-specific resource is a tool kit published by California Childcare Health Program called *Integrated Pest Management: A Toolkit for Early Care and Education Programs*. Find this tool kit in English or Spanish at **www.ucsfchildcarehealth.org**. (Go to Publications & Resources, and then select Training Curricula.)

For guidance about using IPM in schools, go to the Environmental Protection Agency (EPA) website, **www.epa.gov/pesticides/ipm/**. Also see the discussion of IPM in Chapter 10 as a maintenance issue for the whole facility. To manage insects and rodents, follow these steps:

- Store all foods in insect-resistant containers.
- Be sure all doors and windows have screens in good condition. Keep screens closed at all times.
- Close all openings to the outside to prevent rodents and insects from entering.
- If there are insects in the food preparation areas, use only approved pyrethrin-based insecticides or a flyswatter. Do not allow insecticides to come in contact with raw or cooked food, utensils, or equipment used in food preparation and serving, or with any other food-contact surface. Do not use airborne sprays or insect strips that hang from the ceiling.
- Insecticides for crawling insects should be applied only by certified insect control personnel. Because the training and performance of exterminators is highly variable, a staff member should watch where the insecticides are applied to be certain that food preparation surfaces or child contact areas are not contaminated.

Suggested activities

- Assess the menu of a child care facility, matching the menu against your observations of what the children actually receive. Use the CACFP requirements for meals and snacks to see whether the menu and the actual food served meet these requirements.
- Observe the food service for infants and toddlers in a child care center or home-based program, and compare your observations against the guidelines detailed in this chapter. Which requirements are met? Which are not met? What change in practices would be required to meet the requirements? Would this cost the program additional money? What could be changed without additional cost?
- Observe food preparation in an early childhood facility. What sanitation and food handling practices do you see the staff using? Use a thermometer to check refrigerator and freezer temperatures. Use a food thermometer to check perishable foods, including those brought from home. Look at how foods are prepared and stored. Do you see any breaches in sanitation?
- At an early childhood facility, ask how families and staff members are involved in ensuring good nutrition for the children. How could this involvement be improved so that children and families have better nutrition without disrupting the program's operations?

6

Promoting Health with Physical Activity

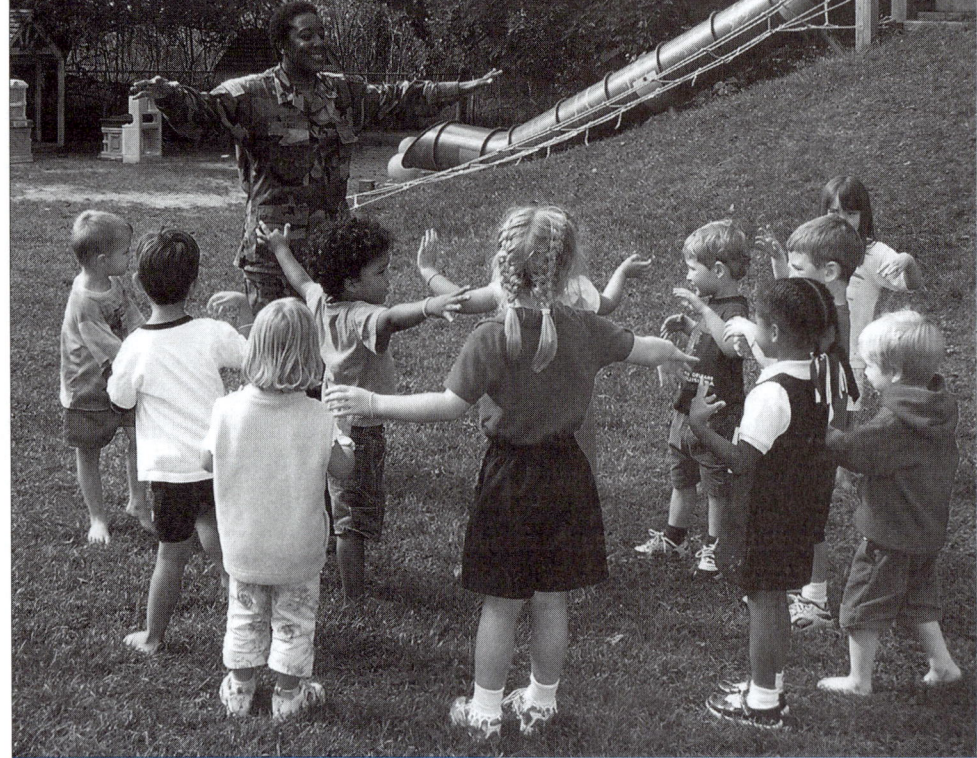

MAJOR CONCEPTS

- Current national recommendations and standards define best practices for promoting health through physical activity.
- Significant health benefits are associated with meeting the national standards for physical activity for children in group care.
- Physical activity is essential for prevention of overweight and obesity.
- Physical activity and movement are essential elements for development and learning from infancy.

Excellent updated resources are available for early educators to use to help implement health-promoting physical activity in their programs.

Researchers are focusing attention on the health benefits of physical activity and the role that early care and education programs play in ensuring that children get the type and amount of physical activity they need. In addition to helping to prevent overweight and obesity, physical activity is necessary for children to acquire motor skills. It also prepares children to be attentive for cognitive learning. (See References in *Caring for Our Children* Standards 3.1.3.1, 3.1.3.2, and 3.1.3.4, as well as Appendix S: Physical Activity: How Much Is Needed?)

The documented health benefits of physical activity for children include:

- Increased muscle and bone strength
- Reduced blood pressure and total body fat
- Better psychological well-being
- Decreased risk of obesity

National standards for physical activity for children in group care

Standard 3.1.3.1 in *Caring for Our Children* requires that children engage in active play every day.

> The facility should promote children's active play every day. Children should have ample opportunity to do moderate to vigorous activities such as running, climbing, dancing, skipping, and jumping. All children, birth to six years, should participate daily in
>
> a. Two to three occasions of active play outdoors, weather permitting (see Standard 3.1.3.2: Playing Outdoors for appropriate weather conditions)
>
> b. Two or more structured or caregiver/teacher/adult-led activities or games that promote movement over the course of the day—indoor or outdoor
>
> c. Continuous opportunities to develop and practice age-appropriate gross motor and movement skills

For each age group, teachers should implement the recommended guidelines in *Caring for Our Children* for the total time allotted for outdoor play of any type. This time outdoors can include less vigorous activities, such as reading stories, planting gardens, painting or drawing with chalk on walkways, and playing in a water table into which a gently running hose adds fresh flowing (and overflowing) water. Children may also spend time outdoors in moderate to vigorous physical activities, such as running, jumping, skipping, hopping, and dancing. Moderate activity is a level where talking is possible, but a bit difficult. Vigorous activity is too strenuous for talking. Follow the recommended guidelines to determine the appropriate amount of these types of activity for all age groups—whether such play occurs outdoors, indoors, or both.

Infants up to 12 months of age should be outside two to three times a day, although the standards do not state how long infants should remain outdoors. Children 12 months to 6 years of age should have 60–90 minutes of outdoor play, allocated in part-time programs as 20 minutes for every three hours in the facility. The time allocated for vigorous activity should be 60–90 minutes per eight-hour day for toddlers and 90–120 minutes per eight-hour day for preschool-age children (see Figure 6.1).

The *Caring for Our Children* standards also emphasize the need for supervised tummy time for infants every day, while they are awake. Tummy time helps very young children develop the muscles they need to sit up, crawl, and walk. At first, infants may tolerate only a few minutes on their tummies. Teachers should interact with infants during this time to encourage their efforts to lift their heads and chests. As the infants grow stronger, they can spend more time on their tummies. Standard 3.1.3.1 suggests ways to encourage infant activity during tummy time. For example, for very young infants, the teacher can lie down on the floor on her back, with the infant's tummy against her chest. In this situation, most infants will try to lift their heads to see the adult's face. Contact with the teacher's body may help the infant tolerate the tummy position for longer than lying on a harder surface. As infants start to reach for objects (around 3–4 months of age), the teacher can place toys around the infant in areas where the infant must reach for them. As the infant's abilities increase, choose challenging but not frustrating placement of these toys so the infant works to reach in all directions.

Caring for Our Children Standard 3.1.3.1 requires that infants not be sedentary while in a child care setting for more than 15 minutes at a time, except during meals and naps. Time spent in equipment such as infant swings, stationary activity centers, and infant seats (e.g., bouncers) should be limited, if these items are used at all. Infants who fall asleep in such equipment should be removed and placed to sleep on their backs in a crib that meets federal regulations. Sleeping while slumped in a seat is associated with decreased blood oxygen, which can harm brain cells. Ideally, environments for infants should be as unrestrictive as possible at all times.

Older children need to learn to take breaks for physical activity, especially after they have been engrossed in doing a project that has kept them physically inactive. Research shows that children are not as physically active while in group care as they should be. (For reports of some of these studies, see the list of references for Standard 3.1.3.1 in *Caring for Our Children*.) Some investigators have measured children's activity through observations; others have used devices that actually measure children's movement throughout the

Figure 6.1.

Physical Activity Guidelines

Type of activity and age group	NASPE[1]	USDA[2] Dietary Guidelines	AAP[3]	USDHHS[4] Physical Activity Guidelines	CFOC[5]
Unstructured time					
Infants	—	—	Focus on age-appropriate play, exploration, safety	Not enough data to recommend lengths of time	2–3 outdoor occasions/day
Toddlers	60 min	—			60–90 min opportunity to be active
Preschoolers	60 min	60 min, most days			90–120 min opportunity to be active
Structured time					
Infants	Promote development	—			2–3 outdoor occasions/day
Toddlers	30 min	—			At least 2 structured occasions, of 5–10 min
Preschoolers	60 min	—			At least 2 structured occasions, of 5–10 min

Type of activity and age group	NASPE	AAP	NAP SACC/ Baby NAP[6]	CFOC
Sedentary time				
Infants	—	—	30 min	Less than 15 min
Toddlers	Less than 60 min	—	30 min	—
Preschoolers	Less than 60 min	—	Less than 30 min	—

Source: Adapted and updated with permission from K. Copeland, "Practical Strategies for Increasing Children's Physical Activity in Child Care." Slide presentation at the National Conference and Exhibition of the American Academy of Pediatrics, San Francisco, October 2010.

[1] National Association for Sport and Physical Education 2002
[2] United States Department of Health and Human Services and United States Department of Agriculture 2005
[3] American Academy of Pediatrics (Council on Sports Medicine and Fitness and Council on School Health 2006)
[4] United States Department of Health and Human Services 2008
[5] *Caring for Our Children*, 3d ed. (AAP, APHA, NRC 2011)
[6] Nutrition and Physical Activity Self-Assessment for Child Care (Benjamin et al. 2007); Baby Nutrition and Physical Activity Self Assessment for Child Care (Benjamin Neelon et al. 2012)

day. One finding is that there is wide variation in how physically active children are from one facility to another. Also, teachers tend to overestimate the amount of physical activity children in their care are doing.

All children need active play opportunities. Withholding active play from children who exhibit challenging behavior is not effective. These children need to spend their emotional energy in an acceptable way until they can restore their self-control and rejoin the group. Children who are exhibiting challenging behavior may benefit from brief periods (one to two minutes) of structured physical activity.

Assessment of children's nutrition and physical activity

To help improve young children's nutrition and increase their physical activity, the Centers for Disease Control and Prevention (CDC) sponsored research that led to the development of valid, reliable training and tools that educators can use to improve this aspect of their programs. The intervention developed by the University of North Carolina at Chapel Hill is called the Nutrition and Physical Activity Self-Assessment for Child Care (NAP SACC). To access the NAP SACC Training Module and associated tools, go to **www.center-TRT.org** and look under Training. To access these materials, you must register on the website. Many of the materials are written in both English and Spanish. Using the NAP SACC tool is an excellent way to identify and remedy gaps in a program's nutrition and physical activity practices.

Playing outdoors

Outdoor time is essential to provide children opportunities for gross motor activities, as well as cognitive and social experiences that differ from those that usually take place indoors. In addition to essential daily physical activity for physical fitness, children can learn about nature and the larger world by being outdoors. Even if the outdoor experience is limited to a fenced terrace, children learn about variations in natural light from day to day and can see more of the world around them than they can view from their usual play areas indoors. Both the children and teachers benefit from a change in environment during the day.

Inclement weather

While indoor physical activity is acceptable when the weather is extreme, outdoor activities—even for brief periods—are preferable. Playing outdoors in cold or wet weather does not increase the risk of illness or make a cold worse, so only severe weather that poses a significant health risk should preclude outdoor play. The guideline for limiting outdoor play because of cold weather is a windchill factor at or below -15° F. In hot weather, children should go outside for play unless the heat index is at or above 90° F. These conditions are identified by the National Weather Service, which also issues warnings about other weather hazards, such as high wind conditions or unhealthy air quality. Children should wear or bring appropriate clothing to the facility so they can go out in the rain or in cold weather.

Experiencing inclement weather provides valuable opportunities to learn about the environment. Playing outdoors may decrease the risk of illness by allowing children to breathe fresh air that has fewer germs in it, and by giving staff members the opportunity to ventilate indoor spaces by opening windows or allowing the air to circulate when people are not in the room. If outdoor playtimes must be shortened because of adverse weather conditions, or because of the need to

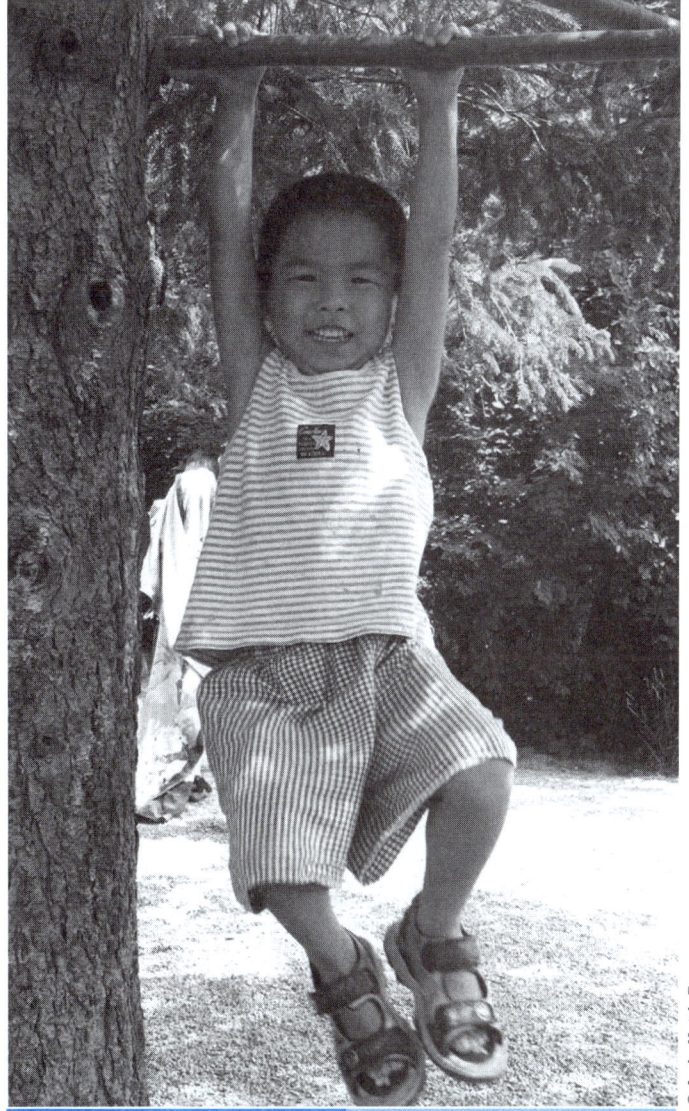

share safe outdoor play space, children should still play outdoors for some time. However it is accomplished, the total amount of exercise time for each age group should meet the requirements for the standard.

Protection from injuries from sun exposure, cold weather, and other environmental hazards

Children need protection from the sun all year, not just when the weather is warm, so play areas should have shade available. In addition, children should wear sun-protective clothing and, if older than 6 months of age, have sunscreen applied to exposed skin at least 15–30 minutes before being in the sun *in all seasons*. Staff members in programs that operate for more than two hours must apply sunscreen before the children go outside in the sun, as any applied at home will no longer be sufficient after two hours. Sunscreen should provide protection from radiation in the UVA and UVB spectrum and have an SPF of 15 to 30. With permission from parents, teachers can apply sunscreen to the children from a bulk supply. Only children who cannot use the bulk product because of a reaction to the product or parent preference need to have their own sunscreen. Alternatively, parents may provide sun-protective clothing that completely covers their children's skin. Children should wear shatter-resistant sunglasses with at least 99 percent UV protection and have shaded areas where they can play out of direct sunlight. For more details about sun protection, see *Caring for Our Children* Standard 3.4.5.1.

Teachers should have clean hands when applying sunscreen to children. If they have performed hand hygiene at the times required in *Caring for Our Children* Standard 3.2.2.1, separate hand hygiene isn't necessary before starting to apply sunscreen. Teachers do not need to wear gloves or practice hand hygiene between applying sunscreen to children unless either they or the child has open sores. Although sun exposure assists the skin in making vitamin D, extensive sun exposure is unnecessary for this process. If sufficient vitamin D is a concern, ask the child's health professional to prescribe supplements rather than put the child at risk of skin damage from the sun.

On hot days, children should have extra water available to drink. Infants who drink human (breast) milk in a bottle can be given additional human milk when it is very warm.

In cold weather, children should wear dry, layered clothing. Since children have more surface area relative to their body weight than adults, they lose heat from their extremities more quickly. Check children's extremities for normal color and warmth at least every 15 minutes when children are outdoors in cold weather.

Children will be warm enough, even in rain or snow, if they are properly clothed (with boots, gloves, hats, etc.) and participate in moderate to vigorous play.

The standards in *Caring for Our Children* address the importance of being aware of environmental hazards in outdoor play areas. These include air, soil, and water contamination; accumulations of water or ice on walkways and riding toy and paved surfaces; places where children could fall more than 36 inches in height; electrical hazards; pest infestations; areas treated with toxic chemicals; poisonous plants; pressure-treated wood containing arsenic; lead in the soil; and other hazards. (See the applicable standards in Sections 5.1 and 5.2 of *Caring for Our Children,* as well as Standard 5.7.0.2.) Children need to be observed closely when playing in dirt or soil to ensure that they do not put their hands in their mouth. Play areas should be secure against intruding animals or people and should not have openings that allow a child to leave the supervised area. Preventing access by animals that carry disease in their urine or feces or by insects requires measures that control the unwanted pests yet are the least harmful to humans. (See Integrated Pest Management in *Caring for Our Children* Standards 5.2.8.1 and 5.2.8.2 and Chapters 5 and 10 in this manual.) Play areas should be located away from heavy traffic and public access areas because of both air quality concerns and the possibility of intrusion of a threatening individual or a vehicle in an accident situation.

Teachers' views of active play

Teachers generally know about the potential benefits physical activity has for children. (Some of these are benefits for teachers, too.) Kristen Copeland conducted focus groups with early education teachers in Cincinnati, Ohio, between 2006 and 2008, to discuss physical activity. The teachers identified the following benefits for children. Physical activity

- Prevents obesity
- Builds lifetime healthy habits
- Enables mastery of gross motor skills (e.g., throwing and catching a ball)
- Develops self-confidence as children's competence increases
- Improves peer relationships during active play
- Is followed by better ability to be calm, pay attention, concentrate, and learn
- Is associated with better naps

Teachers also identified benefits of time spent outdoors. This time

- Provides more room to run

- Provides time away from germs that concentrate in indoor environments, so children are less likely to get sick
- Promotes better moods
- Increases creativity and expression
- Teaches pre-math concepts of distance and time; vocabulary about weather, animals, and plants; and cause and effect
- Provides opportunities to practice taking turns on the playground equipment
- Provides opportunities to learn about community workers, such as the mail carrier or sanitation workers
- Exposes skin to sunshine to make vitamin D (limited to avoid damage to the skin from UV rays)

However, the early education teachers in the study also described what they viewed as drawbacks of physical activity. Some of these concerns echoed the misconception frequently voiced by parents about susceptibility to illness from going outside in cold or wet weather. Parents and some teachers worried that children could get hurt or dirty while playing outdoors. The teachers pointed out that some parents deliberately interfere with their children's ability to play outdoors by sending them in inappropriate clothing for play in cold or wet weather. Some teachers said they do not like being outside themselves because of weather and insects or because of their concerns about their own weight and fitness. Some complained that it takes too much time and work to dress the children, put on sunscreen, and take out play equipment. Many teachers did not think about using the outdoors as an extension of the classroom, a setting in which valuable learning can take place. Some teachers identified the problem of investing in fancy and costly climbers that look good to adults but do not interest the children for long.

Encouraging and modeling physical activity

For many young children, their best opportunity for exercise may be while they are in a group care setting. However, research suggests that children in group care settings spend very little time in moderate or vigorous activity. It also shows that children are more active when they are outdoors and when adults prompt them to be active (Copeland et al. 2012; see also the list of references for *Caring for Our Children* Standard 3.1.3.1).

The active play area should have enough space for children to move freely without running into one another. At all times, children need close supervision while they are playing on equipment intended to foster moderate to vigorous activity. This allows teachers to stop mishaps, promote children's participation in active play, and participate themselves in such play.

Some adults have inhibitions about doing moderate to vigorous activity themselves when they are outdoors with children. Peer support may help them overcome this. For example, more than one teacher could be involved in an activity. Generally, adults are comfortable being purposely involved in children's physical activities if they have planned games with a learning objective. So that teachers actively supervise and participate in gross motor activities, playgrounds should not have places for adults to sit during active play time.

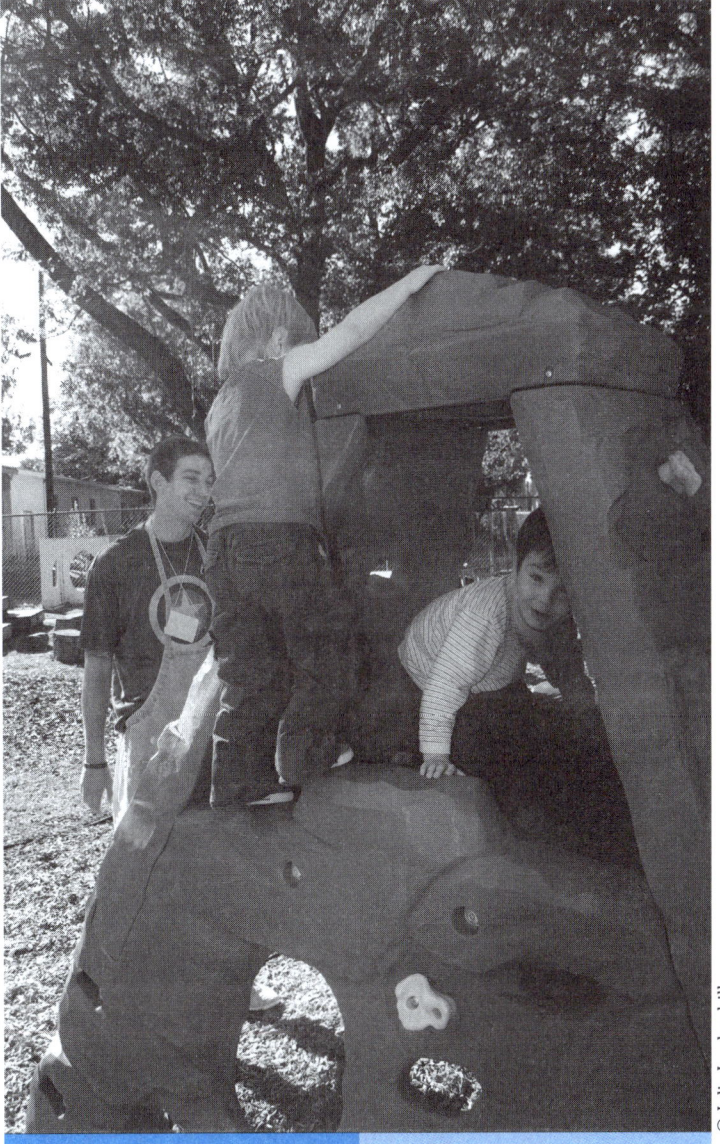

Standard 3.1.3.4 in *Caring for Our Children* states

Caregivers/teachers should promote children's active play, and participate in children's active games at times when they can safely do so. Caregivers/teachers should

a) Lead structured activities to promote children's activities two or more times per day

b) Wear clothing and footwear that permits easy and safe movement

c) Not sit during active play

d) Provide prompts for children to be active (e.g., "good throw")

e) Encourage children's physical activities that are appropriate and safe in the setting (e.g., do not prohibit running on the playground when it is safe to run)

f) Have orientation and annual training opportunities to learn about age-appropriate gross motor activities and games that promote children's physical activity

g) Limit screen time (TV, DVD, computer, etc.), except for 1) school-age children completing homework assignments and 2) children with special health care needs who require and consistently use assistive and adaptive computer technology

Physical activity for children with asthma

Some children with asthma require special accommodations to fully participate in active play. For some, cold air triggers their wheezing, or they wheeze when pollen levels are high. Some may have their symptoms triggered by hot temperatures or physical activity. Solutions are available that usually reduce these problems. For example, during cold weather, children whose asthma is triggered by cold air can wear a scarf to cover their nose and mouth. The child's health care provider may be able to adjust the child's medication to control the asthma or allergy symptoms. Medication used before exercise can reduce the risk of symptoms for children whose asthma would worsen otherwise. During the winter, when indoor allergens may trigger asthma symptoms, properly circulating and cleaning the air may reduce symptoms. Each child with asthma should have a special care plan, as should every child who needs care that differs from that required by a typical child. (For more on special care plans, see Chapter 12.)

Structured physical activities

Usually, preschool children are vigorously active in short bursts of 15–30 seconds and do not sustain vigorous activity for longer than 5–10 minutes at a time. During active play time, if children start to become less active, intersperse short periods (5 minutes or so) of structured activity that allows them to be less active with 10–15 minutes of unstructured gross motor play so they are more likely to be vigorously active during their unstructured time. Then the children are more likely to accumulate the time they should spend in vigorous activity. Structured movement and learning activities can be conducted outdoors or indoors, and they can include playing games such as "Simon Says" or "Mother, May I," moving to music such as "I'm Gonna Shake My Wiggles Out," pretending to move like different kinds of animals, having relay races, and taking community walks. Sources of recommendations differ somewhat for time and type of physical activity children should have. These differences are related to variation in the process of developing guidelines and do not represent significant disagreements among the experts. Figure 6.1 compares recommendations from different expert sources for the appropriate amount of time for unstructured, structured, and sedentary activities for different age groups.

In addition to NAP SACC, other resources for nutrition and physical activity ideas and materials include the following, some of which are free:

- Nemours Health and Prevention Services guide at **www.nemours.org** (search for "Best Practices for Physical Activity: A Guide," then select **paguidelines.pdf**)
- Color Me Healthy Teacher's Guide with 12 circle-time lessons, posters, recipes, activity ideas, and music at **www.colormehealthy.com**
- I Am Moving, I Am Learning, a program developed for implementation and national roll-out in Head Start (find details and materials on Head Start's website, **http://eclkc.ohs.acf.hhs.gov**, or by searching the internet for "I Am Moving, I Am Learning")

Suggested activities

- Plan a week of physical activities for a specific age group, identifying the time, equipment, and learning objectives for each.
- Observe a group of children in an early care and education setting for a day, noting the amount of time and type of physical activity for the children in the group (e.g., structured/unstructured, moderate/vigorous). Compare your observations with the recommendations in Figure 6.1. Did the observed practices meet the guidelines? How could the practices be improved?

7

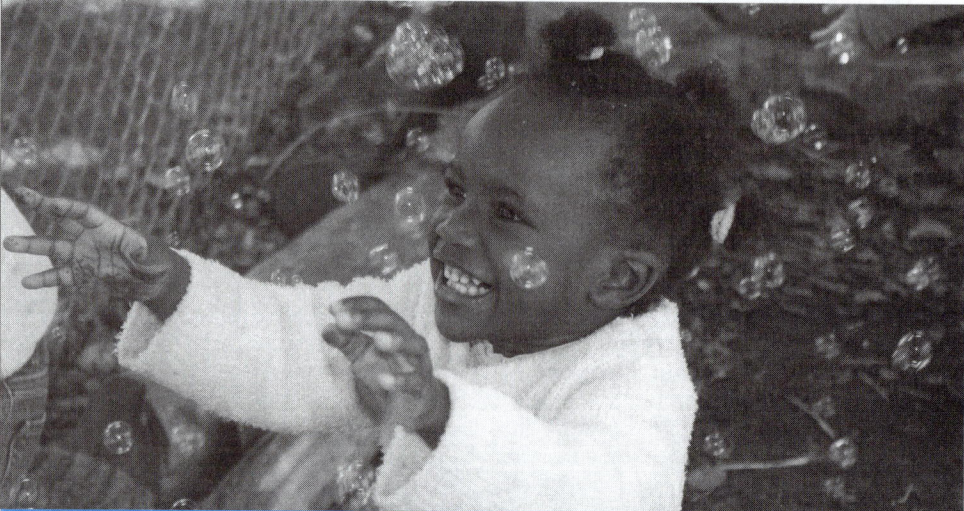

Promoting Health through Oral Health, Mental Health, and Health Education

MAJOR CONCEPTS

- Oral health contributes to good nutrition and speech, a positive self-image, and a sense of well-being.

- Teachers should teach oral health habits as part of the curriculum, including practicing routine oral hygiene activities. For children 3 years of age and older, give developmentally appropriate information about plaque, the process of dental decay, dietary influences on the teeth, and the benefits of routinely scheduled dental care.

- Mental health is monitored through child behaviors viewed in the context of child care arrangements, families, and communities, and its promotion is the cornerstone of child development. Mental health services support children's emotional, cognitive, and social development.

- Early education programs should not suspend or limit services provided to a child or family on the basis of challenging behaviors unless: 1) continued care in the program jeopardizes the physical safety of the child and other children as assessed by a qualified mental health consultant; 2) all supports recommended by that consultant to provide a physically safe environment have been exhausted, or the family is unwilling to participate in mental health consultation provided or arranged by the program; or 3) continued placement in the program does not meet the needs of the child as agreed by the staff and family, *and* a different program that can better meet those needs can immediately serve the child.

- Health education is taught daily through teachable moments, modeling of healthy and safe behavior, and planned activities for staff members, parents, and children. It should address current concepts of nutritional, physical, oral, and mental (cognitive, emotional, and social) health.

- Use credentialed, credible sources for health information to avoid spreading misinformation.

Children depend on adults for protection from harm and for health promotion. Infection and physical injury are commonly recognized as the types of harm from which young children need the most protection. Other health problems, including social-emotional difficulties, may be prevented or best managed when corrective actions are likely to be most effective, early in a child's life.

The roots of lifetime healthy behaviors and emotional resiliency are planted in the early years. Early childhood educators have unique opportunities to include positive experiences for children on a day-to-day basis. In addition, through early identification of health problems and sharing sources of information and services with families, teachers can help families identify and initiate solutions. Nutrition, physical activity, and safety are areas of great importance for lifelong, overall health and were discussed in previous chapters. This chapter addresses three other areas that have a powerful influence on child health: oral health, mental health, and health education.

Oral health

The type of oral hygiene and dental care children receive, along with diet and heredity, determines their oral health throughout life. Child care programs can help prevent dental disease by incorporating the following practices:

- Serve nutritious food, limiting sugary and sticky foods.
- To prevent the spread of germs that cause dental decay, adults should not place a child's pacifier in their own mouths to clean or moisten it or mouth anything that goes in the child's mouth.
- Ensure that children get the right amount (and not too much) of fluoride through an appropriate means (in drinking water, rinses, toothpastes, professionally applied tooth varnish, tablets, or drops).
- Emphasize good oral health care by having children and staff members brush their teeth.
- Identify children with evident dental problems and refer them to oral health professionals.

Healthy foods for teeth

High-sugar foods and frequent eating are clearly linked to tooth decay. Help children preserve their teeth by avoiding or limiting sweet drinks, candy, jelly, jam, cake, cookies, sugared gelatin, and sweetened, canned fruit. Fresh fruit and vegetables make great snack and dessert alternatives.

Mealtimes in group programs can promote oral health. Avoid grazing as a style of eating for children and for adults whom children observe in child care. Infants should be fed on demand, but mealtimes for older children should be at clearly defined intervals. Young children need frequent meals and snacks, most of which include some sugar or some food that saliva breaks down to release some sugar. When a meal or snack is over, the food should be put away until the next planned eating time. Here are some important facts about sugar and teeth:

- Natural sugars (such as maple syrup and honey) are just as harmful to teeth as refined sugar.
- Sticky sweets (such as caramel) are particularly harmful because they remain on the teeth longer than other sweets.
- Eating a sweet all at once is better than eating one over a period of time (e.g., a lollipop) or eating sweets often (e.g., mints or hard candies throughout the day).
- Sweet sticky fruits, such as raisins and dates, should be eaten with a meal so that the other foods help remove the sticky fruits from the surfaces of the teeth.
- Because teeth are attacked by the decay process each time food is put in the mouth, frequent eating or snacking can cause problems.
- Toothbrushing or rinsing with water after eating reduces the time teeth are exposed to the decay process.
- Infants should not be put to bed with a bottle. Milk, formula, sweetened liquids, and fruit juices all contain sugars. Prolonged feeding can result in serious decay, called nursing bottle mouth or baby bottle tooth decay. (Putting babies to bed or in a lying down position with a bottle also increases the risk of ear infection and choking.)
- Rewarding good behavior with candy or other sweets teaches children to reward themselves with sugary foods.

Fluoride

Fluoridation of public water supplies is the single most effective method to prevent tooth decay. When children have fluoride in their drinking water, or fluoride supplements from birth, tooth decay can be reduced by about 50 percent. Know whether your community fluoridates its water and whether the children in your care drink this fluoridated water. Certain types of home water filters remove fluoride; others do not. Many families buy bottled water in the false belief that it is better than their community water source. (Because the bottled water industry is unregulated, the safety and content of any particular container of bottled water is unknown.)

Children also may be consuming other sources of fluoride. Some commercially prepared foods and beverages are made with fluoridated ingredients, a fact usually not indicated on the label. Consequently, it is hard to know whether children who frequently consume commercially prepared or packaged foods (rather than those prepared from fresh ingredients) are receiving significant amounts of fluoride.

Most toothpaste now has fluoride. Adults should monitor the amount of toothpaste that children use. Infants should not use toothpaste. A thin smear of toothpaste no bigger than a grain of rice on the toothbrush, or none at all, is about right for toddlers; a dab the size of a small pea is the right amount for preschool-age children. Excess ingestion of fluoride can lead to staining of the teeth, called fluorosis. While this staining does not make teeth weak, it can be unattractive. Depending on their assessment of a child's individual situation, dentists may prescribe fluoride drops or tablets, or paint the teeth with a fluoride varnish.

Brushing teeth

Very young children can learn good oral hygiene habits that will last into adulthood. Routine brushing at least once in the group care program after a meal or snack has the double benefit of cleaning teeth *and* establishing a good habit. If organized well and performed as a group activity as described below, brushing probably will not take more than five minutes. Few families provide adult-assisted brushing at home at least twice a day. Each child should brush for a total of two minutes while at the program. Participating in this tooth hygiene activity with the group will not harm those who do brush twice a day with adult supervision at home as long as they do not use toothpaste with flouride for their third brushing. CFOC standard 3.1.5.1 allows these children to be exempted from toothbrushing during child care to avoid excess fluoride intake. However, it is difficult to know which children actually brush their teeth twice a day at home, and it is awkward to leave a child out of this important health education lesson.

Here are some points to remember:

- Each child must have his or her own personally labeled, age-appropriate toothbrush. It must *never* be shared.

- A sink is not necessary for toothbrushing. In fact, using a sink for a group of children is very difficult. Instead, give each child a cup of water to wet the toothbrush, take a mouthful of water to swish to rinse any loose food particles off the teeth, and then spit the swished mouthful back into the cup.

- The teacher puts the right amount of fluoride toothpaste on the edge of each child's cup. Occasional swallowing of these small amounts of fluoride toothpaste is not harmful. The child should spit out again

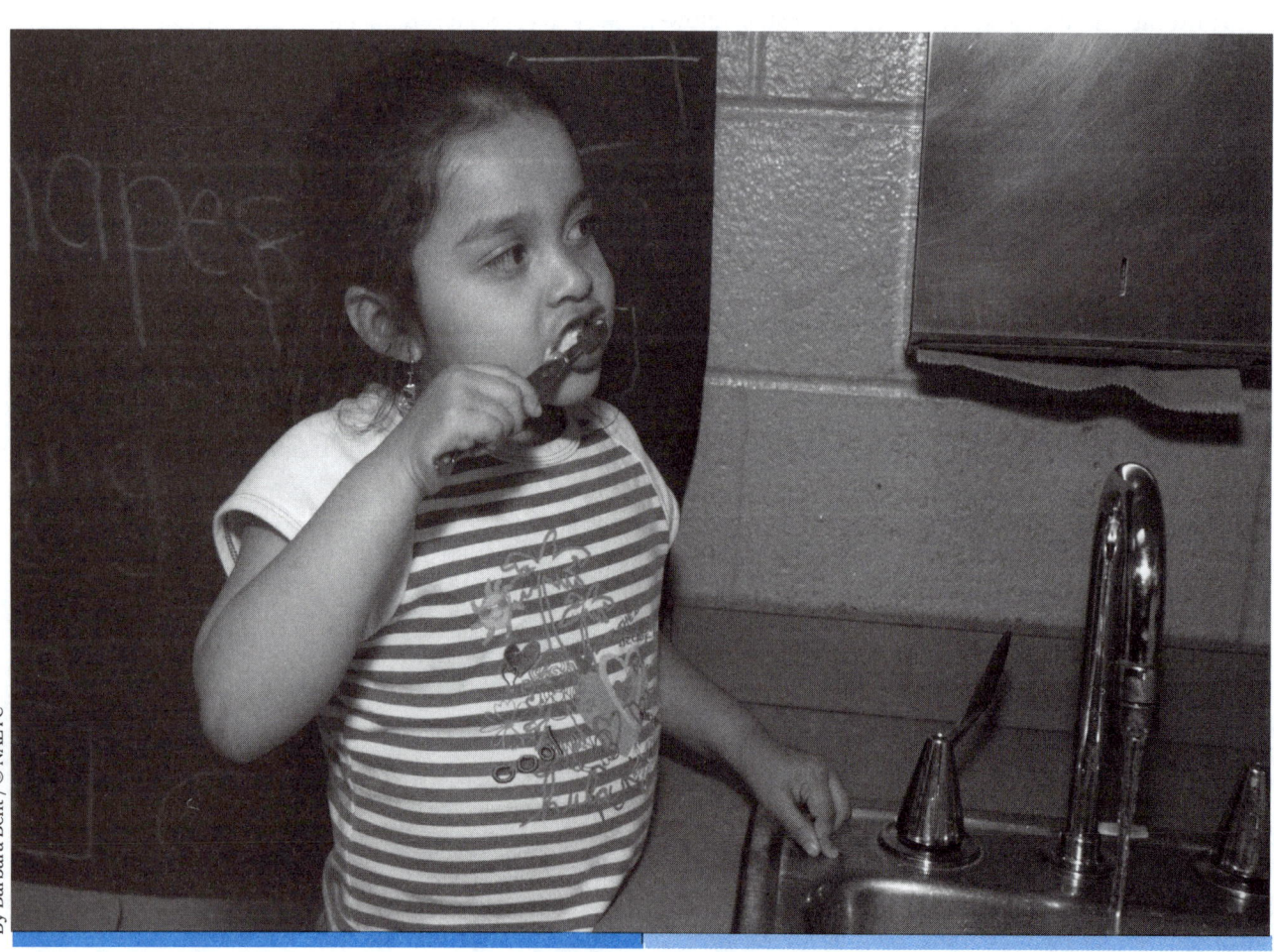

By Barbara Bent / © NAEYC

after brushing, but not rinse again. The child's saliva does the necessary rinsing at this point.

- Until around 6 years of age, children need adult assistance or close supervision to do a good job of brushing. If the teacher actually brushes the child's teeth, then the teacher must practice hand hygiene before and after the brushing. Gloves are needed only if a child has bleeding gums.

- Teachers should offer children water to rinse their teeth after snacks and meals when toothbrushing is not possible.

- Wiping the teeth and gums of an infant who has teeth or using a soft brush to clean the infant's mouth and teeth after feeding removes milk left in the mouth and reduces buildup of decay-causing plaque.

- Store toothbrushes with the bristles end up to allow the bristles to air-dry. The bristles should not have contact with any surface, and the brush should not drip on another toothbrush. Label and disinfect racks and devices used to hold toothbrushes as needed. Children can store their own brush in an individually labeled cup instead of in a rack.

- Many dentists and hygienists recommend a small toothbrush with soft, rounded, nylon bristles. The type should be determined by whatever is easiest for the child to brush every tooth. (At home, parents might invest in an inexpensive electric toothbrush to get the job done better and faster than a young child can manage.) When the bristles become bent, the brush should be replaced. Routinely replace brushes about every three to four months.

- Teachers should brush their own teeth with the children and supervise how the children do this task. When adults model good toothbrushing, children learn the importance of this lifetime habit. Because of limited motor skills, some children may need an adult's help to reach all their teeth. Model proper brushing technique, but don't worry if children do not have the skill to do it well. Use a circular scrubbing motion to cover the teeth from the gums upward over every biting edge—from all directions and on all surfaces. This technique is easy and effective. Scrub back and forth on the chewing surfaces after brushing the surfaces closest to the tongue and those closest to the cheek. Finish by brushing the tongue. You can make up chants and songs to reinforce this pattern of toothbrushing. Remember, the most effective teaching technique is to actually brush with the children.

Oral health education

Children and families must understand the importance of good oral health. Children can learn effectively through integration of oral education activities with their regular routines. Children 3 years of age and older can learn about plaque and the process of dental decay—how sticky and sweet foods and sugary beverages feed the germs that damage teeth, making holes (cavities) in them. Family education can involve posters, newsletter articles, parent handouts about oral health activities the children are doing, or videos. Parents should be encouraged to ask their child's health provider about the correct amount of fluoride for their child, the right way to provide it, and whether/when their child needs dental sealants or fluoride varnish. Brochures describing particular problems, conditions, or resources are frequently available from state or local health departments and local dentists. Many dentists or hygienists are willing to come to child care programs to teach children about oral health and oral health examinations. A field trip to a dentist who enjoys working with young children can be a wonderful introduction to regular dental care.

Dental care

Encourage families to follow recommended oral health routines and get regular dental care. Taking their children for preventive dental care is essential. Some families have dental health insurance, but many do not. Even those with insurance may have coverage for only a portion of treatment services, not for preventive care. Remind parents that painful and expensive dental repair experiences can be avoided with good preventive care. Offer the names of children's dentists (pediatric dentists) or family dentists who work regularly with young children. Some communities have dental health clinics, dental school clinics, and community health centers that provide pediatric dental care. Some children's hospitals provide emergency dental care.

A child's first visit to the dentist for preventive services should occur within six months after the first tooth appears, or by 1 year of age. Pediatric dentists want to examine the child's mouth and provide advice about oral health to families as soon as the first tooth erupts. If there are no pediatric dentists in the community and the general dentists are not prepared to examine and care for young children, encourage families to ask their pediatrician to inspect their child's teeth for signs of decay, need for sealants, and any alignment problems. With so much to do in such a short well-care visit in a pediatric office, the parent's interest sets the priority for issues that will be addressed.

By age 3, most children have all 20 of their primary (baby) teeth showing for an oral health professional to check. Most children need little treatment at this stage, so the dentist can form a friendly and relaxed relationship with a child. Some, however, may be at high risk for dental caries (cavities) and should have fluoride varnish applied to their teeth every three months or so. The dentist will look for early signs of future problems, such

> **Figure 7.1.**
>
> ## Dental Referral Criteria
>
> Listed below are some observations you can make about young children's oral health. If you answer *no* to any of the questions, you should recommend that the family take the child to a dentist.
>
> **Soft Tissues (Tongue, Lips, Cheeks, Gums)**
> - Can the child stick the tongue tip completely out of his mouth?
> - Can the child swallow with the teeth together (without the tongue pushing through)?
> - Are the upper and lower lip the same size?
> - Is there a clear distinction between the lip and the skin of the face?
> - Is the color inside the cheeks even throughout?
> - Are all gum tissues the same color? Are gums free of pimples and/or swelling?
>
> **Hard Tissues (Teeth)**
>
> *Number*
> - Does the child have at least one or two teeth by age 1? At least 12 by age 2?
> - Are the same number of teeth on either side of the middle of the jaw?
> - Are teeth on either side the same shape?
>
> *Bite*
> - When the child closes her mouth, do the top teeth bite over the bottom teeth? Do the back teeth meet?
> - Do all the teeth come in contact when the jaw is closed?
> - Are the teeth spaced out, not crowded?
>
> *Color*
> - Are the teeth milky white? Are they all an even color?
> - Do any stains and colors come off easily with a toothbrush?
> - Are the teeth free of any chalky white or dark spots, or pits on the teeth?
>
> *Condition*
> - Is the mouth free of any broken or unusually shaped teeth?
> - Are all the teeth formed without deep valleys that could trap food?
>
> **Oral Hygiene**
> - Are the teeth clean?
> - Does the mouth have a clean, sweet odor?

as overcrowding or poor dental hygiene. In addition to preventive care, certain observations that teachers can make should lead to a visit to a pediatric dentist. (See Figure 7.1.)

Help families make a dental visit an appealing new experience. A good first trip will help mold children's feelings for many years. Explain to children that the dentist and the dental hygienist are friendly helpers who will help keep their teeth and mouth healthy. Talk about the visit in a positive, matter-of-fact way as you would any new experience. Avoid statements that suggest the visit may be unpleasant, such as "It won't hurt." If you are fearful about dental visits, do not pass on the fear to the children. Most adult fears come from treatment for problems that could have been prevented by routine dental care and good personal oral health habits in childhood.

Common dental problems

- *Broken tooth.* Tell the family about the broken tooth and make sure a dentist is contacted immediately. If a permanent tooth is broken and not cared for in a very short time, it can be lost. Even if a tooth appears to be hanging by a thread, don't pull it out. Get in touch with the dentist right away. Broken baby teeth may require treatment to prevent development of a gum infection.

- *Knocked-out tooth.* Contact the family and dental provider immediately and *save the tooth*. Examination of a baby tooth may reveal a retained fragment. A permanent tooth sometimes can be replanted. If the tooth is a permanent tooth, try to put the tooth back into the socket right away, and have the child bite on a piece of cloth to hold it in place. If the tooth has a lot of dirt on it, hold it by the chewing surface and gently swish in a cup of water or milk, then either put it back in the socket or into a cup of milk for transport to the dentist. (Do not put a tooth that you know is a primary [baby] tooth back in the socket.) Rush the child and the tooth to the dentist (within 30 minutes if possible). The sooner the child sees the dentist, the better the chance of a good outcome. The first permanent teeth usually erupt at around 5–6 years of age. A permanent tooth will have long roots. A baby tooth will have very short roots. If you are unsure whether the tooth is a baby tooth or a permanent tooth, put it back into the socket so that if it is a permanent tooth, it has the best chance of being saved. The dentist will determine what kind of tooth was knocked out.

- *Toothache or swelling, redness, or bleeding of the gums.* Ask the parent to call the dentist at once. The dentist can find the cause of the toothache or soft tissue irritation and reduce the pain. When a child is in extreme pain, you can use the following temporary emergency measures. If a cavity can be seen in the tooth that aches, flush out any food particles with warm water. Parents can give the child acetaminophen for temporary pain relief and should arrange a dental appointment immediately.

- *Thumb, finger, or pacifier sucking.* Sucking the thumb, fingers, or a pacifier often gives an infant a feeling of pleasure and security. During the first several years, it should cause no concern. However, if the child continues this habit beyond the age of 5, or when permanent teeth begin coming in, it can affect the position of the incoming teeth and the shape of the jaws. The pressures of sucking may push the teeth out and narrow the dental arches. Eventually orthodontic care may be needed. Work with the parents and their child's pediatrician or dentist to find a caring way to help the child eliminate this habit.

- *Baby bottle tooth decay.* Baby bottle tooth decay is a condition that can destroy the teeth. It is caused by frequent and lengthy exposure to liquids containing sugars (milk, formula, fruit juice, and other sweetened liquids). The teeth most likely to be damaged are the upper front teeth, but others also may be affected. The tongue lies over the lower teeth and protects them more than the upper teeth from exposure to the sugary liquids.

- *Bleeding around a tooth after an injury.* Apply ice to the area as soon as possible and for as long as possible to minimize bleeding into the tooth and discoloration. Have the child suck on a Popsicle or hold an ice cube with a clean cloth on a fresh injury. Although the sugar content in a Popsicle makes it a less healthful food, in an injury situation, applying cold to the area of the injury is a priority. The family should consult a dentist to be sure the tooth or teeth do not need treatment.

Mental health

Sound child development practice fosters good mental health. Unlike physical health needs, mental health cannot be achieved by focusing on the child alone. The child is a part of a family, a child care group, and a community. All of these entities affect the child's mental health. Teachers often notice or call attention to behaviors that are of concern before parents do; they have the opportunity to compare a child's behavior with that of typically developing peers. Parents are the reporters to the child's health care provider about behaviors of concern. So unless the teacher brings the behavior symptoms to the attention of the family and asks the family to share the teacher's observations with the child's health care provider, the health care provider may not learn about the possible concerns.

Why do children develop challenging behavior?

Sometimes healthy, well-adjusted children experience environmental stress, which leads to challenging behavior. When you are aware of these stresses, monitor the child closely and note any changes in mood or behavior. Children's responses to stress vary greatly, some mild, some severe. High-quality, consistent, and supportive relationships with family and teachers may lessen the effects of stress.

Sometimes children exhibit challenging behavior for no apparent reason. These behaviors can range from mild to severe. As you seek to better understand and handle these behaviors, do not assume that the family is the root of them. Consider all possibilities. The child may be reacting to peer relationships in the group care setting, having upsetting interactions with children or adults in the child's neighborhood, or being troubled by viewing the news or a violent TV show. Listen to what the child says while playing. Look at the child's artwork and listen to what the child says when you say, "Please tell me about it." Often children reveal the cause of their distress through such activities.

Stressful situations that call for closer monitoring of child behavior

- *Changes in the family or teacher.* If a loved one becomes ill, is hospitalized, or dies, or if parents separate or divorce, the child loses physical contact and emotional support. When parents have problems at work or lose their job, both children and adults may feel stress. When a family moves, children miss their old home and friends or may experience stress from adapting to a new culture and language. Even seemingly positive changes can be stressful for children. For example, new siblings—whether through birth, adoption, or blending of families—increase a child's number of playmates but can also be stressful.

- *Problems in family relationships.* Conflict between parent figures or between parent and child are very stressful. Conflict often accompanies problems of communication. Children can become victims of *maltreatment*, or abuse. This maltreatment can be physical, sexual, emotional, or psychological. The child may feel completely rejected or repeatedly terrified. (For more information about child maltreatment, see Chapter 13.)

- *Inadequate care.* Some parents do not adequately supervise a child, respond to his needs, or place reasonable limits on behavior. They may be harsh, too permissive, or inconsistent. Others may overprotect their children and not let them do what other children are doing at that age.

- *Problems of individual family members.* When parents have serious illnesses, the conditions may affect their ability to care for and nurture their children. Similarly, mental health problems or alcohol or drug abuse can impair the competence of adults. A sibling's physical or mental health issues affect the parents and children. When parents have difficulty with reading or do not speak English well enough to be understood, their children may feel stress in situations where the parent cannot do what is expected of them.

- *Community conditions.* Sometimes the source of stress is one or more conditions in the community. Too many families face poverty. Some experience social discrimination or isolation. Housing or schools may not be adequate. There may be considerable violence on the streets or fear of violence. In an unsafe neighborhood, some families do not allow their children to go outside to play. The children cannot interact with peers and get sufficient physical activity. Children become particularly distressed if they witness violence. When a child views violence, the result can be an uncomfortable lifetime memory of the event. The associated stress of living in poverty increases the risk of behavioral and emotional problems.

Common behavioral or emotional problems in young children

Children respond to environmental stress and challenge in different ways, depending on chronological age, developmental stage, and the child's own intrinsic vulnerability. Many children demonstrate challenging behaviors for hours or days at a time. The following behaviors and emotions are cause for serious concern when they occur over long periods of time or are extreme:

- *Extreme emotions and moods.* Children may cry often for no obvious reason. They may have quick changes of moods. They may become sad or withdrawn and refuse to play with other children or talk with adults. They may not seem to enjoy play, or their play may display extreme emotions.

- *Increased activity level and poor attention.* Some children are very active and disorganized. They may not be able to concentrate on games or stories.

- *Negative behavior.* Children may throw frequent temper tantrums or become aggressive, biting and hitting. Some are quick to anger; others remain calm even when anger might be expected. They may fight with their friends. They may refuse to do the things adults ask of them. They may strike out at teachers who are trying to comfort them. These behaviors are particularly of concern in children who are more than 3 years old.

- *Problems in eating, elimination, and sleep.* Some children refuse to eat; others eat too much. Some lose control of their bladder after toilet learning has occurred. Some children may want to sleep more than usual; others have difficulty relaxing for a nap or falling asleep at night. Sleep deprivation may add to other behavioral issues.

- *Problems with relationships.* Children may show dramatic changes in how they relate to others. They may become extremely distressed when a parent or teacher has to leave. This may make it very hard for parents to leave their children at the child care facility. Children may become clingy. They may become afraid of being alone. On the other hand, some children become indifferent. They may go to anyone, whether an adult they trust or a stranger. Some children avoid eye contact, stare, and refuse to let others help them. They may isolate themselves from their friends and teachers.

- *Developmental problems.* Children may not achieve developmental landmarks typically acquired by their age, or they may lose developmental skills they previously mastered. For example, a child who has been using the toilet may need to go back to diapers, a child who can speak in sentences reverts to single words, a child able to feed herself independently suddenly demands adult help, or a child who played independently or with other children is not able to play alone or socialize.

- *Physical aggression.* Many children go through a period in which they bite or are bitten by other children. Some hit other children. Teachers must be ready to handle and prevent these unacceptable behaviors, and help the child find other ways to deal with what is causing them.

What parents and teachers can do

First, it is essential to understand the way children are expected to behave in each stage of development. For an excellent review of these expectations and what to do when children deviate from them, use the tutorial called "Recognizing and Supporting the Social Emotional Health of Young Children Birth to Age 5" on the website of the Center for Early Childhood Mental Health Consultation (**www.ecmhc.org**). This center was created with funds from the federal Office of Head Start. Its website is richly populated with observation checklists for groups of children and for individual children that teachers can use to record their observations. When reviewed in retrospect, such records of observations may reveal patterns that suggest what is causing the behaviors of concern and what might be done about them. To help a child who is showing behavior that is not typical for either the specific child or the age of the child, a teacher can try several approaches, such as the following:

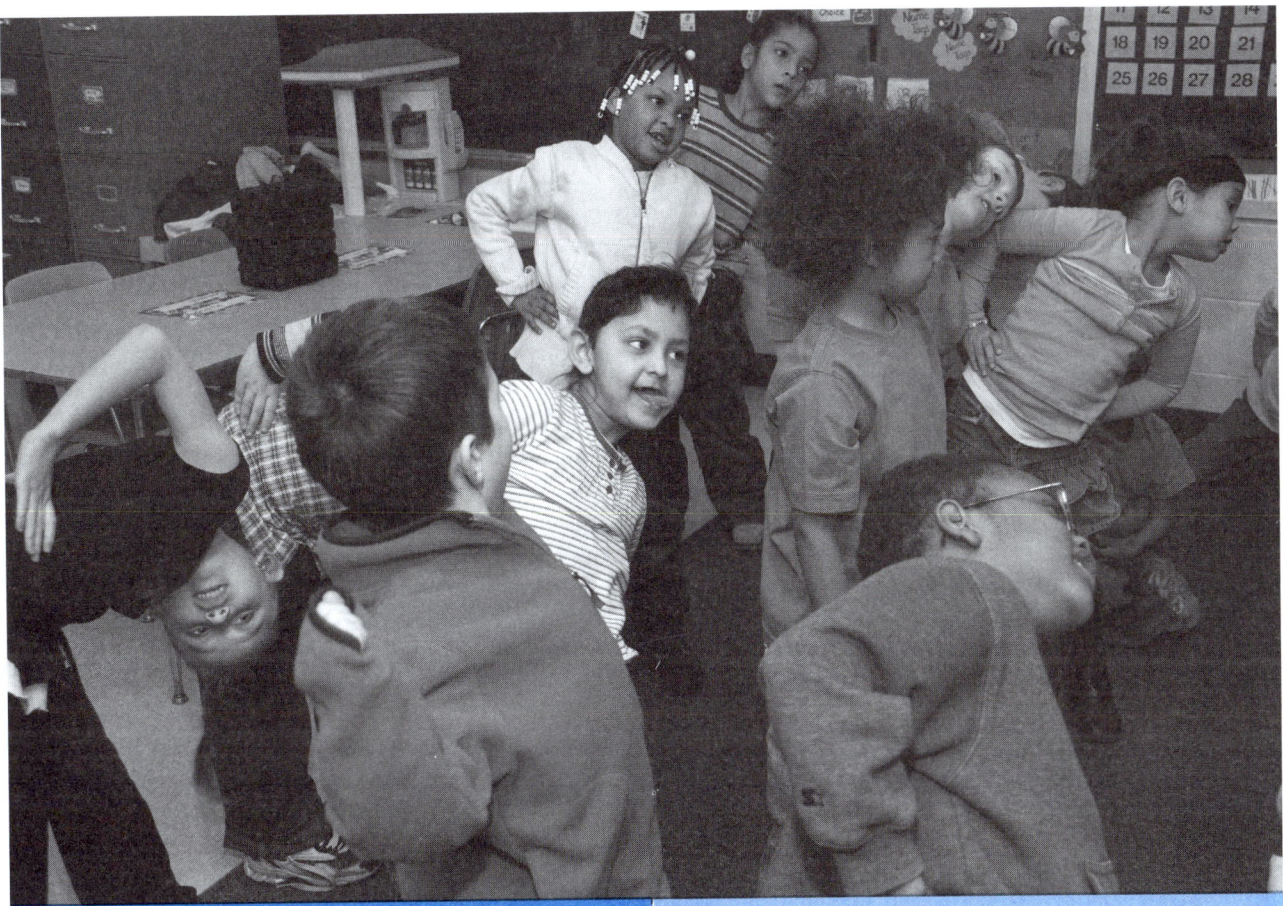

- *Observe the behaviors* and document what seems to precede them, what time of day they occur, and what seems to happen while and after they occur.
- *Discuss the issues with a co-worker, supervisor, or mental health consultant.* Arrange for someone else to observe the child who is not directly involved in providing care so that the observations can be more objective and complete.
- *Talk with the family* about the child's behavior early in the process. Do not wait until the child's behavior or moods seriously deteriorate. Begin with a description of the changes you are observing. You might say to a parent, "I notice that your child is crying a lot at school. It is difficult for me to comfort him." If you know why the child is experiencing anxiety or stress, you might say, "Since her father has been in the hospital, Sarah has been eating poorly at school. What do you see at home?"
- *Be supportive of the child.* Remain calm. Use supportive language: "I know you feel sad, but please try to eat a little." Provide comfort when possible. Comment on the child's behavior when she does something appropriate. Be gentle. It is easy to arouse children who are under stress.
- *Maintain the structure of the program.* Children may find routines and the usual schedules reassuring. Keep a predictable program. Do not insist that the child participate fully. Gently remind the child that she is welcome in the group.
- *Encourage communication.* Invite the child to talk about his feelings. Play is the language of young children. Sometimes a child will act out the stress in play or in an art activity. Use play to demonstrate some ways to handle stress. For example, use a doll to express in words sad or angry feelings. Provide positive reinforcement when the child's behavior is appropriate.
- *Limit dangerous or hurtful behaviors.* Provide clear messages that tantrums, biting and other forms of aggression, and negative behaviors are not acceptable. Be ready to handle this behavior. Give the child acceptable alternatives. Focus on comforting and giving first aid to the child who was hurt as the first step. For biting, remind the biter that biting hurts and is not how we use our teeth: "We bite food, not people." For other types of aggression tell the child, "Use your words to tell *[other child's name]* how you feel. It's not okay to hurt someone."

  Keep the two children separate for a while, allowing them back in the same space but not letting them play with or be close to each other. Shadow the child who showed hurtful behavior to prevent further aggressive acts. Support the child with suggestions for more socially appropriate ways to handle situations and feelings that led to the aggression. This will also help reduce the attention given to aggressive behavior. *Caring for Our Children* Standard 2.2.0.7 describes a step-by-step approach to handle physical aggression, including biting and hitting. These steps include who should be notified when such incidents occur, a list of possible reasons a child would bite or hit, and some strategies for extinguishing aggressive behavior. For example, use positive guidance and create environments that promote positive behavior and minimize the triggers for aggressive behavior.

- *Establish a comfort corner.* Designate a place in the classroom where children can go and spend time alone. A comfort corner is a place where children choose to go. There they can sit on bean bag chairs, pillows, or a carpeted floor. They can relax, reduce stress, and recover their composure. Stock the area with items such as soft balls to squeeze; soft music to listen to through headphones; stuffed animals to hold and talk to; a basket of paper and crayons; and any other items that help children calm down.

- *Reassure children that you will keep them safe and that their needs will be met.* Both the child with the challenging behavior and the others in the group need to know that you are working with all those involved to make the situation better.

- *Make structured observations of behavior.* Record both positive and negative behaviors using checklists such as those in the tool kits from the Center for Early Childhood Mental Health Consultation recommended earlier in the chapter. As soon as possible after a challenging behavior occurs, log when the behavior occurred, what happened before the incident, and what helped the child. You can summarize the data you collect using the Behavioral Data Collection Sheet in Figure A.10 in Appendix A.

The Center on the Social and Emotional Foundations for Early Learning (CSEFEL) (**http://csefel.vanderbilt.edu**) is another excellent resource for helpful strategies and materials. CSEFEL is funded by the Office of Head Start and the Office of Child Care to disseminate research and evidence-based practices to early childhood programs across the country. It focuses on promoting the social-emotional development and school readiness of young children birth to age 5. CSEFEL's Pyramid Model for Promoting Social and Emotional Competence in Infants and Young Children is a widely used framework to target appropriate interventions that enable social-emotional competence (see Figure 7.2). At the base of the pyramid are those who care for children using best practices. Resting on this base are high-quality supportive environments and nurturing and responsive relationships in all settings where the child receives care. For most children, these essentials are sufficient to achieve social-emotional health. Some children need targeted supports beyond what most children require. Mental health consultants can coach those who care for children to provide these targeted supports. A few children require more intensive interventions from mental health professionals.

What comes next if staff efforts do not resolve the behaviors of concern?

Mental health services should be available to early educators when their approaches to handling a child with challenging behavior are not working. Early childhood mental health professionals can help teachers address behaviors of concern and significantly improve the well-being of children, staff members, and families. Many mental health professionals are skilled assessors of individual, group, and organization functioning. They can address the stress the staff members feel in working with the child, observe the child's behavior, and suggest additional strategies to try. They can also help determine whether it is necessary to refer the child for further evaluation and care.

Every facility should identify a qualified early childhood mental health consultant who can develop an ongoing, proactive relationship with staff members and who will visit the program at least quarterly and be on call when help is needed. To identify a qualified consultant, ask mental health and behavioral service providers in the community who does such work. The types of professionals who are likely to be helpful include psychologists, licensed clinical social workers, child psychiatrists, developmental-behavioral pediatricians, and pediatricians with a special interest in behavioral health. Developmental-behavioral pediatricians provide consultation on behavioral issues that a primary care pediatrician would not typically handle. Another approach is to contact nearby institutions where such professionals receive their education and training. Students preparing for mental health careers may provide some service to early care and education staff under faculty supervision. If a mental health professional consultant is not available to work with the program staff, the appropriate staff members must decide when it is time to refer a child to a mental health professional and have the parent arrange for the child to have further evaluation. One or more of the following factors may trigger a referral:

- The problems have lasted several weeks to months.
- The problems are severe or getting worse.
- Your supportive care and interventions have not helped.
- The child is unable to function successfully in the child care setting.

- The child is not achieving age-appropriate developmental levels and tasks.
- The family is extremely distressed, or the stresses are getting worse.

Whom you refer the family to depends on the child's condition and the resources in your community. The child's usual source of health care is always a good starting place. The child's health care provider may understand the family's circumstances and be able to provide additional support. It is also easier, in many cases, to refer the child to a pediatrician or family doctor than to a psychiatrist or psychologist. However, some families appreciate an immediate referral to a mental health professional.

Know the names of professionals in your area who work with young children who have behavioral issues; do not wait until there is a crisis to identify such professionals. If the parent provides written permission to share the notes of your observations and concerns with the professional, be sure to do so. Include any observation checklist data you have gathered (the Behavioral Data Collection Sheet provided in Figure A.10 in Appendix A is written in an easy-to-use format), and fill out the Special Care Plan for a Child with Behavioral Issues provided in Figure A.11. Such information will help the clinician formulate suggestions that the child care program and family can implement. It may be best to arrange a conversation with the clinician, with the parents' permission, to clarify observations and recommendations. If you make a referral to a mental health professional, try to maintain the child in your program. This stability may be very helpful to the child and family.

Fact sheets from reputable sources provide helpful information that teachers can use and also share with families. The CSEFEL website, for example, includes tips and parent training modules, sample scenarios, and professional development tools. Another federally funded resource is the Technical Assistance Center on Social Emotional Intervention (TACSEI). TACSEI works in partnership with CSEFEL to promote adoption of the Pyramid Model. Free products, resources, and links to other useful information are available on the TACSEI website at **www.challengingbehavior.org**.

Adult mental health

Teaching and caring for children is a stressful occupation. Mentally healthy adults may have to defer meeting their own immediate needs so they can provide competent care for children. Just like everyone else, teachers have sources of personal stress outside of their jobs. Family issues, upsets in plans, and the impact of events in the community and in society all take their toll.

Co-workers and administrators in early childhood programs provide an essential support group for one another. Usually this support is sufficient and enables the effective operation of the child care program. Sometimes, however, a staff member may require professional mental health resources. In such instances the administrator or supervisor can help the staff member find and use a competent mental health professional. Insurance coverage for mental health services varies widely. Finding sources of community mental health services for a staff member often requires persistence and patience. Because professional mental health services are scarce and expensive, it may be difficult and frustrating for those around stressed and mentally ill adults to find a way to help.

Community mental health resources

As illustrated in CSEFEL's Pyramid Model, accessing developmental pediatricians, pediatric psychiatrists, and social workers who specialize in working with children who are experiencing social-emotional difficul-

Figure 7.2.

Pyramid Model for Promoting Social and Emotional Competence in Infants and Young Children

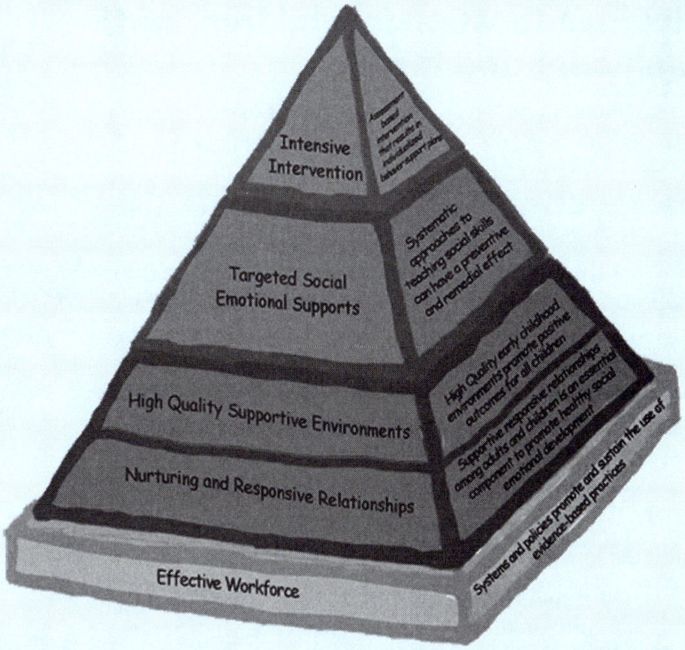

Source: Reprinted, by permission, from the Center on the Social and Emotional Foundations for Early Learning, www.csefel.vanderbilt.edu

ties should be reserved for the most difficult cases. Competent teachers and the child's usual source of medical care are the first level resources for planning and providing necessary interventions. They should work with families to formulate a management plan to modify a child's inappropriate behavior. The first step is to collect observations of the child over a reasonable period. These observations are the basis of decisions about what strategies should be tried and whether to seek a mental health professional's help.

Most mental health professionals are affiliated with hospitals, clinics, and/or mental health agencies. Some mental health professionals for young children are accessible through a referral by the early intervention system or by the child's pediatrician. The United States has been organized into geographic regions for mental health services. Most of these services are targeted to older children and adults. To locate local community mental health services, contact the state, county, or municipal department of health.

Occasionally mental health professionals who are skilled in working with young children can provide training for early educators. However, many of these professionals have long waiting times for evaluation of children and limited time to coordinate implementation of their recommendations, which is frustrating for both themselves and teachers. Teachers and mental health professionals must do the best they can with the resources available to them and continue to advocate on behalf of children for needed services.

Health education for children, staff members, and families

This manual mentions many opportunities and responsibilities for health education. Health education should be integrated into program activities for children, staff members, and families. Everyone can benefit from ongoing learning about current fitness, illness prevention, oral health, social-emotional health, and nutrition information. Your program can promote wellness by providing evidence-based, credible information and activities for children, staff members, and families, addressing the same topic with all three groups at the same time. A child health curriculum is more successful if all adults who are part of the children's lives are involved in the process, reinforcing the ideas and practices being taught. At the same time, the adults themselves will gain valuable knowledge.

Ensure that information shared with families or staff members is reliable and consistent with practices recommended by national government and professional organizations that base their guidance on scientific evidence. Information from the internet or print media is not always credible or based on scientific evidence. It may come from a well-meaning but ill-informed group with a scientific-sounding name. A reliable place to start a search for health information is **www.healthfinder.gov**. This website has links to many reliable sources for current health information.

Health education for children

During the early childhood years, children form habits and attitudes that can last a lifetime. We know that health education can help establish good habits such as eating healthy foods, exercising regularly, wearing seat belts, crossing streets safely, avoiding poisons, and choosing other healthy behaviors. *Caring for Our Children* Standard 2.4.1.1 states:

Health and safety education for children should include physical, oral, mental, emotional, nutritional, and social health and should be integrated daily into the program of activities, to include such topics as

a. Body awareness and use of appropriate terms for body parts

b. Families (including information that all families are different and have unique beliefs and cultural heritage)

c. Personal social skills such as sharing, being kind, helping others, and communicating appropriately

d. Expression and identification of feelings

e. Self-esteem

f. Nutrition, healthy eating (preventing obesity)

g. Outdoor learning/play

h. Fitness and age-appropriate physical activity

i. Personal and dental hygiene including wiping, flushing, handwashing, cough and sneezing etiquette, and toothbrushing

j. Safety (such as home, vehicular car seats and safety belts, playground, bicycle, fire, firearms, water safety, personal safety, what to do in an emergency, getting help and/or dialing 9-1-1 for emergencies)

k. Conflict management, violence prevention, and bullying prevention

l. Age-appropriate first aid concepts

m. Healthy and safe behaviors

n. Poisoning prevention and poison safety

o. Awareness of routine preventive and special health care needs

p. Importance of rest and sleep

q. Health risks of secondhand smoke

r. Taking medications

s. Handling food safely

t. Preventing choking and falls

Health education works best in an environment in which adults consistently demonstrate and promote healthful behavior. Children learn healthful behaviors by observing what others do, experiencing healthful routines, hearing stories, engaging in dramatic play, and using opportunities for acceptable real-life risk taking and practice of risk control, guided by adults who care for them. A child care program must follow healthy routines, such as frequent hand hygiene and toothbrushing. Activities should be safe and organized so that children feel secure and cared for. All people—adults and children—must respect and care for other people and the environment.

To create a healthy environment, all staff members should model the behaviors that they want children to learn. If adults instruct children to take care of their bodies, but they themselves smoke, drink soda, eat candy, spend a lot of time watching TV or using computers and other media, and fail to engage in moderate to vigorous physical activity, children will copy these behaviors. Adult behavior, attitudes, and appearance are the most powerful tools for children's learning.

Health activities should fit into the natural flow of the program throughout the year. An occasional puppet show or video/DVD on a health topic is not enough. Routines such as toothbrushing, hand hygiene, careful food handling, good nutrition, and use of child passenger safety seats should happen every day.

When you know what you want to teach, you can capture the teachable moments when children are most likely to learn. For example, when a child with the sniffles sits in your lap, talk about taking good care of your body when you are sick (rest, drink liquids). When a child is scheduled to go into the hospital, set up a hospital corner and read children's books about hospital experiences. Spring is a natural time to talk about growing and eating good foods; plant a vegetable garden if you can. Talk about avoiding sticky and sweet foods while you're brushing teeth. Before and during time on the playground, ask children to repeat the positive rules about using play equipment and to show how they comply with the rules. Practice the proper use of car seat restraints, then follow through by helping parents make sure they and their children are safely buckled up.

Remember that children learn best when what they are taught is

- Concrete
- Geared toward their skills and interests
- Complementary to whatever else they are learning
- Presented in many different ways—books, conversations, free play, group activities, songs with instructional lyrics (e.g., the handwashing song, singing and performing motions for children's songs about healthful activities), field trips, videotapes/DVDs, etc.
- Tied into all areas of the curriculum—science (e.g., growing food), cooking, dramatic play (e.g., going to the doctor, dentist, or hospital), art (e.g., making a collage of pictures showing children engaged in moderate to vigorous activity), and so on
- Strengthened through practice

Provide children with an opportunity to learn about personal health, the health of those around them, and their world. Expand your pool of ideas and resources by involving other teachers, parents, nutritionists, mental health specialists, professionals who work with children who have special needs, professional organizations, community agencies, and other community resources. Many groups have materials and teaching ideas intended for young children.

Health education for staff members and families

Knowledge is power

Having good information is one of the best ways to feel confident and in control. When you know what to do—whether it is taking a temperature, giving first aid, or keeping a child relaxed while receiving medicine or going to a medical care facility—both you and the child benefit from your knowledge. The result is that necessary and appropriate care is provided while the person receiving the care remains calm and maintains control. Lack of information often leads to panic in emergencies and consequently to less adequate care.

Keys to getting the message across

Some basic ways that program administrators can teach staff members, families, and volunteers about health include the following approaches:

- Model good health behaviors—practice what you preach!
- Establish good health routines (e.g., brushing teeth, serving healthy foods, following hand hygiene practices).
- Post routines and suggestions as reminders (e.g., emergency plans, hand hygiene techniques, diapering instructions).
- Teach children good habits (and then they will remind the adults).
- Use a variety of media and instructional techniques, such as staff meeting discussions, workshops or guest speakers, newsletters, site visits (e.g., to a hospital emergency room), newspaper and magazine clippings, posters, pamphlets, online tutorials, webinars, DVDs, music with healthful messages (e.g., the handwashing song), and other audiovisual materials.

Selecting health education topics

Staff education about health correlates with better implementation of health practices. *Caring for Our Children* Standard 2.4.2.1 indicates that:

> Health and safety education for staff should include physical, oral, mental, emotional, nutritional, physical activity, and social health of children. In addition to the health and safety topics for children in Standard 2.4.1.1, health education topics for staff should include
>
> a. Promoting healthy mind and brain development through child care
>
> b. Healthy indoor and outdoor learning/play environments
>
> c. Behavior/discipline
>
> d. Managing emergency situations
>
> e. Monitoring developmental abilities, including indicators of potential delays
>
> f. Nutrition (i.e., healthy eating to prevent obesity)
>
> g. Food safety
>
> h. Water safety
>
> i. Safety/injury prevention
>
> j. Safe use, storage, and clean-up of chemicals
>
> k. Hearing, vision, and language problems
>
> l. Physical activity and outdoor play and learning
>
> m. Appropriate antibiotic use
>
> n. Immunizations
>
> o. Gaining access to community resources
>
> p. Maternal or parental/guardian depression
>
> q. Exclusion policies
>
> r. Tobacco use/smoking
>
> s. Safe sleep environments and SIDS prevention
>
> t. Breastfeeding support
>
> u. Environmental health and reducing exposures to environmental toxins
>
> v. Children with special needs
>
> w. Shaken baby syndrome and abusive head trauma
>
> x. Safe use, storage of firearms
>
> y. Safe medication administration

Many state licensing agencies require specific teacher training in topics such as approved first aid procedures and fire safety. Staff members may receive health education from the program's child care health consultant or from someone whom the consultant suggests. Often, it is possible to arrange for staff members to earn state-recognized credit for such education. Here are some ideas to help you plan health education for staff members and families:

- Ask a supervisor or health consultant to observe the program, consider families' needs and strengths, and suggest health education topics for immediate and long-term concern.
- Ask staff members and families about what they want to learn. Present a list of suggested topics with an opportunity for them to suggest others as well. You might ask them to set priorities for their choices.
- Find out the most convenient time to meet with families.
- Try to get a sense of parents' and staff members' learning styles, then plan something for everyone (e.g., speakers, written materials, hands-on experience, and videos).
- Plan a yearly training schedule based on the priority topics. Revise and update your schedule each year. In addition to the list in *Caring for Our Children* Standard 2.4.2.1, some specific topics to consider are the following:

• Orientation to your health policies

• Preventive health practices

• Transportation safety and the results of site safety surveys

• First aid

• Management of minor illness

• Child growth and development

• Observation and recording of health signs and symptoms

• Child abuse/neglect

• Cultural views of health

• How to be a good consumer of health services; how to advocate for better community health services

• How to provide health education for young children

• The value and meaning of health screening results

• Chronic illness/special needs

• Parenting

• Acceptable guidance/classroom management techniques

• How to talk with children

Suggested activities

- Visit a child care facility and look for oral health practices and missed opportunities for oral health promotion. What resources would be needed to improve oral health promotion in the program?
- Find a community oral health professional who will work with you to plan an oral health education activity for a preschool group. Ask the staff members to evaluate whether any of the children or adults changed their practices after this activity.
- Call the health department and ask about mental health resources available to families in your area. Call one or two to ask how they would handle a request for mental health assessment of a 3-year-old whose behavior makes inclusion a burden for staff members.
- Ask a program director who has held her position for at least a few years about her experience with managing children who have challenging behavior that is beyond typical developmental expectations. Ask if and how staff members' mental health issues have affected the program in the past.
- Research a health education topic and prepare a presentation for your peers. If appropriate, prepare and present a simplified version of the same topic to a group of children and then to their families.

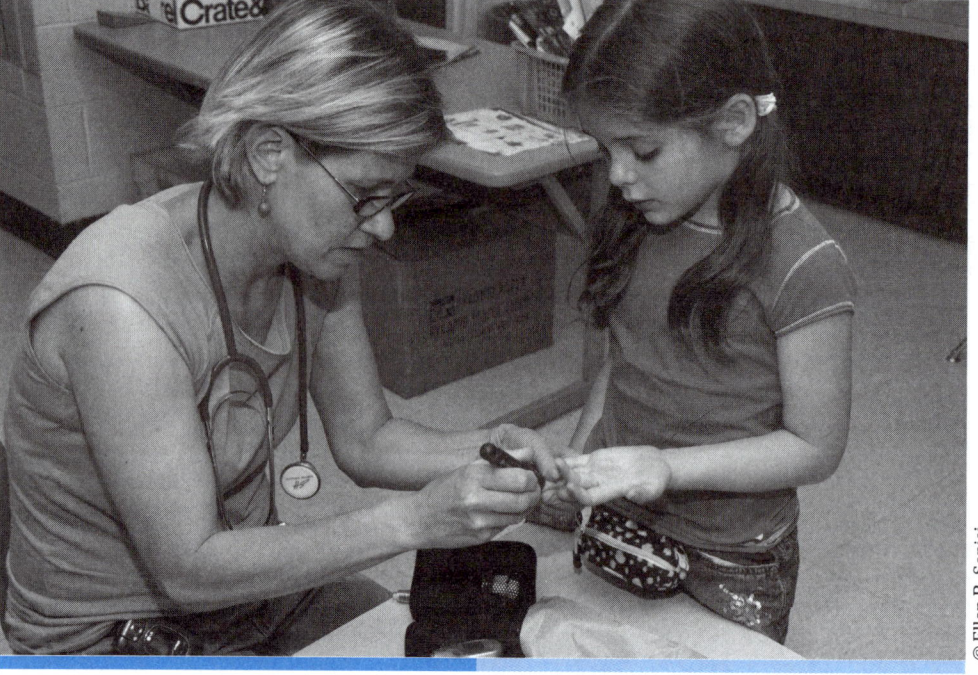

8

Medical Care—Clinical Health Services for Children

MAJOR CONCEPTS

■ Regularly scheduled health care visits are essential to maintain children's health and readiness to learn. They should include a review of the child's health history, a physical assessment, screenings, and immunization to identify and treat correctable child health conditions.

■ The facility should develop and follow a written policy for obtaining, reviewing, and tracking medical care information from each child's regular source of health care. The information should show that the child is up to date for the currently recommended preventive health services. Immunization documentation should be provided by the family at enrollment, preferably before the child physically joins a group at the facility. The rest of the health assessment data should be provided within two weeks of admission, or the family should provide verification that an appointment for the services has been made.

■ Health is assessed through evaluation of a child's health history, screening tests, and selective laboratory examinations.

■ Families may need help to find a medical home in which they can obtain routine preventive care or medical care for illness evident to them or identified by routine health supervision.

■ Teachers are key guardians of a safety net that identifies young children (and families) who need clinical health services or referral to other community resources.

■ Families may need help to find health insurance coverage for their child.

As children grow, their health needs constantly change, particularly during their early years. *Health* is defined by the World Health Organization, according to its website (www.who.int/suggestions/faq/en/index.html), as "a state of complete physical, mental, and social well-being and not merely the absence of disease or infirmity." Wellness is affected by the interrelationships between each area of a person's development. For example, when children are ill, tired, hungry, or poorly fed, they cannot function well; they may be cranky or inattentive. A child who has an undetected medical condition or who is neglected may become depressed or withdrawn. A child with a physical problem also may develop emotional or learning problems; a child who has emotional upsets may develop physical symptoms.

Young children are at risk for developing a number of health problems, such as hearing or vision difficulties, lead poisoning, developmental delay, and injury. The goals of preventive health care are keeping children well and safe, early detection and management of problems, and planning for accommodations that enable children to reach their potential. Early educators play a key role in ensuring that children receive needed health services in a timely fashion. Parents may delay or fail to obtain the health services their children need, putting their children and those who are in contact with them at risk. This may occur because of misinformation about the risks and benefits of services, difficulty in making arrangements for their children to receive the services due to either conflicting priorities for them or the limited availability of convenient appointments, or the cost of care. As indicated in *Caring for Our Children* Standard 9.2.3.4,

> When age-appropriate health assessments and use of health insurance benefits are promoted by caregivers/teachers, children enrolled in child care will have increased access to immunizations and other preventive services. With the expansion of eligibility for medical assistance and the federal subsidy of state child health insurance plans (SCHIP), the numbers of children who lack insurance for routine preventive health care should lessen.

Health care

Every child should have a source of medical care where the child receives preventive and treatment services, including vaccines. A comprehensive, medically and culturally competent source of care that is continuously available, accessible, compassionate, and family centered is called a *medical home*. A medical home is not a place; it is an arrangement for health care that not only responds to requests from families but also reaches out to support them in doing what is in their children's best interests. Ideally, the medical home has procedures to look for children and families who do not come for routine and follow-up visits. Although increasing use of electronic medical records is making such outreach more feasible, currently the gap between the goal and performance remains large.

Lack of comprehensive health insurance coverage for medical home services is a barrier to care for many families. If you find a family lacking such a resource, seek health care providers whose approach for children and/or adults in the community most closely meet the characteristics of a medical home. (See Figure 8.1.) Make a referral to local physicians who offer medical home services or to a health department clinic. Be familiar with the state Medicaid program and state Child Health Insurance Program (CHIP) referral resource telephone numbers to assist families who lack health insurance. If the child is not up-to-date with vaccines and does not have a medical home to provide them, refer the family to public vaccine programs.

The federal government created CHIP as part of amendments to the Social Security Act in 1997. This state-administered program uses a combination of federal and state funds to provide health insurance for children whose family income is high enough to make them ineligible for Medicaid but whose parents are unable to buy private insurance. Implementation of CHIP varies from state to state. Some states have sliding scale co-payment arrangements for CHIP that allow families to buy private health insurance at a premium cost that they can afford. Other states allow CHIP-eligible families to participate in the state's Medicaid program. To find out about your state's CHIP program, contact the office of your state's insurance commissioner or your state's office of maternal and child health, usually located in the state's health department. Federal funds support state governments to provide a telephone help line available to the public to address maternal and child health questions and to provide referrals to appropriate service providers. They give information about where women and children can receive free or low-cost health care and vaccines.

Teachers play an important role in promoting the use of a medical home for every child. By checking whether children have followed the nationally recommended schedule of preventive health services, teachers can identify children who have gaps in health care services. For children who have special needs, it is especially important for teachers to collaborate with families and their children's health care providers to ensure that these children have and use a medical home. (For more about inclusion of children with special needs, see Chapter 12.)

Routine preventive health services:

- Detect medical conditions that may not be easily recognized but require medical attention (e.g., fluid in the ear, anemia, or lazy eye). Early identification and treatment of such conditions may completely

Figure 8.1.

What Early Educators Can Do to Help Families Use a Medical Home

To ensure that health care is

Accessible

- Provide literature on community agencies that offer services to children, including those with special health care needs such as Title V, Department of Public Health, Respite, and Mental Health.
- Assist families who may be eligible to enroll in either Medicaid or the state Children's Health Insurance Program (CHIP).
- Provide a directory of pediatricians who are accepting new patients in the communities where the families live or the child care facility is located—or give suggestions about how to access this information through the website of the American Academy of Pediatrics at **www.aap.org**.

Comprehensive

- Ensure that all children with special needs have a primary health care professional.
- Develop a transportation policy and procedure for transporting children, including children with special needs. Identify a local child passenger safety technician to provide up-to-date transportation safety information, education, and technical assistance support for special transport needs.
- Develop an emergency plan that addresses the needs of every child in the facility, including the accommodation that is required for children with special needs. Review and revise the plan with input from the child's family and primary health care professional.

Compassionate

- Become an advocate for the child by communicating observations and concerns to the family and to the child's health care professional.
- Be aware of and comply with applicable laws and regulations concerning children with special needs.
- Distribute information about the requirements of the Americans with Disabilities Act that relate to quality care in child care and in health care.

Continuous

- Educate all teachers about how to recognize and respond to signs and symptoms of distress and emergencies in a way that relates next steps for involving the child's health care provider.
- Keep updated emergency contact information as part of each child's record.
- Coordinate education for parents related to immunizations, developmental screenings, or other health-related topics presented by a local pediatrician or primary pediatric health care professional.
- Transmit information about observations and concerns to the child's primary health care professional, with appropriately obtained consent from the family.
- Create a system of recording and sharing information within the program so that all teachers are knowledgeable about the conditions and health needs of each child they care for.

Coordinated

- If applicable, participate in each child's Individualized Family Service Plan (IFSP) or Individualized Education Plan (IEP).
- When possible, ensure that children with special needs receive their individual services from specialists in the usual care environment. Teachers and the other children in the group can learn how to help the child benefit fully by using techniques that the specialist demonstrates to help the child. Often, the approaches that help a child with special needs in the least restrictive and most natural environment also benefit typically developing children. Such services include speech, physical, and occupational therapies.

Culturally Competent

- Provide information to parents in their primary language and check whether their health care provider communicates in a language they understand.
- Incorporate family customs, beliefs, or rituals into the child's everyday care when possible. Alert the child's health care provider about these traditions when they relate to how the family will accept recommendations for health care.

Family Centered

- Encourage families to share their family circumstances and concerns when they take their child for checkup visits, even when questions about such concerns are not brought up by the health care provider.
- Ask families to identify their preferences regarding accessibility and developmentally appropriate practices (e.g., floor plans, playground equipment, transportation, activities, and toys) in the health care facility as well as in the child care program.

resolve them, or at least limit later disability, while a delay in attention can result in more—or permanent—damage.

- Identify children who may be at high risk for developing diseases due to hereditary factors, family health habits, or environmental factors
- Identify and follow signs in growth patterns, behavior, or development that provide clues to current or future health problems
- Evaluate the effectiveness of and adjust past or current treatments (e.g., ear tubes, antibiotics, patching an eye, medication for prevention of asthma episodes)
- Promote health through counseling, education, and guidance for anticipated problems
- Provide highly effective preventive measures such as vaccines
- Identify potential health problems through screenings (e.g., growth measurements and those for vision, hearing, lead levels, and red blood cells or hemoglobin [for anemia])
- Provide early detection and treatment of illnesses with symptoms (e.g., strep throat) to prevent complications
- Prevent and reduce disability from chronic diseases

Children need to be seen by pediatric health care providers at recommended intervals. The pediatric clinician who provides this care is often called a primary health provider. Primary health providers for children include pediatricians, family practice physicians, and nurse clinicians or nurse practitioners. Because care of children requires specialized training, families should be encouraged to select a pediatrician who provides a medical home for routine checkups, management of common illnesses, and follow-up care.

The majority of pediatricians in the United States are members of the American Academy of Pediatrics (AAP). Groups of experts organized by the AAP set the nationally accepted, minimum guidelines for routine health care for children. AAP guidelines are usually the same as public health guidelines or have only minor differences. The guidelines are reviewed and updated as new information about valuable preventive health measures becomes available. The periodicity schedule, or table of services by age for healthy children, can be found in Appendix I: Recommendations for Preventative Pediatric Health Care in *Caring for Our Children* and at **http://brightfutures.aap.org/pdfs/Guidelines_PDF/20-Appendices_PeriodicitySchedule.pdf**. This schedule is updated by the AAP from time to time. Check the website at least once a year to be sure you are using the most current version. Note that the guidelines are *minimum* requirements for healthy children receiving competent parenting and having no significant health problems. When a child has a special situation, more frequent visits may be required. Many materials for parents and health care providers are available on the Bright Futures website (**http://brightfutures.aap.org**). Explore this website for handouts related to a wide variety of health promotion topics to give to parents and staff.

Some doctors and clinics do not follow the Bright Futures periodicity schedule and guidelines. Teachers should encourage families to seek health care providers who do follow the guidelines, even if all of the services a child needs cannot be provided at a particular checkup visit or at a single location. Some health insurance does not pay for preventive health care that meets the schedule guidelines. Families should be encouraged to seek insurance coverage that does pay for these services (from their employers or from publically subsidized insurance programs for children like Medicaid or CHIP), seek subsidized care from federally qualified community health service centers usually located in low-income neighborhoods, or pay for services that are not covered. The state maternal and child health help line or local department of health will be able to give contact information about all of these possibilities. The family's concerns and the child's needs may require that at any one visit, the most urgent services for the child are provided, with the remaining needed services delayed until follow-up visits. Families may not return for such follow-up visits, however, and some services may be missed or forgotten. Acting in children's best interests, teachers should encourage families to return for follow-up visits.

Some families fragment their children's health care by using different sources of care without coordination or by using emergency rooms or urgent care centers for minor illnesses. As a result, their children are more likely to have poor health. Information obtained from special screening programs should always be forwarded (with parental consent) to the child's usual source of health care. Coordinating services among health care providers for children is essential to approximate the quality of care that a medical home should provide.

Assessing health status

Many individuals with unique skills and experiences participate in assessing a child's health. The child's physician or another member of the health team should coordinate services of health professionals as the child's special needs or family preference suggests. In many health care settings, the coordinator of services is called a *case* or *care manager*. In private practices, this person may be the office manager or a nurse.

In addition to health professionals, the child's health team consists of the child's family, the child's teachers, and others who regularly observe and interact with the child. Members of the child's health team contribute their perspectives on the child's growth, development, and overall health viewed from their specific areas of expertise. This information should be shared with the person acting as the care manager where the child's health care provider works to create a comprehensive picture of the child's health. Clear designation of the health team coordinator is especially important for children with multiple health and developmental issues who need to visit certain specialists. For example, children who have asthma and/or allergies might receive care from a pulmonologist and/or an allergist in addition to their primary health care provider. For information about different types of specialists, look for a website representing a particular specialty.

Health assessment and follow-up care are often separated into three categories: screening, diagnosis, and treatment.

- *Screening* is the use of quick, inexpensive, and simple procedures to identify children who may have an issue in a specific area. Health screening tests typically produce one of three possible results: 1) the child seems healthy, so no action is needed; 2) the child is possibly at risk, so the screening test is repeated; or 3) the child is at risk, so she is referred for further diagnosis and possible treatment.

- *Diagnosis* is a more detailed evaluation to find out if there is in fact a health condition and, if so, what it is. When making a diagnosis, the health professional may use health histories, dietary information, laboratory test results, family/teacher observations, radiology, and/or physical and psychological examinations.

- *Treatment* includes measures designed to control, minimize, correct, or cure a disease or abnormality (e.g., eyeglasses, dental fillings, or therapy). *Treatment is the key to an effective program.* If care for an individual does not result in whatever treatment is indicated, screening and diagnosis are meaningless.

Health histories

Health histories provide important information about the child's prior health experiences and risks for future disease. The family health history may help predict what illnesses the child may inherit or develop. Competent preventive care requires a detailed health history including information about birth, illnesses, hospitalization, all treatments, immunization status, and current health concerns.

Programs for young children should collect a health history from the family that covers major health

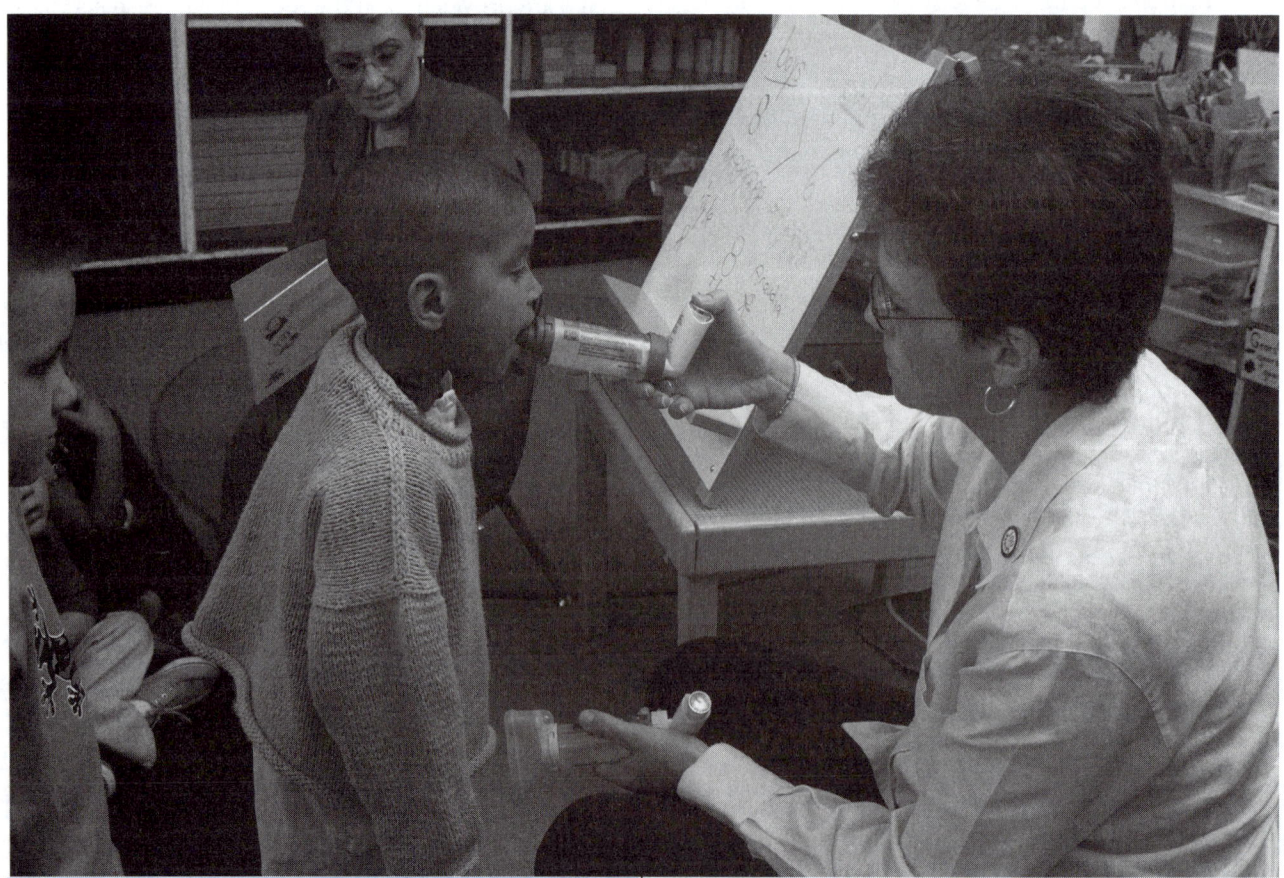

issues and developmental concerns. This information could explain a child's current condition, behavior, and past experience. Most parents can recall many details about their own child. However, the names of health care providers and the chronology of events may be forgotten if they are not recorded. Unless there is a specific request for it, few parents will systematically review the details of their child's nutritional, immunization, health, and family history to identify patterns that suggest a need for attention. Even the most alert parents may innocently overlook the health needs of a rapidly changing and growing child because of other urgent demands in their lives.

When a child care program requests a child's health history, the request helps reinforce the family's role in keeping track of important health information. A form that collects the type of information useful to a child care program is presented in Figure A.12 in Appendix A. Use it as a guide to develop a tool that works well in your facility to gather appropriate information. Check the information you collect against information shared by the child's health care provider on a form such as the Child Health Assessment form in *Caring for Our Children* Appendix FF. The format of the child health assessment forms your program uses may differ from the forms provided by the child's health care provider. What is important is that the program receives all the necessary information, no matter what format the child's health care provider uses.

Filling out forms is time-consuming work in health care offices. Some health care providers charge for filling out forms, especially if it is not requested at the time of the health care visit. With increasing use of electronic medical records, the health care provider may share information as a printout from the electronic file. This reduces the health care provider's burden of transferring information to different forms for a variety of programs that families in one medical home may use. If you cannot understand or use the information you receive, or you notice discrepancies with what you already know about the child, clarify the facts with the parents and, with their permission, with the child's health care provider. Everyone involved needs useful and reliable information.

Observations of physical health, development, and behavior

Opportunities for the health care professional to make valid observations during health care visits are limited by the short duration of the visit with the family and by the health care setting, which may not be familiar or comfortable for the child. Nonetheless, health care providers observe what they can and use these observations as a component of the assessment. Observations made and reported by those who care for children on a daily basis can be very helpful.

Each staff member must be sensitive, conscientious, and systematic in assessing and addressing a child's health needs each day. You probably already notice such things as a new haircut or outfit as you greet a child upon his arrival, but take the time to look closely at the child's appearance. Through daily observation, you can learn a great deal about children as individuals: their typical coloring and appearance, moods and temperament, response to pain and sickness, activity level, and patterns of behavior. Each of these is a vital clue to health. Changes in the child's health from what is typical for a healthy child or for that individual child should be noted in the health record so that the information can be aggregated over time and shared when appropriate to determine a need for medical care.

While you are expected to be observant, you are not expected to be an expert on health. Observe the child, record relevant data, and then report anything unusual to the appropriate person on your staff and to the family. You cannot and should not offer diagnoses or treatment plans, but health professionals will be able to make better judgments using the information you can provide. Health observation is an important first step before screening, diagnosis, or treatment.

Physical health

Physical health observations include observable signs of health or illness (e.g., coughing, vomiting, swelling, limping) and reported symptoms (e.g., nausea, headache, stomachache, refusal to do specific activities). Because young children may not be able to describe how they feel, objective observations provide essential clues. It can be helpful to use a form to record observations and symptoms. (See Figure A.13 in Appendix A for a sample form.) Give a copy to the family to give to the child's health care provider. When communicating your observations, whether in person or in writing, be as specific as you can. For example, say, "Jeffrey has a frequent dry cough, flushed cheeks, and a runny nose with thick yellow mucus," rather than, "Jeffrey is sick." Say, "Jennifer has a sore throat and an oral temperature of 102° F," rather than making assumptions and reporting that "Jennifer has strep throat."

Each observer has a different perspective in obtaining health information. Parents, for example, compare a child's appearance or behavior with what is typical for the child, or with that of the child's siblings or friends. Teachers can observe children in a group setting with many children of the same age. Child health professionals use knowledge and experience from their medical practice. Each view is valuable but limited; to have a total picture of the child, all observations must be shared and seen as a whole.

Use your senses (smell, hearing, sight, touch) when making health observations. Observe clues such as the color, temperature, or texture of skin; breath odor; the appearance of a bruise; or the sound of a cough. Observe the group in general and compare individual children. For example, do most of the children of the same age get out of breath when climbing the hill on the playground? If a child has difficulty doing what the rest of the group does easily, it is worth noting and asking the family to bring it up with their child's health care provider.

Development and behavior

Children's physical health is only one aspect of their lives. Equally important aspects are the development of language, gross and fine motor skills, social-emotional competence, and cognition (thinking). Difficulties in these areas are best managed when they are identified and addressed during the early years.

1. *Developmental milestones.* Knowledge of general child development with in-depth information about children at particular ages provides a general framework to identify children whose abilities fall outside the typical range. These milestones must be viewed flexibly because a child's development is greatly influenced by childrearing styles, culture and ethnic norms, and the child's own temperament.

   Teachers can use developmental and behavioral screening tools to assess children in their care. These tools serve more than one purpose: reinforcing a sense of normal developmental pathways; identifying the child whose development is outside the range for typically developing children; and helping teachers individualize educational activities, some that are comfortable for the child and some that help the child reach for the next level of accomplishment. For information and excellent free materials about developmental milestones and screening, go to **www.cdc.gov/ncbddd/actearly/index.html**. This website of the Centers for Disease Control and Prevention (CDC), National Center on Birth Defects and Developmental Disabilities (NCBDDD), has special sections for families and for early childhood educators, clinicians, and others.

   Increasingly, observers of children are using standardized tools as a framework for assessing a particular child's placement in the range of typical childhood behaviors and developmental skills, then using the same or similar tools to measure the child's progress over time. A teacher's observations over the course of time in the child's daily life yield much valuable information. Teachers should communicate their observations and concerns to the child's family and, with parental consent, to the child's health care provider.

2. *Observation and documentation.* Write down observations that might suggest concerns with a child's development or behavior. (You can keep file cards in your pocket and note on them the day, time, activity, and behavior you observe.) Ask other staff members to also observe and record the child's behaviors. Choose an appropriate developmental screening tool to use in your setting, and apply it to children whose development does not seem in line with their peers'. Document challenging behaviors using the Behavioral Data Collection Sheet in Figure A.10 in Appendix A. Determine the appropriate next steps, and plan a meeting to discuss your concerns with the family. Have the documentation in hand showing your observations.

3. *Communication.* Develop your ability to communicate concerns in a supportive, nonthreatening manner. Parents should be involved in discussions about concerns as soon as possible. Their input can help you identify which of your observations are appropriate for the family and culture and which are not, and which behaviors or traits are of particular concern to them. Often they may have had questions similar to yours but may not have wanted to bother the staff or to appear overly anxious about their child. By addressing these concerns in a respectful partnership, you can be a great help and support.

4. *Referral and consultation.* When concerns suggest the need to consult or make a referral, start with the child's pediatric health care provider. The issue may be solved at that level, or it may be necessary to seek community resources for referral and consultation. Use the Special Care Plan for a Child with Behavioral Issues in Figure A.11 as a guide for reporting behavioral issues. If you have used a standard development screening tool, give a copy to the parent to take to the child's health care provider. If you have not used such a tool, document your observations and concerns succinctly. Many communities have a wide array of experts on every aspect of child health and development. Develop a list of local services that families have found helpful, and keep this list at the center to share with parents when appropriate.

Health screenings

The AAP and the U.S. Department of Health and Human Services recommend the Bright Futures periodicity schedule for all children as described earlier in this chapter, under Health Care. Head Start requires its programs to meet the well-child assessment requirements of their state's Early and Periodic Diagnosis and Treatment Program (EPSDT), which is a component of Medicaid services. Advocates are working steadily to eliminate the differences between the state EPSDT schedules of services and the Bright Futures schedule. By law, states must pay for diagnosis and treatment of any conditions identified in EPSDT screening. To limit spending, some states are reducing EPSDT screening. Other states have expanded screening, recognizing that early identification and treatment ultimately reduces cost. Other forms of child health insurance cover more or less of the recommended screening schedule, follow-up diagnosis, and treatment for conditions identified as a result of screening. What an insurance carrier pays for does not determine the child's need to have services. If insurance or public health services do not cover the costs of needed services, families should be encouraged to pay out-of-pocket for screening, diagnosis, and treatment—just as they do for other necessities such as clothing and food. Sometimes health care providers can identify charities that will help with costs.

Screening tests look for conditions that, if undetected and untreated, may seriously handicap a child for life. Most conditions respond to early treatment, which is often more effective and less costly than later treatment and may also prevent the development of other issues. For instance, children with undetected hearing loss risk developing language, learning, and behavior problems. Children with eyes that are not straight or who have a marked difference in visual acuity between their two eyes are at risk for developing loss of vision in one eye. If decreased vision is not treated during the early years, treatment in the school-age years is slow and often unsuccessful.

Screening generally involves short, simple procedures because it is intended for large numbers of apparently well children. A good screening may identify some children who do not have a problem, but it misses few who *do* have a problem. Without screening, problems may go unnoticed, or if the signs or symptoms are recognized, their significance may not be understood. An abnormal screening test result is a clue that something is wrong, that a further look is needed. Abnormal results should be interpreted by the child's usual source of health care so that appropriate further evaluation can be planned. Premature referral to a specialist may result in overlooking the possibility that the abnormality is part of a multisystem problem.

To be valuable, a screening program must include

- Parent education about the screening
- Family involvement and consent
- Use of a valid, reliable tool appropriate for the child's age
- A competent screener
- Screening and rescreening of children who may have a problem before making referrals
- Written information provided to the family when further examination is suggested
- Family choice of the health professional to follow up
- Information received from the health professional about examination results and treatment plans

Because children are more comfortable and secure in familiar surroundings with familiar adults, screening may be more successful if screeners come to the child care program, as long as the screening is done properly. Prepare the children for what to expect when they will be involved in a particular screening procedure, and follow through on referrals. Be sure to notify the child's usual source of health care about the results of any screening test to avoid duplication and to promote follow-up and coordination of the test results with the rest of the child's health data.

Vision screening

Developmental vision problems may be most effectively corrected during the preschool years. This is especially true in the areas of visual acuity (the ability of each eye to distinguish detail both near and far) and vision skills (the ability to use both eyes efficiently and effectively in a coordinated manner). Some vision problems can interfere with a child's coordination and developmental skills. All children should have an eye examination at birth and at each checkup visit. By 4 years of age, this eye examination should include not only evaluation of general eye health, but also near and far vision acuity as well as the ability to use both eyes together (for depth perception).

Many people believe that preschool children are too young to have their vision tested. Subjective vision screening can be done from birth by covering one eye at a time to see if the child seems to see with the uncovered eye and, by 3–4 months of age, by checking whether the covered eye is out of alignment with the eye being used to see.

At 3 years of age, most children *can* cooperate with a vision screening program that tests for visual acuity and stereopsis (checking if both eyes work together). Objective vision screening is done with an age-appropriate, standardized screening tool designed to identify some of the most common conditions found in young children. A number of tools are available. Picture identification tests are generally considered less accurate than tests with crowded letters or specific shapes, but using pictures is better than not testing. Testing whether the eyes work well together (stereopsis) is essential, yet often not done. The two types of stereopsis tests that are most popular are the Random Dot E and the bug or butterfly test. Vision screening is frequently conducted by volunteers who have received simple training to do the screening correctly. If you are interested in performing vision screening, it is important that you receive training and learn the technique, strengths, and weaknesses of the testing methods you will use. Prevent Blindness America teaches volunteers how to do vision screening of young children and sells the necessary low-cost charts and forms to do the screening.

If possible, it is best for children to receive competent vision screening in a medical home. When this is not possible, you can use the Prevent Blindness America website (**www.preventblindness.org**) to locate a state or regional affiliate or to contact the national office for help to arrange a vision screening program for groups of children that will be conducted by qualified volunteers. Alternately, ask a pediatric vision screening professional (a pediatric ophthalmologist or pediatric optometrist) or a pediatrician to help you find someone who can do competent vision screening, or who will provide training for staff members so they can screen the children. For screening purposes, 3-year-olds are expected to pass at 20/40 line on eye charts; 4-, 5-, and 6-year-olds should pass at 20/30; and 7-year-olds at 20/20.

Any screening program is valuable only if follow-up occurs. The first referral should be to the child's usual source of health care, not to a vision specialist unless the child lacks a usual source of health care to follow up on the vision screening results. *Do not assume that children will outgrow vision problems.* Some problems get worse. Early detection permits early treatment that will correct many conditions more easily and completely and that will cost less than later treatment. Any child who cannot perform well on a basic vision screening by age 4 should be referred to a vision specialist.

Hearing screening

A child who does not hear clearly will have trouble imitating sounds and developing language skills. Behavior also can be affected. Learning to read and write will be difficult and frustrating for the child. Hearing problems may be hereditary or the result of certain illnesses during pregnancy or early childhood. Temporary or intermittent hearing loss may be caused by chronic ear infection, a heavy buildup of wax in the ear, or chronic fluid in the middle ear.

Hearing loss may be readily observed when the loss is fairly severe. Some signs signal milder loss. Infants who do not hear well will not startle at a sudden noise, will not search with their eyes for the source of a noise, will not respond to a musical toy or their parent's voice unless the parent is seen, and will be slow to imitate sounds or respond to simple commands and the sound of their own name. Older children with hearing problems often have smaller vocabularies, use shorter sentences, speak in an unusual voice, and seem to understand less than other children the same age.

Hearing screening for newborns is now being performed in most states. The equipment used measures the brain response to sound. After birth, children need periodic hearing screening because some hearing problems can develop as the child grows. The following are typical hearing tests for young children:

- *Pure tone audiometry* is the typical hearing test used for preschool and older children. It checks a child's ability to hear quiet sounds at four different pitches, or frequencies. The test requires that children perform some specific action, such as putting a toy in a box or raising a hand, when a sound is heard through the earphones.
- *Tympanometry* measures the pressure required to move the eardrum (middle ear) and the way the eardrum moves. Fluid in the middle ear may cause negative pressure and decrease the eardrum's ability to move, affecting a child's ability to distinguish sounds clearly. This test is difficult to do for infants because they have sharply angled ear canals.
- *Acoustic reflex screening* measures the control of a muscle in the middle ear in response to a loud sound. If the contraction (reflex) is absent, there may be fluid in the ear or incomplete healing from a recent infection. This test can be done on very young children.

Measuring height and weight

Height and weight measurements, with determination of the body mass index (BMI) (a calculation widely used to identify children who are underweight, overweight, or obese), should be carried out at each well-child visit. These measurements are one of the best ways to detect physical growth patterns that may indicate a serious problem. They should be graphed over time to show the pattern of the child's growth compared with other children of the same age. Head circumference (measurement around the head at the level of the top of the ears) should also be measured for children from birth to 12 months of age. Growth measurements are usually part of a routine checkup.

Children whose length/height growth percentile differs by more than one percentile curve from their weight/growth percentile, whose growth data are below the fifth percentile curve, or whose BMI is out of the expected range need further evaluation. You should receive this information with the child's physical examination report. If you want to plot the growth data yourself, you can obtain the growth charts online from the CDC at **www.cdc.gov/growthcharts**. To learn more about BMI and access BMI calculators for adults and children, go to **www.cdc.gov/healthyweight/assessing/bmi/index.html**. Using the BMI calculator may increase self-awareness among educators and parents about whether they or the children in their care are a healthy weight or are under- or overweight. You may want to allow school-age children to get the charts, make the measurements, and plot their own weight, height, and

BMI. This activity integrates learning about mathematics, science, self, and health.

Anemia and iron screening

Hematocrit, or hemoglobin measurements, and measurements of *ferritin,* an iron-containing substance in the body, are commonly used to screen children for anemia and problems with insufficient iron during early childhood. Anemia results when the body does not have enough circulating red blood cells to carry oxygen from the lungs to the tissues and/or not enough hemoglobin (the chemical carrying oxygen to the red blood cells) in each cell. An anemic child is likely to appear tired, pale, and inattentive, and to be susceptible to infection. Iron is needed to form hemoglobin and also is a component of many cells in the body. Without enough iron, blood cannot carry the oxygen the body needs. Iron deficiency even without anemia can cause sleep and developmental problems.

Although there are other causes of anemia, iron deficiency is still the most common cause, particularly for children from low-income families or toddlers who did not receive sufficient iron when they were rapidly growing infants. Causes of iron deficiency include

- Overconsumption of milk (more than 24–32 ounces per day), resulting in low intake of other foods, particularly iron-containing foods
- Lack of high-iron, high-nutrient foods in the diet (e.g., meat, fish, beans, and green, leafy vegetables)
- Lead toxicity. Iron deficiency and lead poisoning frequently occur together. Iron and lead compete with each other for the same binding sites in the body. Iron deficiency may increase the absorption of lead from the intestine and make the toxic effects of lead worse. Therapeutic doses of iron are often required to correct the iron deficiency when it is accompanied by lead poisoning.
- Inadequate amounts of the body substance that picks up iron from the digestive system and transports it to places in the body where iron is needed

Normal values for anemia tests and ferritin levels in children vary by race and from one laboratory to another, but laboratories report the normal range for the test the child had along with the test result.

Urine screening

Urine is produced by the kidney and stored in the bladder until it is emptied by urination. Abnormalities in kidney function, infection in the urine, or biochemical problems in the body can be detected by urinalysis. Pretreated paper strips are dipped into urine to determine the presence of any abnormality. Normally, urine does not contain protein, sugar, more than a few white or red cells, nitrites, ketones, or urobilinogen. Routine urine screening for healthy children is no longer recommended.

Lead screening

Lead is widely dispersed in the environment, both in nature and in manufactured products. It is often in layers of interior paint that were put on surfaces before 1978, when lead was banned from paint for buildings. It may be in the soil around buildings painted with lead paint years ago or near highways that were heavily traveled when lead was a routine additive in gasoline. As the painted surface deteriorates or chips, lead dust is released into the air and falls onto nearby surfaces.

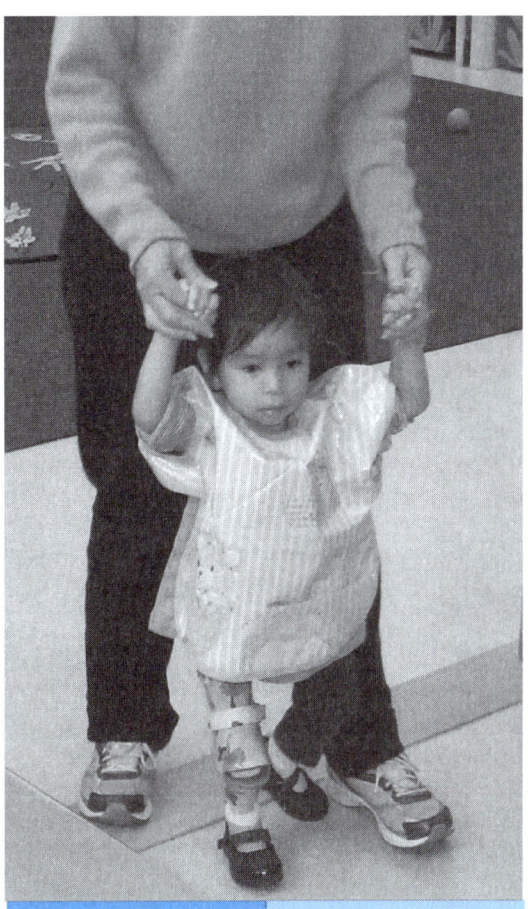
© Meredith Scherrer

Ingestion of a small chip of lead paint or lead dust on unwashed hands can raise the blood lead level. Lead screening is extremely important because even very low elevations of blood lead that do not produce obvious symptoms can cause permanent problems in learning and behavior.

Two major ways to prevent lead poisoning in children are to remove lead in the environment and to conduct lead screening to identify children who must be removed from sources of lead. The current tests for lead recommended by the AAP and CDC are a finger-stick or venous blood test (usually taken from the vein at the inside of the elbow) to most accurately detect elevated lead levels. Blood level screening should be a part of routine health care for children who live, play, or visit in older buildings; who play in the soil where new buildings replaced older buildings; or where the play area has soil that was contaminated by being close to highways that were heavily traveled when gasoline contained lead. According to the CDC, other nonresidential sources of lead include the following: some home remedies, some cosmetics, some candies imported from Mexico, cookware and tableware not certified to be lead-free, some toys and toy jewelry, hot water drawn from pipes in houses with lead-soldered pipes, and stained-glass hobbies. Both the AAP and CDC recommend that risk for possible lead exposure be assessed by at least asking about possible lead exposure at children's health visits between the ages of 6 months and 6 years.

Children should not play in bare soil where old painted buildings stand or stood at one time unless lead testing of soil samples confirms that the soil does not contain lead. In communities where lead is a known environmental problem, lead screening of infants and toddlers should be universal.

Medical examinations/health assessments

A medical examination, or health assessment, is a comprehensive review by a physician or nurse practitioner of all the information gathered from health history, health observations, and screening tests. Although the medical examination is commonly called a "physical," the physical examination—in which the health care provider looks at, feels, and listens to the body—is only one part of a medical examination. The examination includes collecting information from the parent or guardian about any symptoms, concerns, family health problems, the family's social status and stresses, medications being used, nutrition and physical activity, the child's visits to a dentist, and vaccine history. Then, the child health provider performs a complete physical examination and arranges for necessary laboratory and screening tests. The results of a child's health assessment should be reported to the early care and education program. This could be recorded on a form (such as the form in *Caring for Our Children* Appendix FF) or be a printout that includes the necessary information from the child's electronic medical record.

If the information provided by the child's health care provider is incomplete or does not provide a clear picture of the child's needs while in child care, the director or health consultant should obtain parental consent to contact the child's health care provider for additional information. A program's health policies should require that the immunization record be reviewed to ensure it is up to date and that it is on file prior to the child's first day of attendance. Allowing enrollment without proper documents to review may pose some risks. However, the program may offer enrollment as long as the family reports that the child seems to have no health concerns and there is an appointment to obtain the necessary care scheduled within two weeks of the child's first day of attendance. Each child should have a health record maintained in the facility until the child leaves the program. (See *Caring for Our Children* Standards 3.1.2.1 and 9.4.1.2.) The child's health information should be updated at each checkup visit, following the recommended Bright Futures periodicity schedule. The schedule requires updates every two to three months for infants, decreasing frequency of updates for toddlers, and annual updates for children once they reach 3 years of age. Health information should be considered confidential and should not be disclosed without written consent of the parent or guardian.

Tracking and advocating for preventive health care

One of the services early childhood programs provide is acting as an advocate for families by requiring and reviewing children's health data. Documentation from the child's primary care provider should consist of more than a statement that the child is up to date; when requesting documentation, request the specifics of services rendered. Otherwise, burdened medical office personnel may provide information that indicates only that the child has been in the office. This situation may improve with electronic medical record systems that can flag children who are overdue for services. Electronic medical record systems are beginning to be in common use for pediatric care. As stated in the rationale for *Caring for Our Children* Standard 9.2.3.4, "Until tracking systems become more widespread and effective in health care settings, a joint effort by the education system, family, and primary care provider is required to ensure that children receive the preventive health services that ensure they are healthy and ready to learn." Although electronic appointment and immunization tracking and reminder systems are increasingly used by clinicians, many doctors still depend on families to remember when their children are due back. Busy parents may forget or need reminders of when their children are due for their next preventive service. Using the current schedule of preventive care, teachers can advocate for each child to stay up to date with immunization and screening services given at routine checkups. Unless everyone involved with the child's care checks that routine services have been received, temporary delays can become permanent gaps. That is why every child care program should set up a system to review the health records to be sure that the child's services are up to date and that staff members who need to know are informed about any health issues. If you have questions about how to check health records or whether a child is up to date with vaccines and other AAP-recommended preventive care services, seek help from your program's child care health consultant or the public health department.

Reviewing health records and tracking when the next services are due is a tedious task. While some software for child care programs includes a place to record limited health data, such as vaccines, most reminder systems built into commercially available software require that teachers determine and enter the next date when the record needs new data. You can set up an index card system that accomplishes the same purpose, filing an index card with the child's name and the next service due chronologically. However, the schedules are so complicated that it is a job best done by software using a computer.

To help reduce the burden on early educators for checking child health records, the Pennsylvania Chapter of the AAP established and maintains an internet application called WellCareTracker™. This low-cost application stores and tests routine checkup data for up-to-date status and requires a secure, privacy-protected password. It requires no special software, only a connection to the internet, and most users learn how to navigate WellCareTracker™ efficiently within their first hour of entering data.

Users can enter the child's information into WellCareTracker™ within one to four minutes, depending on how many health services the child has received. The application then provides a color-highlighted report that shows for which services the child is overdue, is due now, or will be due in three months. The user can generate aggregate reports that list the status of all the children in the center and can produce letters to give to families and health care providers. A pediatrician who is also a software engineer updates this system whenever the recommendations for routine services change. Go to **www.wellcaretracker.org** to learn more about this useful tool, including the cost of a subscription to pay for maintenance, and to view a demonstration.

With parental consent, both the administrator and staff members who work with the child and family should be familiar with the information in the health record. It is easy to assume that a child who appears healthy has no health needs. However, if staff members do not know that a child is allergic to bee stings, they could face a shocking and life-threatening emergency if the child is stung. If staff members know that a child has had an extended hospitalization early in life, they may observe the child more closely to determine whether she should receive extra support to achieve developmental progress and to overcome separation difficulties and reluctance to become attached to staff members.

In addition to the documentation of the child's health assessment results, the report from the health care provider should include a care plan for any child with special needs. If the care plan for accommodation of special needs is not available at enrollment, then a written plan should be prepared to cover the first two weeks of enrollment while the child's health care professional prepares a more definitive care plan. The facility should have and follow a procedure to review the information on the health record that identifies gaps in service or a need to adapt the child's care. Children must be healthy to be ready to learn.

Children who are up to date do not need a special visit to the health care provider just because the child is enrolling in an early care and education program. Their parents need only obtain the information from their child's health care provider about the services the child has received so the program can check that record against the nationally recommended schedule of services and make sure the program has sufficient information and staff training to address any special needs the child has. For those children who are due or overdue for routine health care, it may take some weeks to get an appointment. If catch-up vaccines are needed, the process may take a matter of months while the child continues to be enrolled in the program. If the child has a special health need, it is not safe to enroll the child without information from the child's health care provider. Teachers must be supportive and persistent to be sure families follow through as quickly and efficiently as possible. When families have been allowed conditional enrollment, it may be difficult to exclude those who are not following through.

Staff members must learn how to address specific special needs. For instance, allergies and asthma are very common in early childhood. If you have a child with allergies or asthma in your program, review the history of treatment and current medications and know when the child is due for the next follow-up visit to the health care provider. Recommendations might change at health visits. Read about asthma and allergy triggers and signs of distress. Ask the parents how the child responds best during an asthma episode or allergic reaction. Ask your health consultant or the child's health provider to give you appropriate information about what you need to know, watch for, and do to prevent and manage an asthma episode or allergic reaction. Let the family and the child's health care provider know about any changes in the child's condition or response to possible triggers. With adequate information, you become part of the child's health team, helping the family and the child manage the situation with confidence.

Health record contents

The health record (or related files) should contain at least the following information:

- Telephone numbers where parents or guardians and at least two emergency contacts can be reached at all times (see *Caring for Our Children* Appendix KK for a sample form)
- Name of the child's regular source of health care (medical home) and any other usual sources of health care, including the name of a specific contact person, address, and telephone number
- Child's preadmission medical examination/health assessment and subsequent updates at each checkup, including immunization status
- Developmental health history (physical and developmental milestones and significant events)
- Results of all screenings and assessments
- Notations about allergies, special diet, chronic illness, or other special health concerns
- Emergency permission for medical care
- All permission slips authorizing nonemergency health care and giving of medications
- Reports of all injuries or illnesses that occur while the child is in the program. (See Figure A.6 in Appendix A.)
- Medication logs
- Reports of referrals and follow-up action
- Notes about any health communication with family or health providers
- Written correspondence about the child's health
- Health observations from staff members

Confidentiality

Confidentiality of health records must be maintained to protect the child and family. *Caring for Our Children* Standard 9.4.1.3 requires facilities to have and implement a written policy on confidentiality of staff and child records. The policy must ensure no disclosure of material in the records (including conference reports, service plans, immunization records, and follow-up reports) without the written consent of parents or guardians for children, or of staff members for themselves. Such consent must specify to whom the information may be disclosed. No discussion or sharing of confidential information should be allowed beyond the limits of the consent. Standard 9.4.1.3 says,

> Consent forms should be in the native language of the parents/guardians, whenever possible, and communicated to them in their normal mode of communication. Foreign language interpreters should be used whenever possible to inform parents/guardians about their confidentiality rights. At the time when facilities obtain prior, informed consent from parents/guardians for release of records, caregivers/teachers should inform parents/guardians who may be looking at the records (e.g., child care health consultants, mental health consultants, and specialized agencies providing services).

Health care providers, but not schools, are required to comply with the requirements of the Health Insurance Portability and Accountability Act (HIPAA). The child's health care provider must have signed consent from the parents that specifies the requested information and to whom it is to be released. When a child care program wants to obtain information about an individual child from a health care provider, it is possible to obtain a form for this purpose from most health professionals' offices. Alternatively, the California Childcare Health Program, together with the Child Care Law Center, developed the Consent for Exchange of Information form, which teachers can download, complete, and have the parent sign. This form can then be sent to a health care provider to obtain health information. The California form is available at: **http://ucsfchildcare health.org/pdfs/forms/CForm_ExchangeofInfo.pdf**.

Early educators have ethical, and often legal, responsibility to maintain confidentiality. Follow these guidelines for confidentiality of records:

- Health records must be kept from public access and unauthorized review.
- Information may not be shared with anyone inside or outside the facility without parental review and consent.
- A telephone request for information from outside parties is not acceptable unless the parent has previously instructed you in writing to release information or gives/has given witnessed telephone consent. This is accomplished by having two people on the telephone with the parent at the same time who listen to the parent authorize release of the information, and then ask identifying questions of the parent to ensure it is the parent who is authorizing the release.
- Information collected by others and forwarded to you with parental consent becomes part of the child's record and thus the responsibility of the program.
- All releases of information should be properly logged.
- Families have a right to see all information in their child's file.
- Families must be made aware of the nature and type of all information collected and how it will be used.
- A family member may ask to speak to you in confidence, but you must receive this information in a responsible manner. This is particularly true if child abuse is suspected. Your primary responsibility is to protect the child.

Make communication with health care providers a two-way street

Each child's health care provider gathers information about the child's medical status, development, personality, and family strengths and needs. When it is appropriate for the benefit of the child's care, and with parental consent, the health care provider can share information with the child's other teachers. Likewise, health care providers can learn more about the child and the family from teachers' daily observations.

To encourage good communication, set up a routine for exchanging information with community health care providers. One system involves sending a copy of each child's periodic reports (always with parental permission) by mail, or hand-carried by parents, to the clinician to share the teacher's observations. The health data request from child care programs for reports from clinicians should request developmental information, specific types of data with relevant details on health issues, and a care plan for any special needs that require accommodation during the program day. Indicate how this information will be used for the child's benefit. Do not send a parent with a blank form with no identifying information about the child or the teacher requesting the information. Form completion is a burden for everyone, but you can indicate a commitment to share the burden by completing all known information before sending a form to the health care provider. Doing so is more likely to produce reciprocal communication.

The following are appropriate topics for communications between the child's health care provider and the child care program staff members:

- Identification of the child's medical home with contact information
- Developmental variations, sensory impairment, or disabilities that may need consideration in the child care setting
- Description of current physical, social, and language development levels
- Current medications
- Special concerns (e.g., allergies, chronic illness, and pediatric first aid information needs)
- Specific diet restrictions, if the child is on a special diet
- Individual characteristics or personality factors relevant to child care
- Special family considerations
- Dates of occurrence of communicable diseases

What if medical experts disagree?

Some recommendations about the health of young children in groups are relatively new, so some health care providers have not yet learned about them. Some approaches for care and treatment are controversial. Thus, one child's health care provider may give families recommendations that differ from the advice of another child's clinician. This can be confusing and frustrating. For example, the evidence-based recommendations are relatively new that children with conjunctivitis do not usually require antibiotics or exclusion from child care or that children who have been treated for lice do not need to be nit-free to return to child care. One health care provider may tell you the now-obsolete recommendation about these situations while another is aware of the changes. When you receive conflicting opinions, follow this procedure:

1. Ask your health consultant to broker differences of opinion for you. Work with the consultant to weigh the facts and rationale for determining what to do, and then make the best decision for your program.
2. If you have additional questions or conflicts (e.g., between your health consultant and a child's pediatrician), contact your local department of health or your state department of public health. They have the legal responsibility to make decisions about health issues for groups of people.

Communicating with families

Teachers and community human service professionals are partners with families to ensure children's optimum development. Families, who provide the continuity of care for children into adulthood, are the primary observers, advocates, and providers of services their children need. However valuable the intervention, all service providers play only temporary roles in the lives of children and their families. Parents need information about health and safety in programs before, during, and after the decision to enroll children in child care.

Communications should be respectful and interactive. Teachers must listen to what families want to do to protect their children's health and safety and determine what families understand (from whatever written or verbal information they have) about what the program requires and does for children. Families should be able to ask questions, express concerns, or suggest changes to improve the program. Teachers and families need to work together respectfully to handle differences of opinion as they arise.

Both teachers and parents of young children function under considerable daily stress. As professionals, teachers must be able to temporarily set aside their own concerns to see situations from the parents' perspective. For example, excluding children from child care puts a burden on families. Helping parents plan for the inevitable illnesses that require exclusion should be a routine pre-enrollment task. On the other hand, programs should not exclude mildly ill children who can participate without making demands on the staff that could pose a threat to the health and safety of other children or staff members.

The requirement to give the early care and education program health data stimulates families to seek the health care their children need—including services they may have overlooked. Having parents seek information from their child's health care provider may empower them to ask what they should learn from health professionals. On the other hand, asking parents to get notes from health professionals to certify children's wellness places an unfair burden on parents and on their relationship with their children's source of health care. To determine the well-being of the child, health care providers ask parents if the child seems well. They trust parents to know when their child is no longer acting sick. Except in the case of diseases that require a laboratory test to determine whether the child is contagious, teachers, too, should base their assessment of the child's readiness to return to child care on what the parent tells them about how the child is behaving.

For many families, child care staff members function as extended family. By reflecting on parental concerns and providing information about alternative approaches, teachers help families navigate their work and home lives more successfully. Communicating about health issues is one way teachers support families as the most important source of continuing care for children.

Just as teachers need to know from parents at the beginning of each day how the child feels and what, if any, problems to watch for, parents need to know similar information at the end of each day in child care. Illness tends to intensify in the evening, when everyone is tired and access to professional medical care is more difficult. When parents call a medical professional for advice, they will be asked how the child ate, drank, slept, behaved, voided, and defecated during the day. Teachers need to establish an effective, routine way to communicate this information to parents daily using oral or written messages. This may require being able to communicate in another language. Passing responsibility for a child from family to teachers and back again requires diligent attention to sharing key information that guides decisions if the child's status changes.

In addition to daily transfer of information about the child's status and routine sharing of information at checkup time, arranging communication among teachers, family, and the child's health care provider is essential whenever significant health concerns arise. This sharing enables competent care not only for the child about whom there is some concern, but also for other children and staff members who may be affected by their proximity to the child. Sometimes the situation may involve a family member's illness—as in a case of hepatitis A in an adult in the family of a child who seems well. This situation requires prompt medical intervention to protect the child, other children in the group, and staff members.

Suggested activities

- Contact the office manager or administrative staff members in the office of a local pediatrician, a public health clinic, and a family practice where some children who are enrolled in an early education program receive their health care. Ask what services are typically provided for a 3-year-old's well-care visit. Compare the responses with the AAP's recommended schedule of routine health services, the Bright Futures periodicity schedule. Are they the same? What might happen to a child who does not receive the recommended services?

- Check the state regulations for what teachers are required to document in children's health records. Compare this to the requirements in the Bright Futures periodicity schedule. Are the state requirements sufficient to ensure that children in child care are fully protected against vaccine-preventable disease and have no detectable disabilities that routine screening would uncover?

- Ask the state licensing agency what inspectors evaluate in health records when they visit child care programs. Are they checking that the documentation shows children are up to date for both immunizations and screening services? Are they selective about which ones they check, or do they check that the child care program gets information on all the currently recommended preventive health services for children in the Bright Futures periodicity schedule?

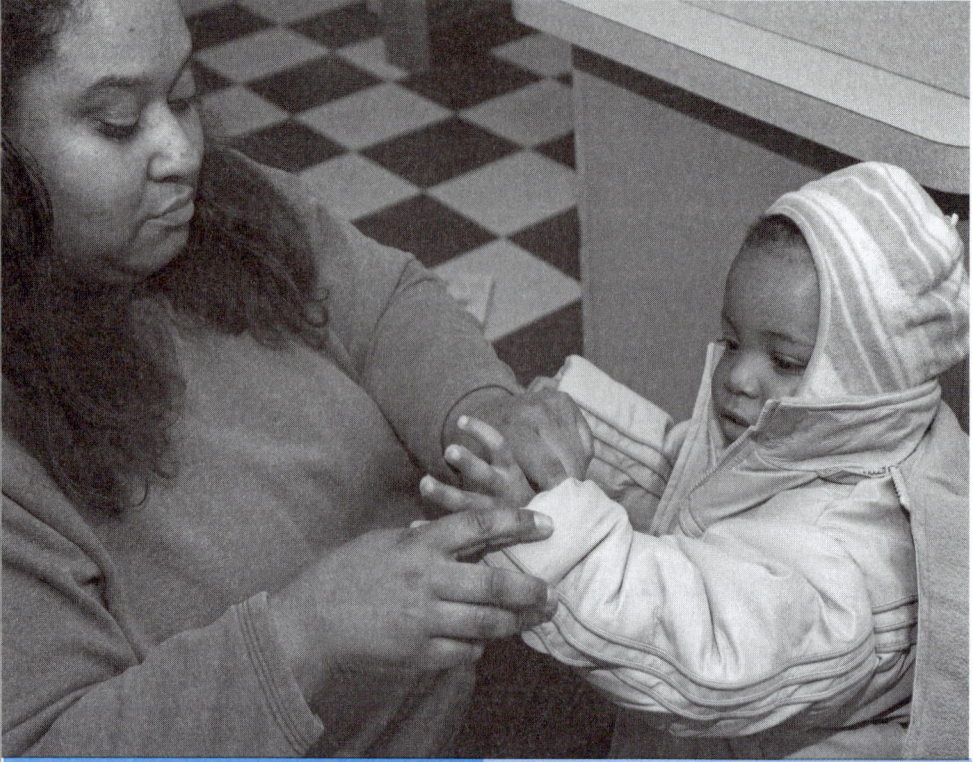

9

Staff Members and Consultants for Safe and Healthy Child Care

MAJOR CONCEPTS

- All staff members have responsibility for ensuring children's health and safety.
- Individual staff members have responsibilities related to their special task area, such as caregiving, nutrition, transportation, maintenance, or administration.
- A health advocate is an on-site staff member empowered to raise health and safety issues and ensure that health is integrated with the other components of the child care program.
- Health concerns play a key role in recruitment, selection, and retention of staff members.
- Paid and volunteer staff members need training to acquire the knowledge and skills to maintain a safe and healthy child care program.
- All early care and education providers should identify and work with a child care health consultant to improve health and safety in the program.

Ensuring health and safety is a basic responsibility of staff members and consultants who work in an early childhood program. Staff members should use best practices. These are described in written standards of nationally recognized organizations and agencies. You will find authoritative written health information on the websites of state and local public health agencies, the American Academy of Pediatrics (AAP), and the national organizations composed of oral health, mental health, and nutrition professionals with a pediatric focus.

Program responsibilities of all personnel

In the press of day-to-day operations, it is easy to overlook important elements of health and safety. Each facility needs written policies and procedures for orientation of new staff and families, routine self-evaluation by staff members, and evaluation by supervisors and peer reviewers. Self-study, such as that included in the NAEYC accreditation process, helps highlight areas in which the program may need to improve. Periodic observations and routine checks for hazards and risky practices in the facility help raise everyone's awareness of best practices and conditions that need to be changed.

Health and safety concerns in recruiting, selecting, and retaining staff members

Program advertisements and job descriptions that are shared with prospective and on-the-job workers should explicitly describe the attributes required for each role. For each role in early education, there are job-related health concerns. While disability laws preclude asking medical questions about a job applicant's health conditions or requiring a medical examination before making a job offer, an employer may specify physical and health requirements to perform a job and ask applicants how they would perform the required tasks with or without reasonable accommodation. If the job description specifies performance that is precluded by certain health conditions, the applicant should disclose this during the recruitment process.

Caring for Our Children Standard 1.7.0.1 lists activities typically required of caregivers:

a. Moving quickly to supervise and assist young children

b. Lifting children, equipment, and supplies

c. Sitting on the floor and on child-sized furniture

d. Washing hands frequently

e. Responding quickly in case of an emergency

f. Eating the same food as is served to the children (unless the staff member has dietary restrictions)

g. Hearing and seeing at a distance required for playground supervision or driving

h. Being absent from work for illness no more often than the typical adult, to provide continuity of caregiving relationships for children in child care

Some physical and mental health conditions would interfere with the formation of warm, positive relationships because they are associated with frequent absence from work for bouts of illness or with limitations that make the applicant unable to perform the tasks required for the job as specified in the job description. Under the Americans with Disabilities Act (ADA), employers are expected to accommodate people with disabilities, but they do not have to employ those who cannot fulfill the stipulated requirements in the job description with reasonable accommodation. For advice about specific situations, consult an ADA expert in one of the 10 regional Disability and Business Technical Assistance Centers funded by the U.S. Department of Education. Find your closest center by calling 1-800-949-4232, or to browse information available online, go to **http://adata.org**.

For more information about the disability laws, see the website of the Equal Employment Opportunity Commission. Pertinent information is available at **www.eeoc.gov/laws/**, **www.eeoc.gov/facts/jobapplicant.html**, and **www.eeoc.gov/policy/docs/factemployment_procedures.html**.

Directors and supervisors

In addition to ensuring they are up-to-date with their own training in health and safety, directors and supervisors have a special duty to orient and monitor all adults who are involved with the program—staff members, parents, and volunteers—in matters concerning health and safety performance. Preservice and inservice requirements must be met conscientiously. When family members assist, or when substitutes who are less familiar with health and safety routines work in the program, directors and supervisors must make special efforts to inform them and to ensure their appropriate performance.

While many health practices are common sense, some of the special precautions required for group care of children are not intuitive. For example, the extra attention paid to avoiding contamination during diaper-changing in group care settings is less critical in a child's own home; usually, only a few people share germs or can be made ill by germs from infected diapers in the home. In early childhood facilities, however, the group is larger. In addition to the children in the group, staff members and their families, as well as families of the children, can be exposed to illness unless all adults who work with children minimize the contamination of surfaces when changing diapers or soiled underwear.

Child care health consultants

Child care health consultants (CCHCs) are health professionals who consult with early educators. CCHCs can contribute expertise, leadership, and motivation to reach for quality in the program's health component. During site visits, they make observations, look at documents, and listen to the people who work in the program to assess strengths and identify hazards and risky practices that need to be improved. Then they collaborate with the program staff members and families to develop plans for change and provide health education. CCHCs bring knowledge of current recommendations and resources to the program for quality improvement. The role of the child care health consultant is discussed in more detail later in this chapter and in Section 1.6 of *Caring for Our Children*. The standards in this section define the role and expertise of child care health consultants, early childhood mental health consultants, early childhood education consultants, and specialized consultation for facilities serving children with disabilities.

Child care health advocates

In addition to having an ongoing relationship with a CCHC, each program should identify someone on the staff as a child care health advocate. The health advocate should be the center director, a lead teacher, social worker, health educator, health professional, or someone with a compatible role in the facility. The health advocate works in partnership with the CCHC to identify concerns and integrate best practices for health and safety into day-to-day operation of the program. The health advocate then works with co-workers to put into practice the advice of the CCHC. The health advocate should be someone who works at least part time in the day-to-day operations at the facility. The role requires spending some time focused on activities related to health and safety during the week. The health advocate should have a special interest in health, safety, nutrition, oral health, and mental (social-emotional-behavioral) health. While health advocates do not need to perform all health and safety activities, their job is to see that health and safety-related tasks are done or brought to the attention of those with the authority and skills to get them done. Very large centers may need more than one health advocate.

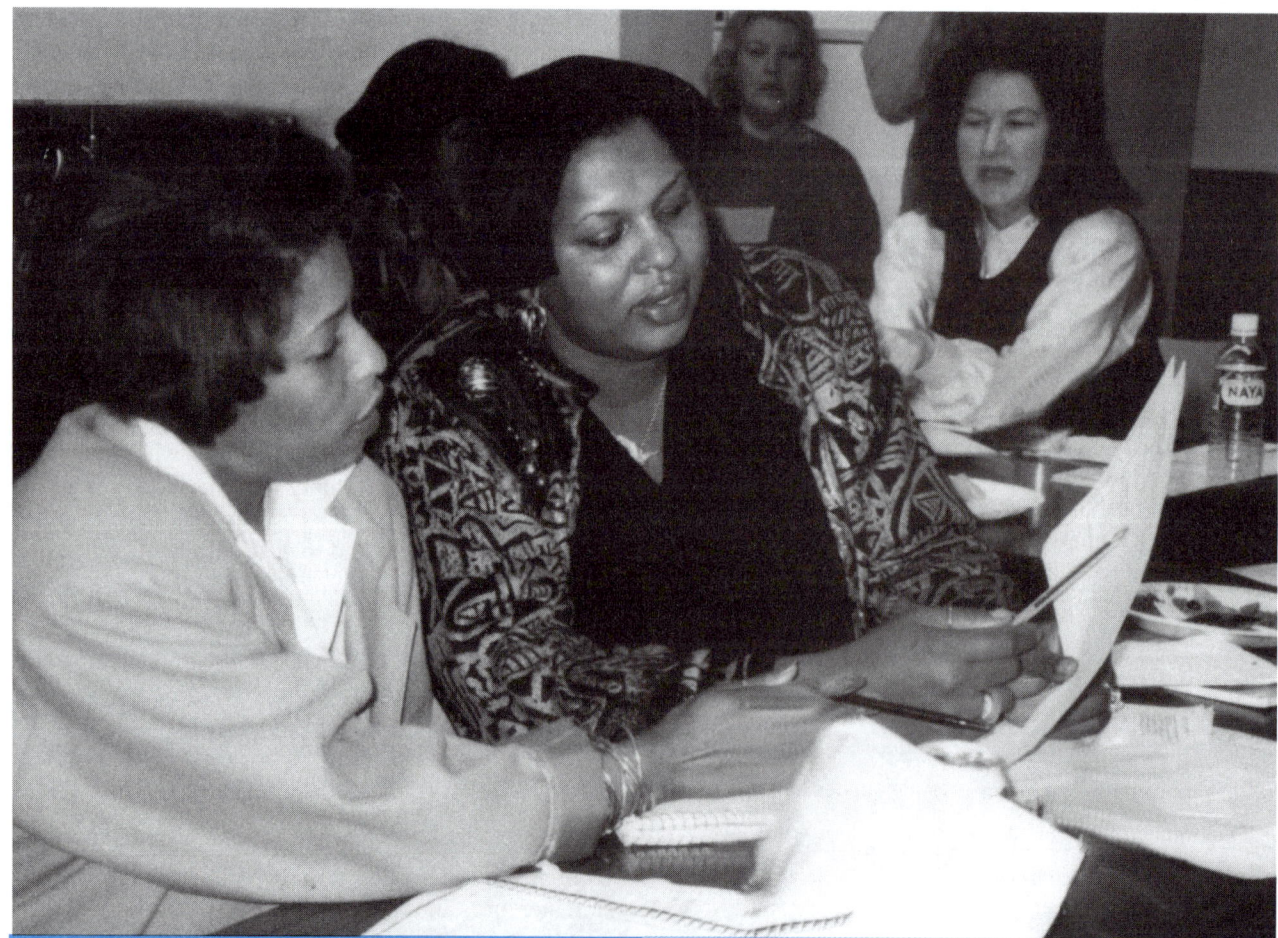

© Paula Jorde Bloom

Caring for Our Children Standard 1.3.2.7 states that the person who serves as the health advocate should receive documented training in the following areas:

a. Control of infectious diseases, including Standard Precautions, hand hygiene, cough and sneeze etiquette, and reporting requirements

b. Childhood immunization requirements, recordkeeping, and at least quarterly review and follow-up for children who need to have updated immunizations

c. Child health assessment form review and follow-up of children who need further medical assessment or updating of their information

d. How to plan for, recognize, and handle an emergency

e. Poison awareness and poison safety

f. Recognition of safety, hazards, and injury prevention interventions

g. Safe sleep practices and the reduction of the risk of Sudden Infant Death Syndrome (SIDS)

h. How to help parents/guardians, caregivers/teachers, and children cope with death, severe injury, and natural or man-made catastrophes

i. Recognition of child abuse, neglect/child maltreatment, shaken baby syndrome/abusive head trauma (for facilities caring for infants), and knowledge of when to report and to whom suspected abuse/neglect

j. Facilitate collaboration with families, primary care providers, and other health service providers to create a health, developmental, or behavioral care plan

k. Implementing care plans

l. Recognition and handling of acute health related situations such as seizures, respiratory distress, allergic reactions, as well as other conditions as dictated by the special health care needs of children

m. Medication administration

n. Recognizing and understanding the needs of children with serious behavior and mental health problems

o. Maintaining confidentiality

p. Healthy nutritional choices

q. The promotion of developmentally appropriate types and amounts of physical activity

r. How to work collaboratively with parents/guardians and family members

s. How to effectively seek, consult, utilize, and collaborate with child care health consultants, and in partnership with a child care health consultant; how to obtain information and support from other education, mental health, nutrition, physical activity, oral health, and social service consultants and resources

t. Knowledge of community resources to refer children and families who need health services including access to State Children's Health Insurance (SCHIP), importance of a primary care provider and medical home, and provision of immunizations and Early Periodic Screening, Diagnosis, and Treatment (EPSDT)

The program administrator should make sure that the health advocate has regular opportunities to report, review, discuss, and follow up on corrective action plans. In some programs, the director nominates the health advocate and then staff members confirm the appropriateness of that person's special (often supplemental) role. The California Childcare Health Program (CCHP) has a free online curriculum in English and Spanish that includes the basic information that the program's health advocate should know. The curriculum, *The California Training Institute Curriculum for Child Care Health Advocates,* is available at **www.ucsfchildcarehealth.org**. In some states, college-level courses are available to teach early educators to be child care health advocates. For more information about child care health advocates, see *Caring for Our Children* Standard 1.3.2.7 and the related rationale, references, and other standards listed there.

Teachers

While seeking teachers with a firm grounding in developmentally appropriate practice, administrators also must be aware of how physical and emotional health can influence job performance. For example, a teacher must hear well enough to distinguish the often difficult-to-understand speech of a young child. Someone with a hearing disability may not be able to foster language development effectively. A teacher must see well enough to read and must be literate to provide developmentally appropriate reading experiences to children. Teachers must be present on a consistent basis to establish trusted, caring relationships with the children. Teachers who have frequent illnesses and absences provide discontinuous and unpredictable care. All staff members must be able to perform frequent hand hygiene and handle the chemicals required for routine sanitizing and disinfecting of surfaces that become contaminated during daily activities. People with skin or respiratory conditions that preclude frequent handwashing and use of the chemicals required to sanitize and disinfect surfaces should not work as teachers for groups of young children. These and other related qualifications should be specified in the job description.

Teachers must be able to pick up infants and toddlers, model healthy eating practices for children, move quickly enough to intercede in a situation where a child is in danger, and evacuate children in an emergency. Unless the program can provide accommodations for these core performance expectations, the quality of care provided by the entire program will be diminished by adults who are unable to perform because of physical or mental health conditions. All of these requirements should be clearly communicated in the written job description so that recruitment and continued employment can relate to the requirements of the job without risk of discrimination against an individual who has a disability. For detailed requirements for recruitment, background screening, preservice orientation, and professional development activities for directors, teachers, teacher assistants, substitutes, volunteers, and health advocates, see the standards in Sections 1.2 through 1.5 of *Caring for Our Children*.

Food service personnel

While some personnel in an early care and education program have unique assignments, each person has a duty to ensure the health and safety of others in the facility. Usually, everyone in the facility is involved in some way in food handling. All staff members must be aware of safe food temperatures, techniques involved in safe food handling, hand hygiene procedures, sanitation of surfaces related to food, and so on. Of course, food service staff members need to know more about food safety and sanitation than other staff members.

People who have never done quantity cooking are unlikely to have the necessary knowledge and skills to plan and prepare food in a way that prevents food poisoning and provides good nutrition. Preparing food for children is also different from cooking in a restaurant. These skills must be learned and practiced under supervision for the individual to work effectively in the child care setting. Food service workers should not have personal health issues such as skin conditions, food or nasal allergies, chronic cough, or gastrointestinal symptoms that increase the risk of their contact with or transfer of their body fluids to food.

Maintenance staff

Maintenance workers should have an appreciation for how the program operates. Even if they do their work after the children and staff members leave the building for the evening, they need to know where children eat, crawl on the floor, have their diapers changed, play with manipulative materials, and so on to give these areas appropriate attention. While written agreements should specify products to use and procedures that maintenance workers are to follow, their work must be monitored by the director or someone the director designates. This should be done whether the maintenance workers are employed directly or by contract with a maintenance service company. The focus of the monitoring is to ensure that they are using the least toxic products that do the required task, that children are protected from contact with any toxic residues, and that the maintenance workers are following appropriate procedures. When these activities occur after everyone has left the building, the director must arrange to review the products the maintenance workers are using and make unannounced observations of what they do.

Maintenance staff must provide the level of service required for sanitation and safety in child care settings. Cleaning of such facilities requires more attention from directors and other staff members to the maintenance worker's performance than does cleaning of office spaces. After cleaning, some surfaces require a separate rinse and sanitizing step. Tables, chairs, other child equipment, floors, doorknobs, toilet rooms, and diapering areas all require special attention. Maintenance staff should be able to safely handle cleaning chemicals, using gloves as necessary. Those who have severe skin, respiratory, or musculoskeletal problems that limit their ability to perform required tasks or make them prone to injury or illness from doing maintenance work should be counseled or otherwise helped to seek a different type of job. Maintenance staff must be able to make prompt repairs, remove broken equipment, or provide barriers to keep children away from hazards that cannot be fixed right away. The requirement for being able to perform these tasks should be in their written job description.

Transportation staff

All staff members should know and use routines to practice passenger and pedestrian safety. Drivers and teachers must be sure children are properly using seat restraints, know how to load and unload passengers safely, count children going into and leaving vehicles, and check all hidden spaces to be sure that all the children are out of the vehicle at the end of the ride. Drivers also need to know about vehicle maintenance and emergency procedures for breakdowns. All staff members involved in transportation should be skilled in pediatric first aid in the event of a mishap. While drivers may not be skilled teachers, they should be developmentally appropriate in their interactions with children.

Drivers must have normal hearing and vision as well as the skills to drive whatever vehicle is being used. They must be mature, capable of making wise decisions in unexpected situations, and tolerant and supportive of age-appropriate behavior of children in their vehicles. Early education programs must be certain that drivers are not using medications or other substances that could affect driving. *Caring for Our Children* Standard 6.5.1.1 specifies the competence and training for transportation staff.

Health assessments of staff members and volunteers

The foundation for adult health in child care is the requirement that all adults (staff members and volunteers) who work or have accepted a job offer to work in the program have a preservice health exam and ongoing exams thereafter. The purpose of the health assessment is to identify any conditions that would interfere with the person's ability to function in a specific role and any reasonable accommodations that are needed to allow that person to meet the requirements for that position. Subsequent health assessments should take place according to the recommendations of the individual's health care provider or when a concern about job performance indicates a need to reassess the individual. The results of such exams are strictly confidential and can be given to the employer only with the staff member's permission. However, sharing confidential job-related health information should be a condition of working in a child care setting.

The program should specify the following elements for occupational health examinations:

- According to *Caring for Our Children* Standard 1.7.0.1, the content of the exam should include such items as
  - A review of the individual's health history related to the performance of the intended role in child care
  - A physical examination, including an assessment of oral health
  - A review and update of vaccines recommended for adults who have contact with children, including Tdap and annual influenza vaccine
  - Vision and hearing screening
  - The results and appropriate follow up of a tuberculosis (TB) screening done once upon entering the child care field and again as determined by exposure or symptoms that suggest a risk for TB

- The professional who can perform the exam should be a licensed physician, nurse practitioner, or physician's assistant.

- The exams should occur before first contact with children, periodically as recommended by the adult's health care provider, when the person's role changes in the program to include new types of duties, and to obtain a health care provider's release to return to work in the following situations specified in *Caring for Our Children* Standard 1.7.0.3:
  a. When they have experienced conditions that may affect their ability to do their job or require an accommodation to prevent illness or injury in child care work related to their conditions (such as pregnancy, specific injuries, or infectious diseases)
  b. After serious or prolonged illness
  c. When their condition or health could affect promotion or reassignment to another role
  d. Before return from a job-related injury
  e. If there are workers' compensation issues or if the facility is at risk of liability related to the employee's or volunteer's health problem

- Special assessments should be required for specific roles, such as teachers and food service personnel

- Who receives and reviews the findings
- Who pays for the exam

For examinations to be effective, the health professional conducting the exam must know the nature and demands of the adult's job. For instance, a chronic lower back problem may not be as critical to the job performance of a social worker as to the teacher of a toddler group. A sample adult health assessment form appears in both *Model Child Care Health Policies* and Appendix E of *Caring for Our Children*.

Ideally, the results of a health exam should be received *before the person has contact with the children*. It is hard to deal with health concerns after an individual has begun to develop relationships or after the children and others have already been exposed to illness or disease. Of course, new health problems may develop after employment. This is why it is important for staff members to have both routine exams as recommended by each adult's health care provider and exams when health problems that interfere with the person's performance of the job requirements are suspected. Reasonable efforts should be made to accommodate an otherwise qualified worker. However, everyone involved needs to understand that some health problems are incompatible with the requirements of a particular job.

The content of adult health assessments for child care work is based on the requirements for job performance and risk. Here are three examples:

- Tuberculosis (TB) screening using the tuberculin skin test (TST) or IGRA (interferon gamma release assay) needs to be done only once before entry into the child care field. Subsequent TB screening depends on the individual's history of high risk for TB, but is not routine for those who do not meet the high-risk criteria of the Centers for Disease Control and Prevention (CDC). Generally, repeated skin testing is required for those who are at high risk because they are foreign-born; have HIV; have chronic cough that could be from TB; engage in foreign travel; have been homeless; or have had contact with homeless people, prison populations, or individuals with active TB. All adults who live in a family child care home who are considered at high risk for TB must have TB screening also.

- Because of the high risk for spread of influenza and pertussis (whooping cough) for those who are involved with the care of young children, all adults in child care should have annual influenza vaccine and should have received Tdap (tetanus–diphtheria–acellular pertussis vaccine). A few staff members may have medical reasons for not receiving certain vaccines. The risk of their exposure and of exposing others to the diseases that the vaccine would prevent must be carefully considered.

- Women of childbearing age or those anticipating pregnancy should discuss with an obstetrician their potential risk of exposure to chickenpox, cytomegalovirus (CMV), and parvovirus (fifth disease). These childhood infections can cause significant problems for the fetus of a pregnant woman who is not immune to them.

Since many early education teachers lack health benefits and earn minimum wage, the cost of health exams can be a problem. Even for those with health insurance, hepatitis B immunization to meet Occupational Safety and Health Administration (OSHA) requirements may not be covered. Ideally, programs should offer arrangements for health insurance for their workers. For valued workers, child care budgets may have to stretch to cover the cost of health services required, such as immunizations and health exams. Otherwise, the adult must be required to pay for these services as a condition for working in child care.

Preservice and inservice training

The program should arrange training for staff members to fill any identified gaps in performance or background. (See Figure 9.1.) The topics to be covered are broad in scope. For example, *Caring for Our Children* Standard 1.4.1.1 says that preservice training should include 30 hours of professional development that covers health, psychosocial, and safety issues in out-of-home group care. The specific topics include

- Child development focused on the ages of children the adult will have in care
- Support of children's developmental progress
- Guidance and discipline
- Relationships with families
- Resources for support services for individual developmental needs
- Procedures to prevent the spread of infectious disease
- Role modeling, as well as environmental measures to prevent infection and injury
- Management of common illnesses
- Occupational health and safety practices
- Procedures for emergencies and threatening situations
- First aid, including CPR for infants and children
- Recognition of child abuse
- Nutrition, including food preparation and age-appropriate feeding
- Physical activity requirements for children
- Care for children with special needs (such as medication administration)
- Health promotion measures

Teaching adult learners may involve small- and large-group discussion and activities, assigned reading, oral review of material, and demonstration of expected skills. The AAP and NAEYC publish videos consistent with *Caring for Our Children* that illustrate how to meet the standards in centers and family child care homes. These videos can be viewed independently by prospective staff members for orientation but are most effectively used as triggers for interactive training sessions. Training may also be obtained from qualified personnel of children's and community hospitals, managed care companies, health agencies, public health departments, pediatric emergency room physicians, or other health professionals in the community. For more information about training opportunities, contact the AAP Healthy Child Care America Project, the National Resource Center for Health and Safety in Child Care, or the National Training Institute for Child Care Health Consultants. For trusted internet links to helpful sources of health information and resources, go to **www.healthfinder.gov** or the website of ECELS-Healthy Child Care PA at **www.ecels-healthychildcarepa.org**.

Figure 9.1.

Caring for Our Children Training Standards

Caring for Our Children provides detailed requirements for preservice and inservice training in the following standards:

1.4.1.1 Preservice Training

1.4.2.1 Initial Orientation of All Staff

1.4.2.2 Orientation for Care of Children with Special Health Care Needs

1.4.2.3 Orientation Topics

1.4.3.1 First Aid and CPR Training for Staff

1.4.3.2 Topics Covered in First Aid Training

1.4.3.3 CPR Training for Swimming and Water Play

1.4.4.1 Continuing Education for Directors and Caregivers/Teachers in Centers and Large Family Child Care Homes

1.4.5.1 Training of Staff Who Handle Food

1.4.5.2 Child Abuse and Neglect Education

1.4.5.3 Training on Occupational Risk Related to Handling Body Fluids

1.4.5.4 Education of Center Staff

1.4.6.1 Training Time and Professional Development Leave

1.4.6.2 Payment for Continuing Education

Health issues related to staff and child turnover

Aside from the obvious emotional benefits of low turnover among the adults and children involved with the program, there are health benefits, too. High turnover constantly introduces new infections. New children and staff members may not be immune to the illness-causing germs carried by people already present in the facility and may become sick more often. Children who leave the program to go to another facility take with them the germs that can cause illness to which they may have developed immunity. Research has shown that when children move from one care site to another, disease spreads across the community. The risk of injury also is affected by turnover. The risk of injury increases until new staff members learn and routinely practice safety measures. Through training and working with co-workers as a team to implement safety routines over a period of time, child care programs can reduce injury risks.

Preventing unnecessary turnover of children requires quality programming that satisfies the needs of children and families. When a program does not provide care during the hours of operation or for the number of days per week needed by families, parents usually seek supplemental wraparound care elsewhere in the community. If children have multiple sources of care over the course of a week or month, these various facilities share a common pool of germs that can cause infectious diseases.

Staff turnover is widespread and difficult to solve. Much of the problem is due to inadequate compensation and lack of benefits for workers in early education and care programs. Sometimes the problem is made worse by difficult working conditions. When advocating for worthy wages for teachers, include the health impact of turnover in your list of arguments for better financing of early childhood programs. The fact that turnover poses disease risks for children and all others in the community may persuade those who do not understand the value of continuous, warm, interactive relationships to support quality early education and care. If your program experiences an unusual level of turnover despite paying wages comparable to those paid by other providers in the area, consider possible causes and solutions.

With large numbers of adults and children arriving and leaving throughout a typical day, programs enrolling 50 or more children or operating more than 10 hours a day appear to be at greater risk for spreading infectious diseases. Such centers should be particularly careful about preventive health routines. Grouping children together in the facility so that one group does not interact with other groups helps reduce the spread of infection. Frequently, providers mix one group of children with another. Many programs mix children from multiple groups when they arrive early or depart late to reduce the number of staff members needed while retaining good ratios. While practical, this mixing of groups fosters the spread of disease across the groups in the facility. Best practice is to separate groups as much as possible at all times of the day, even if it requires more staff at the beginning and end of the day. When the benefits to intermingling groups outweigh the health risks, be sure everyone practices hand hygiene before and after intermingling occurs. Do not allow children to intermingle who have an illness that involves body fluid discharges (e.g., runny nose, eye discharge, coughing, and diarrhea).

When infectious disease is on the rise, programs should be even more vigilant than usual about keeping children within their own groups. Do not admit new children into your program during an outbreak of a serious infectious disease such as hepatitis A. With your health consultant or the advice of the public health department, decide on an appropriate waiting period before allowing new admissions. At all times, but especially during outbreaks, minimize contact and shared use of facilities by children in diapers with older children. Such mixed-age grouping offers developmental learning opportunities but poses special challenges for control of infection. When mixed age-grouping is practiced, staff members must be extra vigilant about following hygiene and surface sanitation procedures.

If you can, avoid having staff members care for different groups of children during the same day. Moving staff members between groups during the day promotes the spread of disease. If this is unavoidable, ensure that staff members who work with more than one group perform good hand hygiene procedures, and consider having them wear a smock that they can change when moving from group to group.

Adult health needs— Occupational risks

Staff members are key contributors to a good program for young children. Most are concerned about personal illness risks, but few recognize specific potential health hazards in their workplace. These hazards include an increased risk of contracting illnesses; exposure to toxic chemicals in art supplies, cleaning agents, and pesticides; back injuries due to frequent heavy lifting and stooping; poor lighting that increases the risk of injury; high noise levels that affect hearing and stress; clutter that affects cleanliness and safety; and job stress in general.

Committed teachers may ignore their own health needs because they lack health benefits and time off and because they feel responsible for meeting children's needs first. Programs can alleviate some of these concerns by doing the following:

Figure 9.2.

Wise Moves to Avoid Injury in Child Care

Challenge	Wise Moves
Lifting children, toys, supplies	Avoid lifting by having children climb steps with help. Pull child or object to be lifted as close as possible directly in front of you; squat and wrap your arms around whatever you are lifting, then tighten stomach muscles and use thigh muscles to raise yourself and your load. Lower objects and children by sliding them down your body to a level where you can squat or kneel to lower whatever you are putting down to its destination.
Inadequate work heights	Reorganize to store frequently used objects where you can reach them easily. Store heavy objects at waist height so you don't have to lift them. Adjust diapering and similar work surfaces to waist height; use adult-sized chairs whenever you can; squat or kneel on a kneepad if you can't sit down next to children to help. Use step stools to reach high places.
Lifting infants in and out of cribs	Do not use cribs with floor-level mattresses. When lifting a child from a crib, get you and the child as close to the crib side as possible before you lift.
Frequent sitting on the floor without back support	When possible, sit against a wall or furniture that supports your back. Sit with a little pillow in the small of your back when you can. Stretch when you get up.
Carrying heavy objects or children	Use carts and strollers. Let children climb up with a step stool. If possible, divide heavy loads into several smaller loads and use carts that can be slid under the load and then tilt the load onto the cart.
Awkward posture to open windows or adjust objects	Move objects away from the window to get as close as possible to it. Put one foot on a step stool for better leverage. Lubricate the window mechanism to make opening it easier. Ask for help from a coworker when the job is hard.
Sweeping/picking up crumbs and small toys from the floor	Use a long-handled dustpan and broom. Keep a separate one for toys (clean) and things going into the trash.
Caring for children with special needs	Get specific training from the child's physical therapist about how to move and carry the child.
Caring for children during active play when sudden moves are needed	Avoid twisting. Practice turning and bending to intercept a running or falling child so the move becomes natural. Bend knees when pushing children in swings. Use good body mechanics to help children on and off equipment.

Source: Adapted, by permission, from A.M. Wortman, "Preventing Work-Related Musculoskeletal Injuries," *Exchange* 140 (July/August 2001): 50–53.

- Promoting adult health as a part of program operations
- Creating a positive, healthful environment for adults
- Helping adults to look after their own health needs
- Providing an adequate benefits package for health care and sick leave

Ways to promote good adult health

Staff members must care for themselves to be able to provide the best care for children. Take the time to look at your environment and program demands. How can you make staff members more comfortable? Does the schedule and coverage provide a long enough break for staff to take a walk to relieve stress and relax? What policies need to be revised to meet adult needs? Are you encouraging good health for yourself and others? Can sick adults stay home without guilt or loss of pay?

When staff members and administration work together, it is possible to adjust a facility and program to the needs of the adults and the children. Here are some examples of solutions to adult health issues. (Also see Figure 9.2.):

- Require initial and ongoing health assessments to identify individual susceptibility to the known occupational risks of early childhood programs (e.g., infectious diseases, back injuries, rashes, stress, environmental exposures).
- Negotiate flexible benefits packages to meet staff needs, including paid leave (annual, sick, and/or personal), medical insurance, and other options.
- Provide high counters with stools, or an adult-size table and chairs, for staff members who do clerical, administrative, or curriculum planning work. Bring in adult-size folding chairs for staff meetings. Place a telephone book on a child-size chair to make it a more comfortable seat.
- Set aside private adult space and provide adequate numbers of substitute staff members to ensure that staff members take breaks to alleviate stress.
- Include staff break time and substitute plans in personnel policies.
- Teach staff members proper techniques for lifting and bending to prevent leg and back strain. (See Figure 9.3.)
- Provide gloves to use with cleaning agents to prevent skin irritation.
- Establish preventive health policies to reduce exposure to childhood illnesses.
- Practice preventive procedures to help keep adults and children healthy.

> **Special Safeguards for Pregnant Women**
>
> Female staff members of childbearing age should be aware that they can be exposed to infectious diseases that can cause significant health problems for a fetus. These infections include rubella, measles, mumps, varicella (chickenpox), hepatitis B, cytomegalovirus, herpes, parvovirus (fifth disease), and HIV infection. Women of childbearing age should discuss these risks with their health care provider. Some of these infections are a risk to the fetus only if the woman did not have the disease in childhood or receive an immunization.

Infectious disease risks for adults

Infectious diseases are common in groups of young children, but most are not serious and would probably spread at a similar rate in a large family. However, because staff members care for a number of young children from different families, many of whom cannot control their body fluids and have not yet learned principles of hygiene, infections can spread to many other employees, children, family members, and—in the case of a pregnant employee or parent—to a fetus. Therefore, all employees need to be familiar with common infections and related prevention measures. The two most important barriers to the spread of infection are immunization and hygiene, especially proper use of handwashing and alcohol-based hand sanitizers. (See Chapter 2 for details.)

OSHA requires that workers in early childhood programs whose activities might expose them to other individuals' blood or body fluids should be offered hepatitis B vaccine within 10 days of starting a job. Any unimmunized employee must be offered gamma globulin and hepatitis B vaccine immediately following a blood exposure.

All staff members should receive training in how to handle blood and other body fluids. (See Figure 2.7 in Chapter 2.) OSHA requirements apply to blood spills, but Standard Precautions cover the exposure that can occur from contact with any body fluid. The specific procedures to follow in these situations are detailed in Chapter 2 of this book, in *Caring for Our Children,* and in *Managing Infectious Diseases in Child Care and Schools* (available from the AAP).

When not to come to work

Children inevitably catch colds and flu. Most will have a bout of diarrhea once a year. Adults working daily with young children are also likely to become ill. Adults need to notify their supervisor immediately about any injuries or illnesses they experience, especially those

Figure 9.3.

Protect Your Back

Most back pain is not the result of a single injury. Even though pain may be felt suddenly, the problem is almost always due to a combination of several factors, including poor posture, faulty body mechanics, stressful living or work habits, loss of flexibility, and a general decline of physical fitness. Back pain can be prevented by improving posture and body mechanics, organizing the ergonomic set-up of the workplace, and exercising regularly to improve flexibility and general fitness.

POSTURE
Having a firm, flattened abdomen and holding your stomach in when you stand and sit provide needed support for the lower spine.

SITTING
When you sit, maintain a normal spine curve. Sitting produces greater loads on the lower back than either standing or walking. Select a chair with a firm seat and adequate lower back support. Keeping your knees bent and resting your back against the chair prevents back strain. Don't sit too long; occasionally get up, stretch, and walk around.

DRIVING
When driving a car, move the seat forward to keep the knees higher than the hips. A small pillow or towel rolled behind the lower back provides extra support.

STANDING AND BENDING
Standing can be hard on your back. Try not to work for long periods in a bent-over position. Muscles and good posture help keep the spine in a balanced, neutral position. Abdominal muscles pull up in front and buttock muscles pull down in back to maintain the natural curve of the spine, allowing you to hold a balanced standing posture for long periods without tiring. Another technique is to stand with one foot elevated to a comfortable level. Switch feet every so often.

SLEEPING
Sleeping rests the back. When you are lying down, your back doesn't have to support your body weight. It is important to use a firm mattress. Sleep on your side with knees bent or on your back with knees elevated.

LIFTING TECHNIQUES
Everyone has a lifting technique that seems most comfortable. But there are basic rules that apply to all. These rules will help control and prevent back pain.

- Step up close to your work area or to a load. Don't overreach to grasp or lift.
- Get a firm footing. Keep your feet parted: one alongside, one behind the object.
- Grip the object with the whole hand. Get a firm grip with the palms of your hands because the palms are stronger than the fingers alone.
- Draw the object close to you, with arms and elbows tucked into the sides of your body to keep your body weight centered.
- Bend knees, lift with your legs—let your powerful leg muscles do the work of lifting, not your weaker back muscles.
- Avoid lifting above the waist, but if you must, reposition your grip to keep the weight centered. Arching your back during a lift makes nerve roots susceptible to pinching and can cause weak muscles to be strained.
- Twisting during a lift is a common cause of back injury. If you have to turn with a load, change the position of your feet. By simply turning the forward foot out and pointing it in the direction you intend to move, the greatest danger of injury by twisting is avoided.

MOVING
Use the suggestions in Figure 9.2. to avoid injury while doing child care work. For a week or two, think about each move before you make it. Moving to avoid injury soon becomes a habit.

Source: Adapted, by permission, from the National Safety Council.

---

that might affect their health or the health and safety of the children. Sometimes, because of the difficulty of arranging for and keeping dependable substitutes or because of inadequate sick leave policies, adults believe it is their responsibility to show up or to stay at work when ill. No ill employee or volunteer should be required to stay at work; supervisors must insist that an ill employee go home. It is the responsibility of the administration, not the ill or injured staff member, to arrange for a substitute provider. The supervisor will need to make staff adjustments to cover the duties of an adult whose ability to function is impaired. Someone in the facility should have responsibility for observing adults (staff members and volunteers) every day for any sign of ill health so these individuals can receive the support they need to go home.

The guidelines for exclusion of children who have infections that pose a risk to others apply equally to adults who work in early education and care programs. Staff members and volunteers should not come to work when they cannot participate in the program at the level they would normally or if they have a disease that poses a risk to others in the group care setting.

Caring for Our Children Standard 3.6.1.2 lists the conditions for which a staff member should be excluded unless that staff member does not have contact with the children or anything with which the children come into contact.

The staff member should be excluded as follows:

a. Chickenpox, until all lesions have dried and crusted, which usually occurs by six days

b. Shingles, only if the lesions cannot be covered by clothing or a dressing until the lesions have crusted

c. Rash with fever or joint pain, until diagnosed not to be measles or rubella

d. Measles, until four days after onset of the rash (if the staff member or substitute is immunocompetent)

e. Rubella, until six days after onset of rash

f. Diarrheal illness, stool frequency exceeds two or more stools above normal for that individual or blood in stools, until diarrhea resolves; if *E. coli* 0157:H7 or *Shigella* is isolated, until diarrhea resolves and two stool cultures are negative; for *Salmonella* serotype Typhi, three [negative] stool cultures collected at twenty-four hour intervals and resolution of diarrhea is required

g. Vomiting illness, two or more episodes of vomiting during the previous twenty-four hours, until vomiting resolves or is determined to result from non-infectious conditions

h. Hepatitis A virus, until one week after symptom onset or as directed by the health department

i. Pertussis, until after five days of appropriate antibiotic therapy

j. Skin infection (such as impetigo), until treatment has been initiated; exclusion should continue if lesion is draining AND cannot be covered

k. Tuberculosis, until noninfectious and cleared by a health department official or a primary care provider

l. Strep throat or other streptococcal infection, until twenty-four hours after initial antibiotic treatment and end of fever

m. Head lice, from the end of the day of discovery until after the first treatment

n. Scabies, until after treatment has been completed

o. *Haemophilus influenzae* type b (Hib), prophylaxis, until antibiotic treatment has been initiated

p. Meningococcal infection, until appropriate therapy has been administered for twenty-four hours

q. Respiratory illness, if the illness limits the staff member's ability to provide an acceptable level of child care and compromises the health and safety of the children

Caregivers/teachers who have herpes cold sores should not be excluded from the child care facility, but should

a. Cover and not touch their lesions

b. Carefully observe hand hygiene policies

If a staff member's or volunteer's condition is an ongoing one that could affect her ability to do her job or require an accommodation to prevent illness or injury to others, the individual should be required to have a health professional's note indicating any needed accommodations or limitations to return to work. For example, a pregnant employee who is not immune to infections that are commonly found in group care settings and could damage the fetus might need to be reassigned from an infant/toddler group to other work. Someone with a back injury might hurt himself again if he has to lift children or objects. A teacher or food handler who had bacterial diarrhea might need to have negative cultures before returning to work.

Substitutes

Even though creating a reliable substitute policy can be challenging, substitute coverage is critical to a well-run program. Here are some suggested policies and procedures:

- Consider hiring a flexibly scheduled, part-time permanent substitute or joining with other programs to hire rotating substitutes. This allows each program some guaranteed coverage and provides dependable employment for the substitute. Even when nobody is absent, a sub can fill in while regular staff members take breaks or attend parent conferences, planning sessions, or other meetings.

- Set an appropriate salary for substitutes.

- Regularly evaluate your substitute procedure to see if it needs to be updated, and keep the substitute list active.

- Call substitutes periodically to make sure they are still available.

- Let parents know about the procedure for using substitutes.

Breaks

Due to the cost of hiring additional staff members, most programs accommodate staff breaks by shifting assignments among regular personnel. Remember that whenever staff members enter or leave an area occupied by a group of children, they should perform hand hygiene. Here are some suggestions for arranging breaks:

- Nonteaching staff members can cover breaks on different days of the week.

- Assign family members, students, and community volunteers as floaters who can work with a regular member of the staff while a co-worker takes a break. The key to making this plan work is regular scheduling and dependable volunteers. Volunteers should receive a thorough orientation to their duties and have the same monitoring skills and health responsibilities as regular staff members. (Be sure to monitor their hand hygiene for proper handwashing or use of an alcohol-based hand sanitizer.) In a well staffed program, one volunteer is designated as a floater during break time for a week at a time. This person can become familiar with each classroom and also gain perspective on the program. Again, before moving to a new group, this person must perform careful hand hygiene and may need to put on a clean smock or some other overgarment to reduce the risk of spreading infection.

- Overlap staff shifts. Afternoon shifts, for example, can begin during the last half hour of the morning shift of the person they are replacing. The other teacher with the group can take a break during the overlap time, returning when the teacher being replaced leaves. Although this model is more expensive, it covers breaks and also allows teachers time to communicate.

- Provide a quiet, separate, and relaxing space for staff members. Even if space is limited, a comfortable chair placed in front of a window can serve as a place to relax. If at all possible, the program should provide nutritious refreshments for the staff and enough break time so a staff member can take a short walk, preferably outdoors, to reduce the stress of the day.

Child care health consultants

Child care programs are affected by many technical health and safety issues. Even the most conscientious early childhood professional cannot be fully informed about all health matters that affect the program, staff members, children, and families. Scores on the Environmental Rating Scales (ERS), which assess process quality in programs, show that the health- and safety-related items that are sampled in the ERS instruments usually score lower than other items. Generally the scores are at minimal or inadequate levels, even in high-quality programs. All programs therefore need regular visits and interactions with a CCHC, who makes informed observations and can collaborate with facility staff members to improve quality by offering access to updated health and safety information and resources.

An overall CCHC who can handle most program needs is usually a licensed health care professional with experience in child and community health and child care, such as a pediatric nurse, pediatric nurse clinician, community health nurse, pediatrician, or family practice physician. In addition to a general consultant, programs may need to use other consultants with specialized knowledge in a variety of fields.

Caring for Our Children Standard 1.6.0.2 specifies that

> The child care health consultant (CCHC) should visit each facility as needed to review and give advice on the facility's health component. Early childhood programs that serve any child younger than three years of age should be visited more frequently than early education and child care programs that serve children three to five years of age.

Be sure that the vagueness of this standard does not lead to insufficient attention to health consultation. In states where regulations require health consultant visits, the frequency required varies from once a week for programs serving children younger than 3 years of age to twice a year for programs serving children 3–5 years of age. Research shows that CCHC visits and follow-up services are associated with improved measured performance of health and safety practices. In states where CCHC involvement is not required, limited use of CCHC services occurs. This is especially true if programs must pay for the services from their budgets.

Caring for Our Children Standard 1.6.0.3 requires a minimum of quarterly visits by an early childhood mental health consultant (ECMHC). An ECMHC is someone with professional credentials and training in young children's mental health, experience working in early education settings, and consultative skills. The ECMHC focuses on improving staff skills for mental health promotion, including helping staff members learn how to minimize and manage challenging behavior and mitigate and manage stress. The ECMHS also helps link program staff members and families with community mental health resources when they are needed.

Caring for Our Children Standard 1.6.0.4 requires visits from an early childhood education consultant (ECEC) a minimum of semiannually. This consultant should have at least "a Baccalaureate degree and preferably a Master's degree from an accredited institution in early childhood education, administration and supervision, and a minimum of three years in teaching and administration of an early care/education program." This consultant should have the knowledge, skills, and materials related to fostering healthy child development, including screening, assessment of individual children and classrooms using recognized standardized tools, and curriculum development. As for all consultants, consultative skills are essential so that the ECEC's coaching and mentoring of adults is effective. The ECEC should review the written documents that the program is using, make observations of program operation, follow the NAEYC *Code of Ethical Conduct and Statement of Commitment,* and be available to provide advice requested by program staff members.

These visits by a general CCHC, an ECMHC, and an ECEC are appropriate for all early care and education programs. When there are children with special health, behavioral, or developmental needs, visits by consultants with expertise in the area of the child's needs should be more frequent and focused to help manage and adjust the program services on an ongoing basis.

Knowledge and skills of child care health consultants

Health professionals who serve as CCHCs do not always have a public health perspective or the full range of knowledge and skills required for a group program. For example, a pediatrician caring for many of the children in the program may not be able to provide advice about food safety and sanitation, but a sanitarian may provide excellent health consultation on food safety, hygiene, and infectious disease control. Other health professionals may need to be consulted about medication administration or playground safety. Figure 9.4 defines the knowledge and skills that the CCHC must have or obtain by involving other health professionals.

Seeking a child care health consultant

Federal support for states to implement projects under the Healthy Child Care America Campaign significantly increased community resources for health consultation to early care and education programs of all types. When the federal subsidy to states to continue the work was withdrawn, however, the programs began to wither. The comments that accompany *Caring for Our Children* Standard 1.6.0.1 suggest ways to find a CCHC in your community:

> CCHC services may be provided through the public health system, resource and referral agency, private source, local community action program, health professional organizations, other non-profit organizations, and/or universities. Some professional organizations include child care health consultants in their special interest groups, such as the AAP's Section on Early Education and Child Care and the National Association of Pediatric Nurse Practitioners (NAPNAP).
>
> CCHCs who are not employees of health, education, family service, or child care agencies may be self-employed. Compensating them for their services via fee-for-service, an hourly rate, or a retainer fosters access and accountability.

Chapter Child Care Contacts with health professional expertise are available from many state chapters of the AAP. These individuals may be able to help early educators find a CCHC to work with them. To identify the Chapter Child Care Contact for your state, go to **www.healthychildcare.org**. (Select Chapter Child Care Contacts and view the roster that shows the name and contact information available for those states where someone has filled this position.)

Graduate students in a discipline related to child health can provide acceptable child care health consultation as long as they are supervised by faculty knowledgeable in early care and education and have a schedule that allows them to establish and sustain a relationship for at least six months to a year. Students come and go fairly rapidly, and rapid turnover of a consultant may not fit well with a program's efforts to improve operations. However, by providing continuity of relationship with the early childhood facility over an extended period of time, the supervising faculty can develop trust, mutual respect, and understanding of the program's needs, which are essential to an effective CCHC's role.

Programs also should not overlook parents of children enrolled in their facility who are health professionals with pediatric and health consultant experience. However, involving parents as health consultants requires caution to avoid crossing boundaries of confidentiality and conflict of interest. Some state regulations limit the roles a parent who is a health professional can fulfill.

Health consultants should have specific training in the child care setting. Such training is not yet commonly included in health professional curricula but is being provided in special courses offered by health professionals who have become involved in child care health consultation. Trainers of CCHCs may be graduates of a federally funded program at the University of North Carolina called the National Training Institute for Child Care Health Consultants (NTI). Every state has CCHC trainers who are graduates of NTI. To learn more about this training and to ask to be connected with an NTI graduate, visit **http://nti.unc.edu**. You can send email to NTI at nticchc@unc.edu or call 919-966-3780.

Few child care staff members are trained as health professionals, and few health professionals have training about community child care programs. As a result, relationships between these professionals must be built sensitively. Health professionals and early educators need to patiently help one another to understand differences in their vocabulary and approaches. When physical, mental, social, or health concerns are raised about a child or family, staff member, or program, they need to be addressed appropriately, with mutual respect for the value of contributions by all concerned to promote a good outcome.

Figure 9.4.

Child Care Health Consultants

The child care health consultant should be knowledgeable in the following areas:

a. Consultation skills both as a child care health consultant as well as a member of an interdisciplinary team of consultants
b. National health and safety standards for out-of-home child care
c. Indicators of quality early care and education
d. Day-to-day operations of child care facilities
e. State child care licensing and public health requirements
f. State health laws, federal and state education laws (e.g., ADA, IDEA), and state professional practice acts for licensed professionals (e.g., State Nurse Practice Acts)
g. Infancy and early childhood development, social and emotional health, and developmentally appropriate practice
h. Recognition and reporting requirements for infectious diseases
i. American Academy of Pediatrics (AAP) and Early and Periodic Screening, Diagnosis, and Treatment (EPSDT) screening recommendations and immunizations schedules for children
j. Importance of medical home and local and state resources to facilitate access to a medical home as well as child health insurance programs including Medicaid and State Children's Health Insurance Program (SCHIP)
k. Injury prevention for children
l. Oral health for children
m. Nutrition and age-appropriate physical activity recommendations for children including feeding of infants and children, the importance of breastfeeding and the prevention of obesity
n. Inclusion of children with special health care needs, and developmental disabilities in child care
o. Safe medication administration practices
p. Health education of children
q. Recognition and reporting requirements for child abuse and neglect/child maltreatment
r. Safe sleep practices and policies (including reducing the risk of SIDS)
s. Development and implementation of health and safety policies and practices including poison awareness and poison prevention
t. Staff health, including adult health screening, occupational health risks, and immunizations
u. Disaster planning resources and collaborations within child care community
v. Community health and mental health resources for child, parent, and staff health
w. Importance of serving as a healthy role model for children and staff

The child care health consultant should be able to perform or arrange for performance of the following activities:

a. Assessing caregivers'/teachers' knowledge of health, development, and safety and offering training as indicated
b. Assessing parents'/guardians' health, development, and safety knowledge, and offering training as indicated
c. Assessing children's knowledge about health and safety and offering training as indicated
d. Conducting a comprehensive indoor and outdoor health and safety assessment and ongoing observations of the child care facility
e. Consulting collaboratively on-site and/or by telephone or electronic media
f. Providing community resources and referral for health, mental health, and social needs, including accessing medical homes, children's health insurance programs (e.g., CHIP), and services for special health care needs
g. Developing or updating policies and procedures for child care facilities
h. Reviewing health records of children
i. Reviewing health records of caregivers/teachers

j. Assisting caregivers/teachers and parents/guardians in the management of children with behavioral, social, and emotional problems and those with special health care needs
k. Consulting a child's primary care provider about the child's individualized health care plan and coordinating services in collaboration with parents/guardians, the primary care provider, and other health care professionals (the CCHC shows commitment to communicating with and helping coordinate the child's care with the child's medical home, and may assist with the coordination of skilled nursing care services at the child care facility)
l. Consulting with a child's primary care provider about medications as needed, in collaboration with parents/guardians
m. Teaching staff safe medication administration practices
n. Monitoring safe medication administration practices
o. Observing children's behavior, development, and health status and making recommendations if needed to staff and parents/guardians for further assessment by a child's primary care provider
p. Interpreting standards, regulations, and accreditation requirements related to health and safety, as well as providing technical advice, separate and apart from an enforcement role of a regulation inspector or determining the status of the facility for recognition
q. Understanding and observing confidentiality requirements
r. Assisting in the development of disaster/emergency medical plans (especially for those children with special health care needs) in collaboration with community resources
s. Developing an obesity prevention program in consultation with a nutritionist/registered dietitian (RD) and physical education specialist
t. Working with other consultants such as nutritionists/RDs, kinesiologists (physical activity specialists), oral health consultants, social service workers, early childhood mental health consultants, and education consultants

The role of the CCHC is to promote the health and development of children, families, and staff and to ensure a healthy and safe child care environment.

The CCHC is not acting as a primary care provider at the facility but offers critical services to the program and families by sharing health and developmental expertise; assessments of child, staff, and family health needs; and community resources. The CCHC assists families in care coordination with the medical home and other health and developmental specialists. In addition, the CCHC should collaborate with an interdisciplinary team of early childhood consultants, such as early childhood education, mental health, and nutrition consultants.

In order to provide effective consultation and support to programs, the CCHC should avoid conflict of interest related to other roles such as serving as a caregiver/teacher or regulator or a parent/guardian at the site to which child care health consultation is being provided.

The CCHC should have regular contact with the facility's administrative authority, the staff, and the parents/guardians in the facility. The administrative authority should review and collaborate with the CCHC in implementing recommended changes in policies and practices. In the case of consulting about children with special health care needs, the CCHC should have contact with the child's medical home with permission from the child's parent/guardian.

Programs with a significant number of non-English-speaking families should seek a CCHC who is culturally sensitive and knowledgeable about community health resources for the parents'/guardians' native culture and languages.

Source: Standard 1.6.0.1, *Caring for Our Children*. Reprinted with permission.

Paying a health professional for consultation and training

To foster access to and accountability of health consultants, programs should offer some form of compensation to consultants who do not perform this work as part of their regular job. Consider various approaches and choose one that will work best for the program and the consultant. A yearly retainer entitling the program to unlimited telephone advice and a specified number of on-site visits and training sessions is best for some providers. For others, a contractual arrangement based on a fee-for-service payment is compatible with the uncertain availability of the consultant and the precarious finances of the child care program. In fee-for-service arrangements, it is easier to set a cost per hour of service, or a specific fee for each service the program might request, than to negotiate the fee each time.

Public health professionals do not usually charge a fee for their services, or they charge only a nominal fee. Even when there is no fee involved, programs should define the expectations with the health consultant in writing so that both parties are clear about the other's expectations.

There is clear evidence of the contribution of CCHCs to program quality improvement. In one study, within one year of establishing a relationship with a child care program, the CCHCs had a positive effect on health policies and practices, child health status, children's access to health care, reduction of absences from the program, fewer outbreaks of infection, less emergency room use, lower medical costs, and fewer absences of parents from work (Kotch & Isbell, 2007). These findings of the efficacy of CCHCs in improving health and safety in child care in North Carolina were echoed by similar work conducted in California by Abbey Alkon, Director of the California Childcare Health Program, and in Pennsylvania by Susan Aronson and Richard Fiene for the ECELS–Healthy Child Care PA, a program of the Pennsylvania Chapter of the AAP.

These findings show that it is well worth the effort for programs to locate and use the services of a CCHC. Some programs raise funds to pay for child care health consultation. Strategies for such fundraising include asking a local business or foundation to partially or wholly sponsor CCHC services. In Pennsylvania, a United Way grant subsidized a fee paid by a number of child care programs to receive CCHC services. This type of shared funding arrangement gives the funding source more confidence that the facility is committed to making good use of the CCHC's services.

Another approach is to discuss with parents the benefits of having a CCHC involved with the program and to ask parents whether they would accept a small increase in their fees to have this service. CCHC services generally cost $1–2 per week per child. Consider contracting with a CCHC as a shared service of a group of centers, so all facilities get at least a minimum number of visits and then have phone or email access for advice. Encourage your state quality improvement program to subsidize CCHC services as a proven method of achieving better performance on otherwise low-scoring health and safety items in quality rating assessments. If the state adopts a regulatory requirement for CCHC involvement, these fundraising efforts are likely to gain credibility with potential funding organizations and families who pay fees for their children's care.

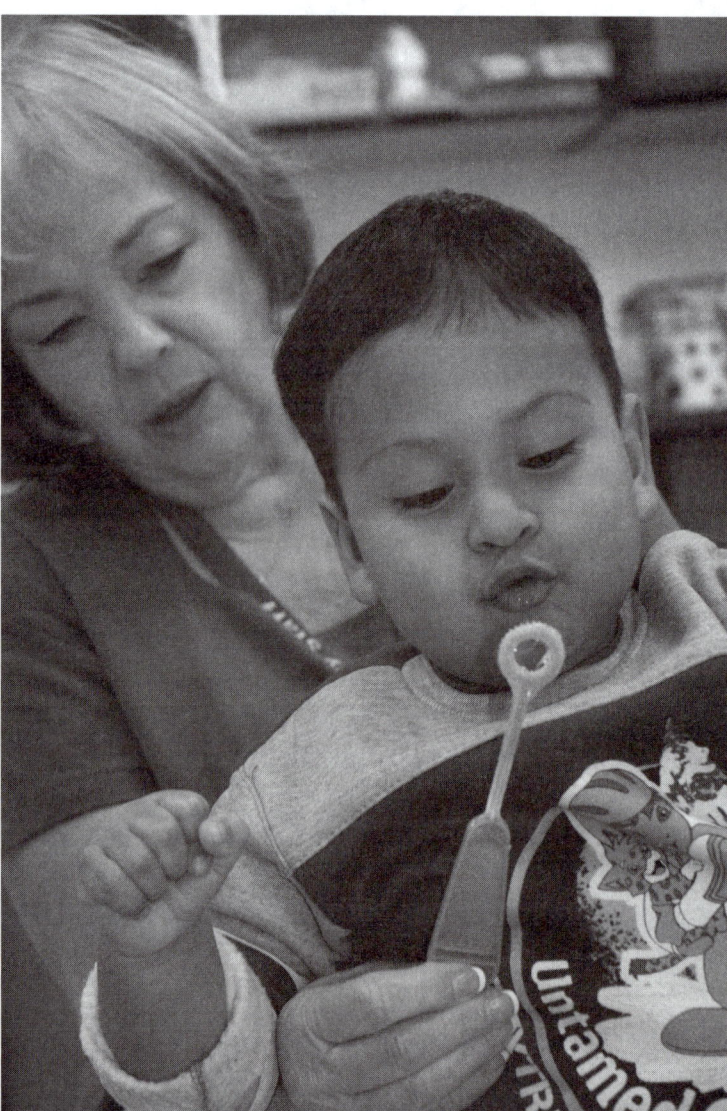

By Peg Callaghan / © NAEYC

Using a health professional as a consultant or an instructor

For both center-based and family child care facilities, the health consultant should review all of the facility's written policies, which should cover the topics listed in Chapter 13 as well as in Chapter 9 of *Caring for Our Children*.

When their busy schedules permit, many health professionals enjoy offering educational sessions for teachers, children, and families. This service is often provided by the program's CCHC, but other health professionals such as dieticians, dental hygienists, sanitarians, fire safety professionals, and child development specialists might be able to provide instructional services in their areas of expertise. Program administrators can help health professionals be more effective instructors in the following ways:

- Suggest some hands-on demonstrations that would be welcomed by the group (ask the health professional to plan some and offer to help with the setup).

- Prepare a list of questions that staff members and families would like to have answered. The questions will help the health professional focus on appropriate concerns and the level of sophistication of the staff members and families who will participate in the educational experience.

- Offer instructional supports, such as flip charts/markers and media (e.g., DVDs, YouTube videos, posters, slides with photographs taken in the facility that are related to the topic, and vignettes). These tools help orient everyone to the topic. Many health professionals are comfortable using slides as they talk.

- Some health professionals need to be reminded to spend some time getting to know the audience, letting participants ask questions of concern to them, and having some type of interaction or activity that interrupts passive listening by participants at intervals. (The recommended interval for interaction that promotes effective adult learning is an interaction no less than every 8–10 minutes.)

All too often, child care programs receive seemingly conflicting recommendations from varied sources. In health-related matters, equally authoritative sources may differ. An issue that affects just one child or one staff member can be decided by that person's physician, but if the issue involves more than one child or adult in the program, the opinion of the program's health consultant should prevail after he or she consults with the sources of the differing opinions. In matters of public policy about health actions, the public health officer in the health department with jurisdiction has the final say. Once an action plan is set, the program administrator should inform all who were consulted so that they know about the decision and the rationale for rejecting the opinions that are not being followed. This feedback leaves the door open for future input and helps generate support for the action plan.

Suggested activities

- When was your last health assessment? What was addressed in the assessment that would be an appropriate concern for working in an early childhood setting? What was not addressed that might affect occupational health concerns in such a setting?

- What health concerns should be addressed with a volunteer? With a colleague, role-play an interview with a volunteer for whom you use a job description to determine whether the volunteer has any condition or issue with doing what you would expect a volunteer in the classroom to do. How do you feel about conducting such an interview? How does your colleague feel about it?

- Think about a time when you or someone you know suffered a back injury. What could have prevented the injury? What has been done since to prevent the person from being reinjured?

- Look in the community for possible sources of child care health consultation. Follow up on one or two leads and ask the agency or individual if telephone advice, on-site observations, and training for staff members are offered. If these services are not currently provided, ask what would be required to arrange for them. If service is being provided, ask about arrangements and the amount and type of services actually provided in the past year.

- Use the list of topics on which staff members should have training to think about resources for obtaining such training in your community. Who would you ask to do it? How would you prepare the trainer to understand what staff members need? What methods of training work best for a group of early education and care providers?

- Review the policies and procedures currently in use in an early childhood facility, checking for the items listed in this chapter that a CCHC should review and approve. Are some missing? Which have been reviewed and approved by a CCHC?

144 Healthy Young Children Chapter 10

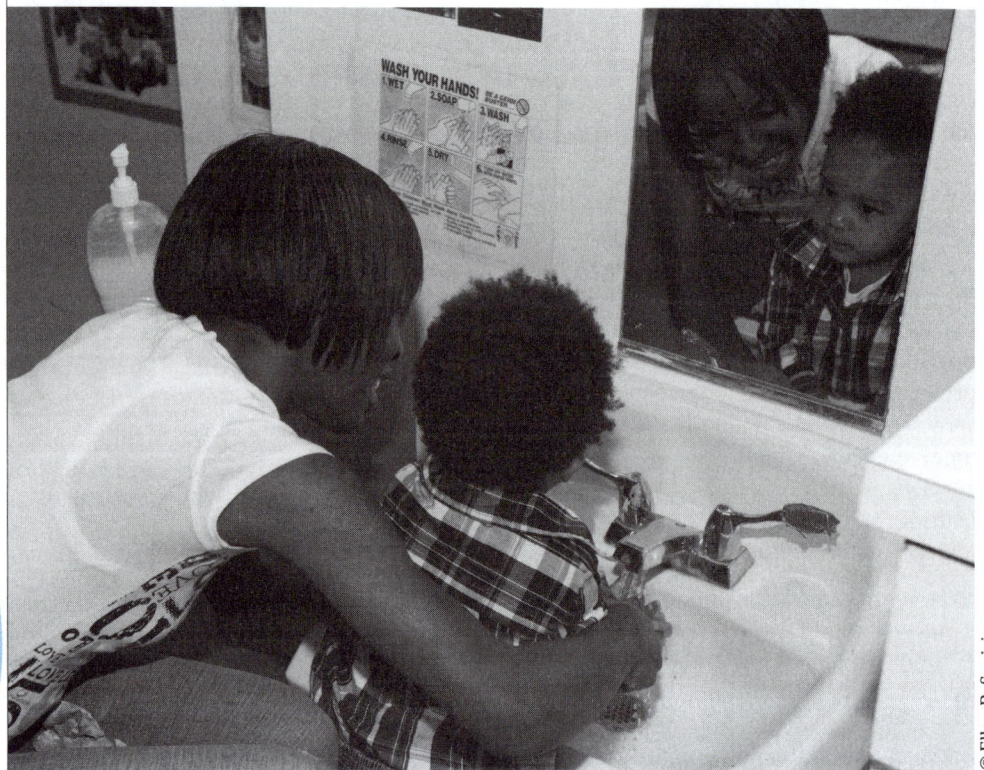

Facility Design and Support Services for Safe and Healthy Early Care and Education

MAJOR CONCEPTS

- The physical environment of an early care and education program influences the behavior of those using it.
- Too little or poorly designed free space creates risks for injury and disease.
- Experts in engineering, fire safety, plumbing, heating and cooling, ventilation, and lighting can contribute significantly to the quality of a program.
- Routine cleaning, sanitation, and disinfecting schedules and procedures are key elements in a safe and healthy setting.
- Controlling exposure to toxic substances is essential to the health of children and adults.
- Transporting children to and from facilities is a universal activity, whether it is done by families or the program.
- Transportation-related injuries are the leading cause of death for young children, about half as passengers and the other half as pedestrians. Most of these deaths are preventable.
- Field trips, which usually involve transportation, require special planning to ensure everyone's safety.

This chapter of *Healthy Young Children* provides a general overview of facility, transportation, and maintenance issues. Some of these issues have been identified in other chapters, but others are addressed here for the first time. Protecting children from harm requires risk reduction in many areas that are beyond the knowledge of early education experts. However, a program administrator must be aware of these issues and know where to find experts to help address them when needed. In *Caring for Our Children* you will find standards that specify the required routines for maintaining safe and healthful facilities and equipment in child care programs. The references that accompany the standards include expert resources that teachers will find helpful.

Space and structural design

The design of areas that children and adults use influences how they behave and feel in those spaces. Open spaces accommodate activities that require the use of large muscles to move around, while object-filled spaces confine movement and offer a smaller frame of things to be seen, touched, or used in some way. Odors, sounds, sights, textures, temperatures, and aesthetic preferences all play a role in the experience that an environment provides.

Many early childhood facilities are located in buildings that were not designed for young children in group care, such as churches, stores, warehouses, and office space. Some large, old homes that were intended to house more than one generation of a single family have been converted into child care centers. Such buildings are often available because they have no other economically useful purpose. While they may be available at relatively low cost, many of these structures are not easily made suitable for child care.

Usually, the health and safety concerns in these buildings rise to top priority when government inspectors call attention to code requirements. Areas with high levels of air pollution, loud noises, heavy traffic, deep excavations, toxic materials in the indoor and outdoor paint and surrounding soil, and radiation hazards are undesirable for child care facilities. The buildings may lack necessary plumbing, electrical, and fire safety fittings. An environmental audit is essential before choosing a site. If one has not been done at the site of a facility already being used for child care, it should be arranged so that hazards can be identified and abated.

Amount of indoor space per child

Many early education professionals have used 35 square feet of free space per child as a guide to meeting the space needs of a group of children younger than school age, and 40 square feet per child for children with special needs. *Caring for Our Children* Standard 5.1.2.1 cites research that these commonly used space requirements are inadequate and recommends a minimum of 42 square feet of usable floor space per child, preferably 50 square feet per child. This does not include space used for walkways, staff work areas for classroom support, furniture, administrative areas, restrooms, food service areas, storage, laundry, mechanical equipment, or rooms for care of ill children. Lack of space is associated with challenging behavior and increased density of air pollutants, including disease-causing germs. Space for school-age children, space for children who have special needs, and spaces with low ceilings are addressed in *Caring for Our Children* Standards 5.1.2.2 and 5.1.2.3. The best layout is one that ensures that the teachers can monitor all the children from wherever they or the children are at any moment. For school-age child care, space must include a separate area where children have tables and chairs to do their homework.

Structural design

Child care facilities should comply with all applicable building codes. When these codes conflict with one another, the rationale for each should be examined to see how the intent of the conflicting requirements can be met simultaneously or with the least risk. The entire building should be structurally sound and weather-tight, with easily cleaned finishes that control mold, dust, and pest entry. Windows and doors should be suitable for children's environments—fitted with safety glass and guards, allowing for views at children's eye level, and designed for easy exit in an emergency.

As much as possible, design safety features into the building. Windows in walls that allow other adults to see into the room reduce the potential for child abuse and accusations of child maltreatment. Vision panels in doors allow adults to see a child who is near the door on the opposite side and allow the child to see someone coming into the room before the door is opened. For finger-pinch protection, doors should have finger-pinch preventing gaskets and slow-closing devices. Windows should open to ventilate rooms with fresh air, or some other system should be installed to provide the required volume of fresh, outdoor air to dilute odors and germy respiratory droplets that accumulate when a group of people use a room (see ventilation specifications in The Role of Ventilation, Temperature, and Humidity in Resistance to Infectious Disease in Chapter 2).

Exit routes must lead to a sheltered place if children and staff members cannot reenter the building. Alternate exit routes should be available in case the most convenient way out is blocked. Consideration should be given to how nonambulatory or less cooperative children can be evacuated to an area where they may need to stay for long periods in an emergency.

Surfaces

The finishes used on room surfaces and the type of furnishings placed in rooms should be chosen based on consideration of where nonporous surfaces are needed for sanitation and where it makes sense to use soft elements that are covered with washable fabrics to absorb sound and provide comfort. For example, an upholstered chair or love seat should have a washable slipcover and should not be next to the diaper-changing table. It might be placed in the reading area of the room next to a washable rug. Avoid large area carpets that cannot be laundered. To help control sound, you can use carpets that are easily vacuumed, washable fabrics on walls, and tiles made for sound absorption on ceilings. Sleep equipment may be placed in areas used at other times for play, and against furniture or walls, but the total area must be sufficient to provide three feet of space between sleep equipment of adjacent children who are resting.

Outdoor play areas

The outdoor play area must be ample and well designed for the intended users. Playgrounds designed for school-age children should not be used by preschoolers and toddlers. Plan for 75 square feet of space per child using the playground at any one time. Then plan enough space so that each group of children can use the playground area for the recommended outdoor time. Usually, this means that no more than two groups can take turns using the same space during the day.

The outdoor space should be designed for play value and safety. Because the greatest number of serious injuries occurs during active play, playgrounds deserve special attention. Playground safety has so many technical issues that program directors should be sure that a Certified Playground Safety Inspector (CPSI) reviews existing playgrounds and any plans for new ones. As mentioned in Chapter 3, the cost of an inspection by a CPSI is usually reasonable and the results very helpful. To find a CPSI near you, follow the online instructions at the National Recreation and Park Association's website, **www.nrpa.org**.

Additional space outdoors may be needed to accommodate children with disabilities. Indoor play areas should augment outdoor space and be sufficient to meet the needs for physical activity when inclement weather limits outdoor play. The same issues apply to indoor areas used for active play; for example, the need for cushioning surfaces under climbing equipment is often overlooked, but it is just as important inside as it is outside.

Equipment and furnishings

The type and placement of furnishings in a space helps to direct people to activities they will attempt in that space. If chairs and tables are put in an area, children and adults will tend to sit down to do an activity there. If wide-open spaces are left unfurnished, children will be tempted to run across them. If furniture is placed near windowsills, children are more likely to climb up on it to look out the window or climb on the windowsills. The types of activity centers and tools that are available determine how well children and adults carry out the program's philosophy. Whatever is chosen should incorporate principles of health and safety. Sinks must be located where handwashing should take place. Food preparation surfaces must be totally separate from surfaces used to change diapers so nobody is tempted to put food on the diapering surface or diapers on the food preparation surface. Diaper-changing tables should have nothing on them that can't be disinfected easily after each diaper change. To avoid injury, equipment used for play should be sized to children's developmental abilities. All equipment, materials, furnishings, and toys should be sturdy, safe, and in good repair and meet the recommendations of the Consumer Product Safety Commission (CPSC) for control of known hazards.

More stringent requirements apply to furnishings in early care and education facilities than to what parents might choose to use in their homes. For example, communal water tables have a high probability of spreading infectious disease in a child care facility, although siblings can use a wading pool at home. Using communal water tables in a child care facility requires considerable attention to detailed arrangements. It is permissible only if the children are closely supervised. The table should be filled with fresh water right before use or supplied with freely flowing water. To provide clean, slowly flowing water indoors, set up a hose that is connected to the sink tap so it empties into the inside of the water table. Then put a bucket under the table drain or attach another hose connected from the drain in the bottom of the water table to a waste water drain. To set up a water table outside, use slowly flowing clean water from a hose and connect another hose to the table's drain to take the waste water to the ground away from under the table. If the water is not free-flowing, only a few children should be allowed to use the water table at a time; then, before another few children use the table, empty the water and then sanitize all the surfaces and objects. Only children free of cuts and runny noses should be allowed to play in the water. Children should wash their hands before water play. No child is allowed to drink the water from the table. As an alternative to a communal water table, use separate basins with fresh water from the drinkable water source for each child to engage in water play. The bins can be put on a table, although putting each child's bin into the water table to catch the splashes might cause fewer slippery floors and smaller messes to clean up.

Equipment should be organized to reduce the risk of back injuries for adults wherever possible. Select furnishings that enable teachers to hold and comfort children while minimizing the need for bending, lifting, and carrying heavy children and objects. Teachers should not routinely be required to use child-size chairs, tables, or desks. See Figure 9.3 in Chapter 9 for guidelines about how to avoid back injury in child care.

Air quality, ventilation, heating, and cooling

A draft-free temperature of 68–75° F at 30–50 percent humidity should be maintained in the winter months, and a temperature of 74–82° F at the same range of humidity should be maintained in the summer months. Rooms that children use should be heated, cooled, and ventilated not only to achieve the desired temperatures but also to prevent accumulation of disease-causing germs, odors, and fumes. Air exchange should be a minimum of 15 cubic feet per minute per person of outdoor air. Heating and air-conditioning equipment should be inspected and maintained by qualified contractors, usually those who follow the guidelines of the national standard-setting organizations. Heating devices should not expose children to surfaces hot enough to burn them or expose them to toxic fumes. For details, see the standards in Section 5.2.1 of *Caring for Our Children* and the accompanying references to national standard-setting and credentialing organizations.

Lighting

Studies on school performance suggest that children learn better in classrooms with daylight and the opportunity for natural ventilation. Natural lighting should be provided in rooms in which children work and play for more than two hours at a time. Where possible, install windows at children's eye level so they can see the outdoors while inside. Visual stimulation is developmentally appropriate practice. Natural lighting provided by skylights exposes children to variations in light during the day that is less perceptually stimulating than eye-level windows but is still preferable to artificial lighting. Section 5.2.2 of *Caring for Our Children* covers specific levels of illumination by type of activity in a particular area, safety precautions for light fixtures, and limitations on the use of certain types of lamps.

Noise levels

Noise in child care spaces should not exceed 35–40 decibels at least 80 percent of the time. In practical terms, this means that it should be easy to hear and understand a conversation spoken without raising one's voice. Use of noise-absorbing materials can help, such as acoustical tiles on ceiling or walls. While it is best not to have carpeted floors, it is acceptable to put carpeting on walls, partitions, and other vertical hard surfaces to absorb sound. All sound-absorbing materials should be cleanable (by vacuuming) and installed to meet fire safety requirements.

Electrical items

Electricity is a potential source of injury. All outlets in areas where children are developmentally younger than kindergarten age should be of the tamper-resistant type or have screwed-on safety covers that accomplish the same objective. Some contain a shutter mechanism that prevents children from sticking objects in them. Others have internal design that prevents current flow unless a two- or three-pronged plug is inserted. Safety covers and shock-protection devices are essential where young children are in care. Safety plugs are not acceptable because children can remove them, and adults often forget to put them back after using the outlet.

Water and electricity pose special hazards and must be kept separated. Ground-fault circuit interrupter

(GFCI) outlets should be installed in all areas where electrical appliances or wires might come into contact with water. These GFCIs need to be tested by pushing on the test button every one to three months. Electric cords must be kept beyond where children who are mouthing objects can chew or bite into them. Avoid electric extension cords whenever possible. If they are used, they should bear the listing mark of a nationally recognized testing laboratory and should not be frayed, overloaded, or placed under or behind anything that touches them. All cords should be inaccessible to children. If a cord must be put behind furniture to make it inaccessible to children, put the cord into the special commercially available rubber holder that encases the electrical cord in a protective channel. Inspect all electrical fixtures and appliances, wiring, and outlets to be sure they do not pose a fire or shock hazard.

Plumbing

We generally take safe water for granted or make assumptions about safe sources of water that are not necessarily correct. For example, many people prefer to drink bottled water even though the bottled water industry is essentially unregulated and the content of water bottles, even from the same company, has been found to vary substantially. Water should be from a source approved by the local public health authorities and should be tested by public health authorities to be sure it contains no unhealthy bacterial or chemical contaminants.

Handwashing sinks are critical to infectious disease control in child care settings. If plumbing is unavailable to provide a handwashing sink, facilities should use a portable water supply and a sanitary catch system approved by the local public health authority. The water in handwashing sinks should be at a temperature of at least 60° F and no hotter than 120° F. The water should flow for at least 30 seconds without having to reactivate the faucet. Hands-free faucets are widely available and provide a significant reduction in hand contamination.

Handwashing sinks should be adjacent to the surface used for changing diapers and soiled underwear. Use of hand sanitizers is permissible only for adults and children over 24 months of age and only when there is no visible soil. Visible soil will be present sometimes with diaper changing, so using hand sanitizers does not eliminate the need for a sink in these areas. Provide step stools that allow children to use the sinks comfortably. Handwashing sinks should be separate from those used for preparing food or washing out contaminated items.

Drinking water should be freely available to children indoors and outdoors—preferably in fountains but acceptably from a portable water supply or faucet with single-use drinking cups. Drinking water, including the output at drinking fountains, should be tested for lead and copper content.

Swimming and wading pools pose special hazards. Pools should be enclosed with child-resistive fences and gates. Also, they must be monitored for water quality and have equipment that is routinely used for sanitation. Few child care facilities can undertake safe maintenance of swimming and wading equipment. Those that choose to do so should check standards in *Caring for Our Children* for detailed requirements and guidelines for working with local public health authorities.

Portable sink equipment or camp-type sinks make availability of sinks with running water possible wherever handwashing should take place. To find sources of this equipment, search the internet for "portable sinks." Toilets and sinks with running water for handwashing should be located no farther than 40 feet from the perimeter of all areas that children use and should be on the same floor as the children unless the children are always escorted to the toilet. The ratio of toilets and handwashing sinks to children should be at least 1:10 for toddlers and preschool-age children and 1:15 for school-age children. Non-flushing equipment (potty chairs or pots) used for toilet learning does not count in

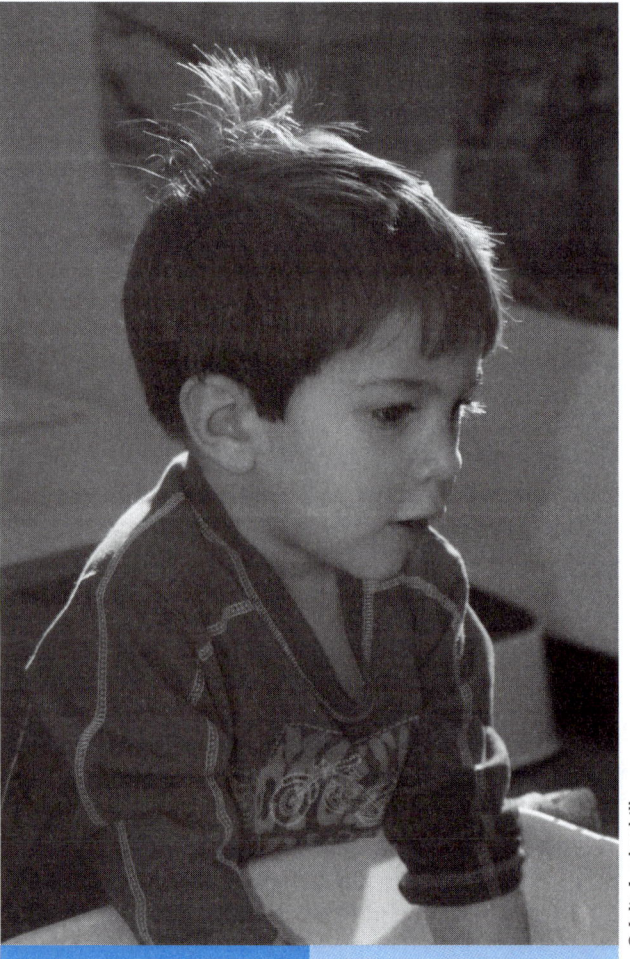

these ratios. This type of equipment poses a significant sanitation hazard, so their use is strongly discouraged.

Fire warning and safety systems

All facilities should have a smoke detection system that is hardwired or is a battery-operated wireless system that signals an alarm when batteries are low or a hazardous situation exists. The system should be monitored by off-site private or public personnel who can alert the child care program if the system malfunctions and notify the fire department if an alarm signal is received. The detectors should be placed in front of doors to stairways and in corridors, adult break and meeting rooms, and areas that children occupy at any time. Generally, local fire or building inspectors will specify how these systems must be installed and how they should be tested and maintained. Portable fire extinguishers should be installed and properly maintained. They should be accessible to adults, but not to children. Staff members must be taught how to use them correctly. Fire extinguishers vary by the type of fire on which they should be used. Some are specifically designed for fires that involve electrical equipment, some are for use on flammable liquids, and others are for fires involving wood, cloth, or paper. (See Chapter 3 for more discussion about fire safety.)

Maintenance of the facility

Early childhood programs should have written policies and procedures for the routine cleaning and maintenance of the facility. These policies and procedures should specify the type of cleaning and chemicals used, as well as the method and schedule for cleaning and sanitizing. They should also name the person responsible for supervising and monitoring cleaning and other maintenance activities.

Use a cleaning, sanitizing, and disinfecting schedule

The routine frequency of cleaning, sanitizing, and disinfecting in the facility should follow the timeline in Figure A.3 in Appendix A. Increase the frequency whenever there is an outbreak of illness, when there is known contamination or visible soil, or when recommended by the health department to control certain infectious diseases. Take out of service any surfaces, furnishings, and equipment not in good repair or that have been contaminated by body fluids until they are repaired, cleaned, and (if contaminated) sanitized or disinfected as required in *Caring for Our Children*. When the hazard cannot be removed, install a barrier that keeps children and adults away from it.

Keep the facility neat, clean, and free of rubbish

- Clean the facility in a way that avoids contamination of food and food-contact surfaces.
- Keep soiled linens or aprons in laundry bags or other suitable containers.
- Wash all windows inside and outside at least twice a year.
- Do not use deodorizers to cover up odors caused by unsanitary conditions or poor housekeeping. Instead, ventilate and clean to eliminate the smell.
- Keep storage areas, attics, and cellars free from refuse, furniture, old newspapers, and other paper goods. These items are a fire hazard and may provide a home for vermin.
- Keep flammable cleaning rags or solutions in closed metal containers in locked cabinets.
- Label each waste container to show its intended use. The containers should be cleaned daily to prevent buildup of soil in them.
- Follow the guidelines in Figure A.2 in Appendix A to select products to use for cleaning, sanitizing, and disinfecting, as discussed in Chapter 2.
- Be aware that techniques that some people recommend as "green" approaches for cleaning, sanitizing, or disinfecting may require more labor and may not be effective. Look for products that bear the United States Environmental Protection Agency's (EPA) Design for the Environment (DfE) logo on their label to quickly identify and choose products that have been tested as "green" products. The DfE logo on a product means that the DfE scientific review team has screened each ingredient for potential human health and environmental effects and that—based on currently available information, EPA predictive models, and expert judgment—the product contains only those ingredients that pose the least concern among chemicals in their class. Product manufacturers who display the DfE logo on recognized products had to invest heavily in research, development, and reformulation to ensure that their products are on the green end of the health and environmental spectrum and that their products effectively perform their intended function. Thousands of products, including cleaners and disinfectants, are listed on the DfE website at **www.EPA.gov/dfe**. Follow the manufacturer's instructions for use. Most often, the product is to be used to remove visible soil and then rinsed from the surface with water to remove any chemical residue.

Keep equipment and cleaning supplies clean, in good working condition, and stored safely

- Keep on hand wet and dry mops, mop pails, brooms, cleaning cloths, and at least one vacuum cleaner.
- Store housekeeping equipment in a separate, locked space, such as a closet or cabinet—not in bathrooms, in halls, on stairs, or near food.

- When possible, use a separate sink to clean equipment (not the same one used for food preparation) that has hot and cold running water.
- Use disposable rags rather than reusable sponges. Sponges allow germs to grow in trapped organic material. If you must use sponges, store them in bleach solution between uses.
- If potty chairs are used, use a separate sink to wash, rinse, and disinfect them. This sink should not be used for handwashing or any other purpose. Because potty chairs pose a significant sanitation hazard, their use is strongly discouraged.

Containers for soiled diapers

Containers for soiled diapers should be washable, plastic lined, tightly covered, and hands free (i.e., a container with a motion-sensor lid or a step can). These containers should be located within arm's reach of changing surfaces. Individual bagging of soiled diapers is unnecessary unless they will be sent home for laundering. Do not use containers that require pushing the diaper through a narrow opening or touching the exterior surfaces with a hand or with the diaper. Do not use those that have exterior surfaces likely to be touched while discarding contaminated/soiled material or those that have lids with handles.

Separate containers should be used for disposable diapers, cloth diapers (if used), and soiled clothes and linens. All containers should be placed away from areas where children are allowed to go without close adult supervision and should be tall enough to prevent children from reaching into the receptacles or from falling into them headfirst. Do not use short, poorly made domestic step-cans because the foot pedals break easily, requiring teachers to use their hands to open the lids. Instead, invest in commercial-grade step-cans big enough to hold all soiled diapers before they are taken out to a trash receptacle. These cans are used by doctor's offices, hospitals, and restaurants. A variety of sizes and types are available from restaurants and medical wholesale suppliers. Electric-eye-operated and other types of hands-free containers can be used as long as users can place diapers into the receptacle without touching the exterior of the container with their hands or with the soiled diaper.

Use an Integrated Pest Management (IPM) program

Pests can pass along disease-causing germs by biting (e.g., mosquitoes and ticks) or by spreading contamination from one surface to another (e.g., flies that land on feces and then on food surfaces). They can damage property (e.g., termites and rodents) and disrupt learning when people become upset or get sick when infestations occur indoors (e.g., lice, ants, cockroaches) or outside (e.g., mosquitoes, stinging insects, weeds). Many pesticides are toxic and especially hazardous for children because children's bodies are still developing. Pesticides enter children's bodies through their mouths, skin, and lungs, and even through their mother's exposure during her pregnancy.

Integrated Pest Management (IPM) is the safest approach for controlling pests that minimizes harm to people and the environment. The first step is to use measures that keep pests out of the facility and outdoor play areas. For example, all the exterior openings of the building should be tightly caulked or otherwise sealed. Any foods brought into the facility should be checked to be sure no pests are hiding in the packaging or in the food. IPM focuses on reducing pest access to food, water, shelter, and hiding places. IPM requires keeping areas clean and uncluttered, using tightly closed waste receptacles, plugging holes and cracks, using traps and fly swatters, using bacteria that are harmless to humans or insect-eating animals like birds and frogs to control specific pests, and choosing the least toxic pesticides when a pesticide is needed.

By monitoring for pests, IPM pest control focuses any necessary pest treatment only where it is needed. Monitoring is usually pest-specific—for example, using roach traps or looking for rodent feces. When pests are found during monitoring, IPM treatments such as enclosed baits, gels, diatomaceous earth, and dusts (e.g., boric acid) are used. Aerosols, concentrates, foggers, bombs, and sprays—especially those labeled DANGER or WARNING—are not first-line IPM approaches. For more information, fact sheets, and guidelines for hiring a pest management professional who is likely to practice IPM, see the Integrated Pest Management tool kit (*Integrated Pest Management: A Toolkit for Early Care and Education Programs*) on the website of the California Childcare Health Program (**http://ucsfchildcarehealth.org**). (Go to Publications & Resources, and then select Training Curricula.)

Animals

Not all animals are suitable for contact with children. Animals permitted for contact with children and adults in group settings include dogs, cats, ungulates (e.g., cows, sheep, goats, pigs, horses), rabbits, and rodents (e.g., mice, rats, hamsters, gerbils, guinea pigs, chinchillas), as long as they meet the criteria in Standard 3.4.2.1 in *Caring for Our Children*. Fish are permitted only if they are inaccessible to children. Some animals should not be allowed as pets in early education programs: bats, hermit crabs, poisonous animals (e.g., spiders and venomous insects), reptiles, amphibians (snakes, turtles, salamanders, etc.), psittacine birds (e.g., parrots, parakeets, budgies, and cockatiels), ferrets, wolf-dog hybrids, stray animals, chickens, ducks, animals less than a year of age, female animals in heat, aggressive animals, or any wild or dangerous animals.

- Before having an animal come to visit or stay in the facility, check with a veterinarian about what risks a particular animal might pose to humans, especially children. Any farm animal or zoo programs that bring animals to children's facilities should be inspected and licensed by the U.S. Department of Agriculture. Review the inspection reports before making any arrangements.
- Any animal coming into the facility or with which children have contact must be adapted to be with young children, be in good health without fleas or ticks, be fully immunized and maintained on an intestinal parasite program, and have a current (time-specified) certificate from the animal's attending veterinarian on file in the facility. Check other pet health and care requirements with a veterinarian before arranging to bring any animal into a facility with young children.
- Before allowing children to have any contact with animals, teachers must explain and demonstrate how to have safe, humane interactions. Because children may forget these lessons, all child contact with animals must be supervised by a teacher who is close enough to remove the child from the animal if the animal is mistreated or shows any sign of distress.
- Do not allow any animals in areas used for preparing, eating, or storing food; areas where children wash their hands; supply rooms; or areas where children play.
- Do not allow adults or children to carry toys, use pacifiers, or have any food or beverage item in animal areas.
- Do not allow children to feed animals directly from their hands, kiss an animal, or put an animal close to their faces. Animals' food dishes should be inaccessible to children. When feeding animals, separate the animals from one another and from children with barriers that prevent interaction. The barrier may allow children to observe from a safe distance.
- Be certain that no child is allergic to the animals in your program. Because it may be traumatic to remove an animal after an allergy is discovered, consider the risks and benefits of having an animal that is likely to cause such problems (e.g., rabbits, guinea pigs, and other furry animals).
- Be sure that animals are friendly and have an appropriate temperament to be around children.
- Clean animal areas frequently. Keep all animal litter boxes out of children's reach. Do not use food service facilities to clean anything related to a pet. Children and adults who touch animals or their equipment should use hand hygiene immediately afterward.
- To protect young children from exposure to disease-causing germs, do not let them assist with pet cleaning or maintenance.
- Separate animal food and cleaning supplies from food service supplies.
- Pregnant women are at risk from infections carried by apparently healthy cats and rodents. They should discuss these risks with their obstetrical health providers.
- Visits to a zoo or local pet store pose significant risk of injury, infection, and allergic reactions to a group of young children. Plan these visits carefully to prevent risky behavior and risky interactions between children and animals.

Use special procedures in the kitchen

Make sure food is handled and used properly. See Chapter 5 for more information about food preparation and service.

Procedure for washing dishes and mouthed toys

The easiest way to wash dishes and mouthed toys is with a dishwashing machine. Commercial dishwashers should meet the requirements of the National Sanitation Foundation (NSF) and be used according to the manufacturer's instructions. The dishwashing machine must incorporate a chemical or heat-sanitizing process.

Three types of household dishwashers are capable of producing the cumulative heat factor to meet the NSF time-temperature standard for commercial, spray-type dishwashing machines. Two of the three are capable of doing so only if the temperature of the water coming into the machine is 155° F or higher, but this temperature exceeds what is considered a safe temperature to prevent scalding of skin. One way to manage this conflict is to install a separate, small hot water heater for the dishwasher. The water in the dishwasher must reach 170° F. Because this temperature is higher than that allowed for most hot water heaters, you may have to adjust the heater for the water in the dishwasher so that it raises the water to 170° F. Periodically check the temperature that the water reaches when dishes are being washed by using special test strips or a thermometer made for this purpose that is held by a rubber band to a glass or cup during a dishwasher cycle.

Washing dishes by hand requires more diligence in group care facilities than doing so at home because of the risk of sharing germs across multiple families. First, you need a three-compartment dishwashing arrangement. This can be a combination of dishpans and sink compartments to wash, rinse, and sanitize dishes. (If this is not possible, and you don't have the required type of dishwashing machine, use paper cups and plates and plastic utensils that are thrown away after every use.)

Using the three-compartment setup to wash reusable food service equipment and eating utensils requires the following procedure:

1. Scrape off any leftover food.
2. Use the first compartment to wash all surfaces thoroughly in hot water containing a detergent solution.
3. Rinse all surfaces in the second compartment.
4. Sanitize all surfaces by one of these methods:
   - Immersion for at least two minutes in a lukewarm (not less than 75° F) chemical sanitizing solution (bleach solution of 100 parts per million, made by mixing 1½ teaspoons of domestic bleach per gallon of water) and then air-drying the sanitized items
   - Immersion in an EPA-registered sanitizer following the manufacturer's instructions on the product label
   - Complete immersion in hot water and maintenance at a temperature of 170° F for not less than 30 seconds, followed by air-drying
   - Another method approved by the local department of health

These procedures provide for proper sanitizing and control of viruses and bacteria. Instead of using a sponge for washing dishes, use a cloth that can be laundered. The structure of natural and artificial sponges provides an environment in which microorganisms thrive.

To manually sanitize dishes and utensils in hot water at 170° F, a hot water booster is usually required. To avoid burning the skin while immersing dishes and utensils in this hot water bath, use special racks designed for this purpose. If dishes and utensils are being washed by hand, the chemical sanitizer method using household bleach is usually a safer choice.

Handling clean dishes and utensils

Pick up and touch clean spoons, knives, and forks only by their handles, not by any part that will be in contact with food or put in someone's mouth. When children help set the table, be sure they have washed their hands thoroughly and remind them not to touch the parts of the tableware that will have contact with food and go into the mouth. Handle clean cups, glasses, and bowls so that fingers and thumbs do not touch the inside or the lip-contact surfaces.

Managing toxic substances

Be sure that all potentially toxic items remain in their original labeled containers except for diluted solutions. Label diluted solutions with the product name, dilution, date the dilution was prepared, and place to find the container (with the manufacturer's label on it) of the concentrate from which the dilution was made. Substances that are likely to be toxic include cleaning materials, detergents of any sort (general, for use in dishwashers, for cleaning rugs, etc.), aerosol cans, pesticides, medications, landscaping chemicals, and any other products labeled with warnings about their toxicity. The Occupational Safety and Health Administration (OSHA) requires that Material Safety Data Sheets (MSDS) must be available on site for each hazardous chemical present. The MSDS is a standard document that describes the product's properties, hazards associated with using it, and instructions for using it safely. Manufacturers are legally required to prepare and make the MSDS documents available for their chemical products.

When toxic substances are used, they must be handled and applied so they do not pose a hazard to staff members or children. They should be stored in a locked closet or cabinet that is inaccessible to children and separate from substances that could be contaminated by them. Staff members should be informed about the presence of toxic substances in the facility. The EPA requires that toxic products regulated by the agency have labels that provide one of its signal words: CAUTION, WARNING, or DANGER (in ascending level of risk). Always choose the least toxic product that will accomplish the task.

Monitoring radon and carbon monoxide

Facilities should be monitored for the presence of hazardous levels of radon and carbon monoxide. For radon, there are protocols to test facilities that follow EPA specifications. Facilities that have any fuel or product that can produce carbon monoxide should have detectors that monitor for this odorless, invisible gas on a continuous basis. Check with local building inspectors for information on types of detectors to install and how to maintain them.

Monitoring asbestos and other friable materials

A facility with asbestos, fiberglass, or any other friable (easily crumbled) material must monitor its condition and arrange for removal when there is a dangerous condition. Removal or repair requires a certified contractor who can do the work in compliance with EPA regulations. Children and staff members should not be present in the facility when such work is being done.

Storing and disposing of garbage

Keep the facility free of accumulated garbage. Garbage containers attract animals and insects. When trash contains organic material, decomposition creates unpleasant odors. Therefore, facilities must choose and use garbage containers that control sanitation risks, pests, and offensive odors. Lining the containers with plastic bags reduces the contamination of the container itself and the need to wash the containers. Washing garbage containers can spread the contamination into the environment.

Trash and garbage should be removed from all occupied spaces of the facility every day and from the premises at least twice a week. Use plastic-lined, durable metal or plastic containers that keep out pests, do not leak, and do not absorb odors. Enough containers should be present to hold all waste properly until it is removed. Using plastic bags as overflow waste storage without an outer rigid metal or plastic container is not acceptable; this practice invites pest infestations. Store toxic wastes and infectious wastes separately from other refuse, in clearly labeled containers. Dispose of these materials according to instructions from your local department of health.

Each trash/waste and diaper container should be labeled to show its intended contents. Clean these containers daily to keep them free from buildup of soil and odor. The wastewater used for cleaning should be discarded by pouring it down a toilet or floor drain. Wastewater should not be poured onto the ground or into handwashing sinks, laundry sinks, kitchen sinks, or bathtubs.

Laundry

Many articles of differing fabrics are used in child care facilities. Sheets, pillowcases, cot covers, dress-up clothes, furniture covers, and other soft articles accumulate soil and become contaminated by drooling, emissions from skin sores, toileting accidents, and vomit. Centers should have a mechanical washing machine and dryer on site or a contract with a laundry service. The laundry equipment must wash or dry at above 140° F, or an approved sanitizer must be used in the rinse cycle. Dryers must be vented to the outside. Store soaps, bleaches, and other laundry supplies in locked cabinets.

Transportation

Transportation is an important aspect of all early childhood programs. Whether you drive the children to and from their homes each day, have them dropped off and picked up by their families, or schedule only an occasional field trip, the cars or buses and walkways that participants in the program use are part of your environment. Motor vehicle pedestrian and passenger injuries represent the greatest threat to a child's life. You can reduce the chances of vehicle-related injury to children and staff members by being alert to potential dangers, eliminating or avoiding these dangers, and knowing what to do when an emergency occurs. Detailed resources about vehicular safety are available from the National Highway Traffic Safety Administration (NHTSA) at **www.nhtsa.gov**. This regularly updated website has information about selecting, installing, and using appropriate seat restraints, as well as information about how to prevent injury to children.

Many children play in and around cars—often while their supervising adult is engaged in conversation or doing something while leaving children "only briefly." Children can be injured when they are trapped in trunks or hot vehicles, run over by vehicles backing up or rolling away, caught by power windows that are used improperly, and entangled in seat belts. Too many adults do not lock their cars; some leave the key in the ignition or elsewhere in the car. A child left in the vehicle with the key can activate the accessory mode, and then open and close power windows, catching fingers, hands, wrists, and arms. The child can also be strangled by the window closing around his neck, which can happen easily if the child climbs on an arm rest that has power switches. Hide-and-seek can turn deadly if a child gets trapped in the trunk or in the passenger compartment, where temperatures can rise very quickly. One positive development in vehicle safety is that since 2010, new cars are being fitted with safety technology to prevent shifting into gear unless the driver's foot is on the brake (brake transmission safety interlock).

The facility should have and communicate with everyone a plan for safe, supervised drop-off and pickup. The locations allowed for these transitions should be protected from traffic and have designated pedestrian pathways. Someone should be assigned to make sure that children are not in the path of moving vehicles. Family members and staff members must ensure that responsibility for each child is clearly transferred from one adult to another.

Transport should be limited to use of vehicles that can be fitted with seat restraints that are appropriate for children's development/age and size. Each child should be securely and correctly fastened in a seat restraint according to the manufacturer's instructions and federal and state motor vehicle safety standards. For details of current recommendations for seat restraint use, go to **www.nhtsa.gov**. School buses are designed to contain school-age children in the space between the seat the child is using and the back of the next seat forward when the child is properly seated. This helps prevent injury of school-age children. However, this containment mechanism does not work for younger, smaller children who need age- and size-appropriate seat restraints often not found in school buses. Vans intended for 12–15 passengers have the highest risk of

> **Figure 10.1.**
> ### Transportation Safety Rules
>
> - Make sure all vehicles used to transport children have the most recent federally approved safety seats and/or safety belts. Follow the manufacturer's instructions, then contact local police, state police, or other public safety officials to arrange for an NHTSA-certified car seat technician to check the installation and planned use.
> - Plan travel so that no child spends more than one hour in the vehicle.
> - Check staff-to-child ratios to be sure that they meet the requirements for indoor spaces (do not count the driver in the ratio).
> - Secure all children and adults in their own safety seat or safety belt. Never put two or more children in the same safety belt. Always adjust a car seat for the child sitting in it.
> - Daily check vehicles for any problems with seat restraints.
> - Immediately before each trip, the driver should conduct a quick five-minute check to ensure that the vehicle is working well and contains nothing that could harm the children. If the day is warm, the vehicle's air conditioning system must be capable of keeping the temperature below 82° F during the ride; if the day is cold, the heating system must keep the temperature above 65° F.
> - Ask drivers to remain alert to changes in the vehicle while driving. Unusual odors, sounds, or vibrations can be warning signals for a breakdown. No loud radio or other noises should interfere with hearing traffic alerts or mechanical problems.
> - Never transport children or adults in the cargo area of a station wagon or van.
> - Never leave children alone in a vehicle, even briefly.
> - Keep sharp or heavy objects out of the passenger compartment. They can become deadly projectiles in a sudden stop or accident.
> - Load and unload young children only where they will not be exposed to traffic. Pull the vehicle up to the curb, up to the side of the road, or into a driveway, releasing children only to an authorized adult.
> - Do not let children put their arms or heads out of the vehicle's windows.
> - There should be no smoking in the vehicle.
> - Drivers should be at least 21 years of age and not use alcohol, drugs, or medications that could impair their judgment within 12 hours of driving.
> - Always do a final check of the vehicle to be sure that all children are safely out.

rollover accidents and should not be used to transport groups of children.

No child younger than 13 years of age should ride in the front seat. Before using a seat restraint, an adult should check all metal parts to be sure they are not hot enough to burn the child. Interior temperatures should be controlled with fresh air, air conditioning, or heating so that the temperature is in the range of 65–82° F. Drivers must know the quickest route to the nearest emergency medical facility along the route to be traveled.

Decisions to transport children involve consideration of family needs and legal, regulatory, moral, and ethical concerns. By learning about safe transportation, providers can reduce their liability and teach families and children how to avoid injury related to transportation by foot, car, bike, and bus. See Figure 10.1 for additional safety rules.

Legal requirements

Research and follow all state laws and licensing regulations pertaining to your program's transportation. Next, develop a written policy clearly stating the rules, responsibilities of staff members and children, and emergency procedures to be followed. Written policies and guidelines do not guarantee safety, but if everyone knows and uses them, they reduce the likelihood of injury. Whenever motor vehicles are used to transport children, special safety measures are necessary. The driver must be experienced and licensed with an excellent driving record and no history of substance abuse, criminal record, or any medical condition that could impair driving ability. The driver must be mature enough to assume responsibility for passengers' safety.

Ratios and supervision during transport

When transporting children, use, meet, or exceed the facility's staff-to-child ratios set by state requirements. Keep in mind that these ratios are minimum standards. Drivers must be able to focus entirely on driving tasks, leaving supervision of the children to other adults in the vehicle. They should not be counted in the staff-to-child ratios.

Staff members are responsible for supervising every child all the time, including when the children are going to or coming from vehicles, and getting in or getting out of them at the facility. Parents may become distracted while chatting with a staff member or another parent. Someone must be paying attention to the children at all times. When volunteers assist with transportation, they must follow the program's policies. After each trip, be sure that family members and volunteers escort children into the building and stay with them until responsibility for the children is transferred to another adult. It is essential to do a careful name-to-face attendance check of children entering and exiting vehicles. There have been more than a few cases in which children have died after staff members inadvertently left them asleep in vehicles.

Carefully assess all pickup and drop-off locations. Each facility is unique in its proximity to local traffic, parking lots, driveways, and pedestrian areas. Drivers of vans and school buses cannot see children who may be walking close to the vehicle; some children have died as a result. The danger zone for pedestrian injuries is 10 feet in front and beside the vehicle. Teach children to take the number of giant steps required to move them 10 feet from the vehicle as soon as they exit it.

All drivers and staff members must be familiar with emergency plans, the use of safety restraints, supervision requirements, and pediatric first aid in the event of an injury.

Transporting children with special needs

Automotive safety devices have been designed to protect children with special physical and behavioral needs when they are riding in motor vehicles. Devices are available for children of various weights and heights with conditions such as prematurity, muscular and skeletal problems, head and spinal cord injuries, temporary orthopedic conditions (e.g., a fracture), neurological diseases, developmental disabilities, recent surgery, obesity, and emotional/behavioral issues that might distract a driver.

Wheelchairs should face forward, not sideways, during transport. Crash-tested wheelchair tie-downs, *not* homemade devices, should be used to secure wheelchairs in a van.

Devices must be easy to use, or they will not be used correctly, if at all. Special devices tend to be expensive, so it is best to choose one that can be used for a number of years and adjusted as a child grows or used for children of different sizes. All restraint systems must be crash-tested according to federal safety standards and retested even if only a small modification is made. Other equipment, such as an oxygen tank, should be secured so that it does not become a projectile should a collision occur. The child's physician, the public health department, or organizations such as Easter Seals may be helpful resources in locating appropriate safety devices.

Drivers and adult passengers who will transport children with special needs should receive training related to the needs of the children they are transporting. All vehicles should be equipped with a two-way radio or mobile phone.

Emergency procedures

Always expect the unexpected, no matter how efficient and safe your transportation system may be. Prepare by taking the following steps:

- Be sure that children, families, driver(s), and staff members all know what to do in an emergency. For each of the following issues, develop a procedure using suggestions from older children, families, and staff members. Use discussion groups and/or handouts to inform everyone of these procedures. Transportation emergency topics to be shared include
  - How to safely evacuate the vehicle
  - How to assess injuries and provide first aid
  - How to explain the situation to the children and reassure them of their safety
  - What staff members still in the building are to do
  - When, who, and how to call for emergency support
  - What to do in bad weather
  - What to do when a child or an adult becomes ill or injured during transport
- Teach drivers the specific steps to follow under various emergency conditions.
- Make sure that staff members who remain at the facility know what to do when they are notified of any emergency on the road (e.g., contact parents or provide alternate transportation).
- Annually, remind families of emergency procedures. Collect and test their contact information by trying to contact them when there is no emergency.
- If you use a bus, practice emergency evacuation drills so the children will be familiar with what they may be asked to do.

Emergency situations must be handled calmly, efficiently, and with constant attention to the children's fears, concerns, and safety.

What to have in the vehicle

A well organized transportation system is important even if you do not transport children regularly. Special trips mean special circumstances. First of all, drivers may be traveling an unfamiliar route or transporting children who may not ordinarily ride with them. Drivers may be sharing responsibility with volunteers who are themselves new to the situation. Finally, the children may be overly excited, tired, or even frightened.

Certain information and equipment kept in vehicles are helpful in various circumstances.

Information

Specific information about the children and the route should be kept in a notebook or similar secure holder in the vehicle. Make sure the information is up-to-date and the driver and other staff members can find it easily. Include the following:

- A map of the route with estimated mileages and travel times and the names and addresses of children in the vehicle
- An information/emergency card for each child that describes how to reach parents and emergency contacts and contains special medical or health information
- Information regarding children with special needs, including descriptions of the condition and medications, behavior patterns, and warning signs for medical attention
- Telephone numbers of emergency services (e.g., local police, fire station, hospital, and ambulance service) and the name and telephone number of the child care program and a contact person who should be called in the event of any difficulty
- Pen and paper to record information from the families at pickup so this information can be passed on to teachers

Equipment to be kept in the vehicle

- *First aid kit.* Use the list of suggested items in Figure 4.2 in Chapter 4 to assemble your kit.
- *Wireless communication device such as a cell phone.* Use this only for emergencies and then only by an adult passenger or the driver when the vehicle is stopped.
- *Emergency supply of toys.* Bring along songs, books, and other activities to help keep children occupied during an unscheduled wait.
- *Travel rope.* Use this for children to hold on to for easy evacuation or for walks from the vehicle to a safe place.
- *Fire extinguisher, extra water, flashlight, and tools for minor repairs.* These may be indispensable in the event of a breakdown.

Field trips/car pools

The following suggestions can help staff members safely transport children during special trips. Refer also to Chapter 3 for other information about pedestrian safety and field trips.

- When the destination is known in advance, review the route mentally (or with a map if the distance is great). Practice the route if you have time and the vehicle is available. When using a GPS device to assist in navigating the route, the driver should also carry a map to serve as a backup.
- Make sure you have a signed authorization for every child and a list of all adults who will be traveling. Check your insurance coverage for car pools.
- Make sure both the driver and other adults (e.g., volunteers and staff members) know who is responsible for providing behavioral guidance to children. Let the children know who is in charge and what the rules are.
- Make sure that all children and adults use age- and size-appropriate safety restraints (e.g., child car seats and safety belts).
- Never have more passengers than seat restraints.
- Help the driver concentrate by keeping children occupied with soft books or toys, songs, and conversation.
- Use travel time to talk about rules for safe riding or other important concepts.
- If children become unruly or remove their safety restraints, stop and pull off the road to calmly address the situation. *Do not attempt to provide behavioral guidance while the vehicle is moving.*
- Make sure all passengers know when and where they are supposed to return to the vehicle.
- If more than one vehicle is used for the trip, make sure all passengers know which vehicle they are to ride in during the return trip.
- On field trips, make sure that no child enters the vehicle alone or plays on the vehicle while the others are visiting the site. *Never leave children alone in the vehicle.*
- Use a trip sheet to record destination, mileage, times of departure and return, and a list of passengers. For field trips with larger numbers of participants, the latter is particularly important.

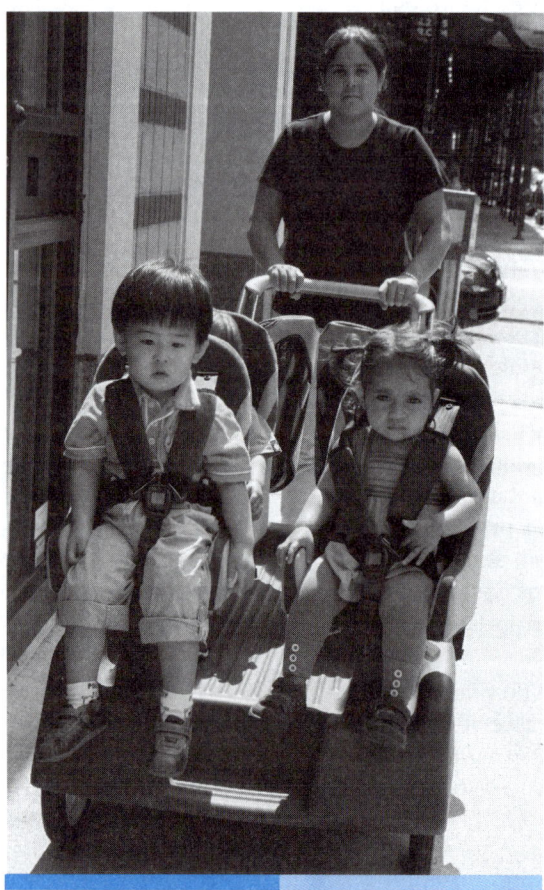

By Susan Woog Wagner / © NAEYC

- Ensure that all participants in the car pools understand and agree to follow the established guidelines.
- Provide enough staff assistance to ensure that every child is buckled, unbuckled, and removed from the vehicle. People who are in a hurry may make unsafe "just this time" decisions.

Passenger safety education

For children

Preschoolers are old enough to understand simple concepts of passenger and pedestrian safety. Consistent use of safe behaviors helps children continue to practice them in later years. There are four major messages to emphasize with children and parent passengers:

- Everyone in the car must buckle up—including drivers and passengers in the front and back seats—no matter how short the trip.
- Safety belts go across the hips, not the stomach, with the shoulder portion across the chest.
- The back seat is the safest place for child passengers.
- Good passengers ride quietly.

The *Risk Watch®* curriculum available from the National Fire Protection Association at **www.nfpa.org** includes child passenger safety activities. It also includes materials for use with parents. You might make pretend cars out of cardboard boxes and make chairs, seats, and safety belts from fabric scraps. Practice in the classroom or on the playground by playing games such as Simon Says to encourage the use of safety belts and entering/exiting vehicles correctly. Practice taking giant steps after exiting the vehicle and count how many steps are needed to reach 10 feet, which is the distance that allows the driver to see a child. These games are fun role-playing and dramatic play activities. Invite the safety officer from your community to come to the program to talk about traffic safety.

Teach pedestrian safety to children from infancy onward. Adults who discuss and personally practice these rules consistently effectively teach children how to walk safely. (See Pedestrian safety in Chapter 3.)

Teach children to safely use riding toys that are pedaled and have a wheel base over 20 inches in diameter. Start teaching these rules when children first learn to ride any riding toy with pedals (e.g., big wheels, tricycles, bicycles):

- Always wear a properly fitted helmet.
- Ride only on something that is the right size for you.
- Ride on the right side of the road.
- Learn hand signals to let others know what you will do (e.g., turning right and left, stopping) as soon as you can.
- Stop before crossing any street to look left-right-left, scanning for cars. Use your eyes like a flashlight to sweep the area to look for cars.

For families

It is important to involve families in all educational activities; they can promote concepts presented in the classroom. Keep them informed through letters, parent education meetings, and personal contacts. With transportation topics, send home suggestions and activities that parents and children can work on together (e.g., counting the number of seat belts in the car). Focus on three main issues:

- Children must use child safety seats and safety belts for every ride.
- Select a suitable child safety seat.
- Use child safety seats and seat belts correctly. Children younger than 2 years of age should be seated facing the rear of the vehicle. Newer seat restraints are being sold to allow this positioning.

The American Academy of Pediatrics (AAP) regularly updates materials on family transportation safety. Go to **www.aap.org** and use the search terms "child passenger safety" and "child pedestrian safety."

Suggested activities

- Visit a child care facility and check how well the facility meets the guidelines in this chapter. Where there are differences, could modifications be made at reasonable cost and with available time and personnel resources?
- What compromises that increase health and safety risks have you seen made in facilities? Why were these compromises made? Were better alternatives possible?
- Observe passenger safety restraint use by standing at the curb outside a child care facility during an hour when the largest number of children in the program are arriving or leaving. What proportion of the adults are wearing seat belts? Are all of the children in seat restraints? Are all of the children younger than 2 years of age seated facing the rear of the vehicle?
- Ask a child care center director about the facility's cleaning routines. Use Figure A.3 in Appendix A to check how each item is cleaned and how often, as well as whether and how it is sanitized.
- Contact the licensing agency in your area to see if you can accompany a licensing inspector to see what maintenance issues get checked and how they are observed. Are any problems overlooked?

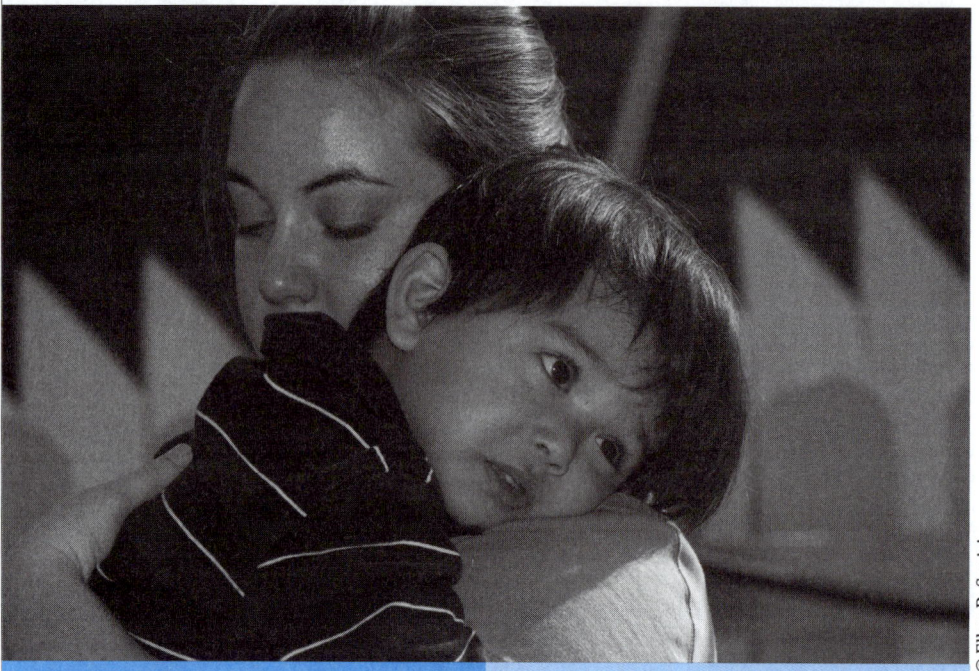

Caring for Children with Short-Term or Chronic Health Needs or Disabilities

MAJOR CONCEPTS

- Because all children inevitably experience illness, mostly mild infectious disease, all early education programs must be prepared to recognize and respond appropriately to minor illness.

- The daily health check, used before the child is left in the care of staff members for the day, is an essential practice for detecting illness and collecting information that will help meet the child's needs during the day. In addition, the daily health check procedure is a valuable tool to use when the child becomes ill while in care.

- Communication at drop-off and pickup about the child's eating, drinking, sleeping, and participation in activities is essential to ensure that care is appropriate in the time that follows.

- Specialized programs that provide care for ill children who are excluded from typical program care require specific facilities, procedures, staff training, and access to consultants so that they can provide such care safely.

- Staff members who will give medication to children must receive training and follow procedures to do so safely.

- Teachers should be able to follow currently recommended practices to provide temporary care for children with common symptoms and frequently occurring chronic health needs, whether this care is needed only until the parent can pick up the child or the program provides ongoing care for mildly ill children.

The most common childhood illnesses are caused by mild infections. Chapter 2 discussed prevention, detection, and the need to plan for management of these inevitable—but usually short-term—mild illnesses. Almost every early childhood program includes several children with special needs, such as developmental disabilities or chronic health conditions. For example, more than 1 in every 10 preschool children has some type of allergy. Asthma occurs in approximately 7 percent of all children. Skin conditions such as eczema are fairly common. Other less common conditions are heart problems, epilepsy, and diabetes. This chapter will discuss caring for children with common minor illnesses that may affect typically developing, healthy children; it will also discuss children with the most common types of chronic health problems and special needs. More detailed information about caring for children who have special needs, including chronic health conditions, can be found in Chapter 12. For information about managing a wide range of chronic health conditions, consult the Quick Reference Sheets in *Managing Chronic Health Needs in Child Care and Schools: A Quick Reference Guide,* a publication of the American Academy of Pediatrics, available from the AAP bookstore at **www.aap.org**.

The daily health check

Every day, someone on the facility staff who is familiar with a child's behavior and appearance should check the child on arrival at the facility or wherever the care of the child transfers from the family to the staff (i.e., when picked up from home if transportation is provided by the program). The staff member should talk with the parent about how the child has been while at home. This staff member should repeat this assessment anytime the child does not seem well. The purpose of this check is to identify conditions that might require exclusion of the child or special care while the child is in the facility. The procedure is best done as part of a warm greeting of the child and family that shows interest. The staff member who conducts the check should respect the feelings and concerns of the child and family. A similar procedure should be followed when transferring the child back to the family. Face-to-face communication is best, but if it is not possible, the staff observation and communication with the family must occur when responsibility for the child's care transfers from or back to the family. Alternate means of communication include notes, electronic communications, health checklists, and/or daily logs. Use the list of items in Figure 11.1 to guide the daily health check until the procedure becomes routine.

If you have concerns about what a family member tells you or how a particular child looks or feels, discuss these concerns before accepting care of the child. Be clear that it is the program's decision, not the family's, whether the program will accept responsibility for the ill child that day. The child cannot stay at the program if the responsible program staff member decides that the child should not stay. If the child can stay, be sure to discuss how the program staff will manage the situation and at what point you will call the parent. If an ill child stays in the program all day, be sure to document any symptoms the child has. The notations can be made on the Observation and Symptom Record provided in Figure A.13 in Appendix A. When the ill child leaves for the day, staff members must let the family know what happened during that day—preferably in written form. Simple information about activity level, appetite and food intake, naptime, and bowel movements that seems inconsequential at the time can be invaluable to the family and to the health care professional if the child becomes more ill after leaving the program for the day. Written reports kept by a staff member about the child's illness, such as the Observation and Symptom Record, help overcome the natural tendency to forget to pass

Figure 11.1.

Items to Include in the Daily Health Check

Take the following information into account:

1. From what the family and the child tell you:
   a. Any complaints about not feeling well
   b. Any symptoms of illness or injury reported by the family such as a runny nose, cough, difficulty breathing, having loose stools, being cranky, not sleeping well, not eating or drinking normally, having any problem with urination, and skin rashes or itchiness
   c. Last time child ate, drank, and had a diaper change or used the toilet
   d. Any illness in the family, exposure to someone else who is ill, or experience of an unusual event

2. From what you see:
   a. Appearance or behavior that is unusual for the child
   b. Symptoms of illness or injury as in 1.b. above and flushed appearance, warm or unusually dry skin, shivering, or discomfort or bruising noted while gently touching the child. (Check the child's temperature with a thermometer only if the child seems unusually warm or ill.)
   c. Any odors suggesting the need for a diaper change or some other condition that needs attention

Source: Adapted, by permission, from S.S. Aronson, ed., *Model Child Care Health Policies,* 5th edition (American Academy of Pediatrics, forthcoming).

along some of the details when the child is picked up at the end of the day.

At drop-off and during the day, use a cumulative log to record symptoms for the group over a period of time, such as the Enrollment/Attendance/Symptom Record form provided in Appendix F of *Caring for Our Children*. Attendance can be documented on this form, too. This type of record allows easy identification of trends for an individual child, for a particular group of children, or for the program as a whole.

Care of the mildly ill child

The care of ill children in group programs can be viewed from many perspectives: the child's needs, the family's needs, the teacher's needs, and the needs related to the parents' employment. Parents' need to prepare for inevitable illness is addressed in *Managing Infectious Diseases in Child Care and Schools*. All families should have a backup plan for when the child must be excluded from the child care program. Families need to understand the program's exclusion policies, especially the rule that designated program staff members will decide when exclusion is necessary. As discussed in Chapter 2 and reviewed briefly in this chapter, some specific conditions *require* exclusion. For other conditions, only the staff members who are authorized to make exclusion decisions know the actual circumstances of the program on any given day and can therefore decide whether the child can be accommodated—even when the family thinks the child is well enough to participate and does not require much extra care. Staff members will consider the family's description of the child's behavior, the results of their own findings from the daily health check, and the circumstances of the program to determine when a child may need to be excluded and when the child may return to care.

Basic issues for decision making about caring for ill children

Many health policies concerning the care of ill children have been based upon common misunderstandings about contagion, risks to ill children, and risks to other children and staff members. Research clearly shows that certain ill children *do not* pose a health threat to others. Research also shows that keeping certain mildly ill children at home or isolated at the facility *will not* prevent other children from becoming ill. Usually, the other children have already been exposed to the illness-causing germs while the ill child was becoming sick. For many viral diseases, the amount of germs the ill child is shedding is already decreasing when the child develops symptoms.

Children with common colds who feel well enough to participate in the program do not need to be excluded. Children receiving antibiotics for a specific bacterial infection usually are not contagious after a day's treatment and can return. Refer to Chapter 2 of this manual and Appendix A: Signs and Symptoms Chart in *Caring for Our Children* to know when to exclude children with specific symptoms and conditions and when children who have been excluded can return.

Issues for programs

When deciding whether to keep a mildly ill child at your facility, ask these questions:

- Are there sufficient staff members (including volunteers) to change the program for a child who needs some modifications, such as quiet activities, staying inside, or extra liquids?

- Are staff members willing and able to care for a sick child (e.g., wiping a runny nose, checking a fever, providing extra loving care) without neglecting the care of other children in the group?

- Is there a space where the mildly ill child can rest? Is there a space that might be used as a get-well room so several children could be cared for at once? Is the child familiar with the staff member(s) who will be providing the child's care?

- Is the family able or willing to pay extra staffing costs for sick care if other resources are not available?

The essential question is this: Can the child participate with *reasonable comfort* and receive appropriate care without interfering with the care of the other children? One child with a low fever and cough may still have a high energy level, good appetite, and good mood, but another child may be droopy, whiny, uninterested in any activity, and very unhappy. *Every case is different and should be decided for each child by the designated staff members with family input, using guidelines and procedures developed in consultation with health professionals.* The focus of policies for all children should be on what conditions and symptoms the program can include and manage.

When a child becomes ill while in the program, the family should be notified. Discuss the issue with the family sensitively. Demonstrate concern for the child's health and the family's situation, refer to the program's health policies, and do the best you can to meet the needs of everyone who is involved. The most common—and usually best—alternative care arrangement is for the parent to care for the ill child at home. For children who are excluded from their usual care arrangements, one or more of the following alternative care arrangements may be available:

- Care by a family member in the child's home or in the family member's home

- Care in the child's own home by a caregiver who is not a family member

- Care in a small family child care home
- Care in the child's usual group
- Care in a separate space in the child's own center if there are special provisions designed for the care of ill children (sometimes called the infirmary model)
- Care in a separate center serving only children with illness or temporary conditions

Whether or not the child needs to be excluded, the program must plan how the ill child will be cared for until the family picks up the child. If the program provides care to ill children, there must be a plan for what the program will do while the child is getting well. (See the section later in this chapter, Temporary care for children with common minor illnesses.) The program can protect others from the spread of a contagious disease by maintaining at least a three-foot separation between the child and other children, practicing hand hygiene, and cleaning and disinfecting surfaces that the ill child has used. The specific requirements for facilities that provide care for children who are temporarily excluded from their usual group care setting can be found in *Caring for Our Children* Section 3.6.2.

Excluded children and staff members may come back when they are well enough to participate in the program. When anyone has an infection, continue to follow strict hand and surface hygiene for a while afterward. Being lax in following these precautions can easily lead to an outbreak. Some bacterial diarrhea requires a specific number of negative cultures before the infected person can return. Sometimes a person who had diarrhea continues to have looser and more frequent stools, but otherwise seems well. After a week or so of waiting for the diarrhea symptom to go away, unless this person has an infection that requires negative stool cultures to return, the facility can assume that the increased number and looser consistency of stools is that person's new normal pattern and allow the individual to return to the facility. The details for when to allow return for most infections can be found in *Caring for Our Children* Standards 3.6.1.1 and 3.6.1.2 and in *Managing Infectious Diseases in Child Care and Schools*.

Issues for families

When families decide whether to send an ill child to group care, they must weigh many factors, such as how the child feels (physically and emotionally), the program's ability to serve the child's needs, and the potential for income lost if the parent stays home with the child—even the potential for job loss. Employers put both overt and implied pressure on workers to come to work every day, and they want their employees to find ways to manage illness that do not affect work performance. Parents facing a disruption of their work obligations may bring the child to the program in the hope that he is not ill enough to be excluded from care. They may take an ill child to work with them if they think the child will be excluded and they have no alternative care available.

Although many families may honestly try to consider all the facts and decide what is best for the child, this is hard to do when the facts are fuzzy. Parents are often unaware of a child's illness when they drop off the child at the program. A child may awaken cranky at home but show no signs of illness, or the child may have vomited after dinner the night before but slept well and seemed cheerful on waking up. The child may have an unexplained low-grade fever but seem absolutely fine.

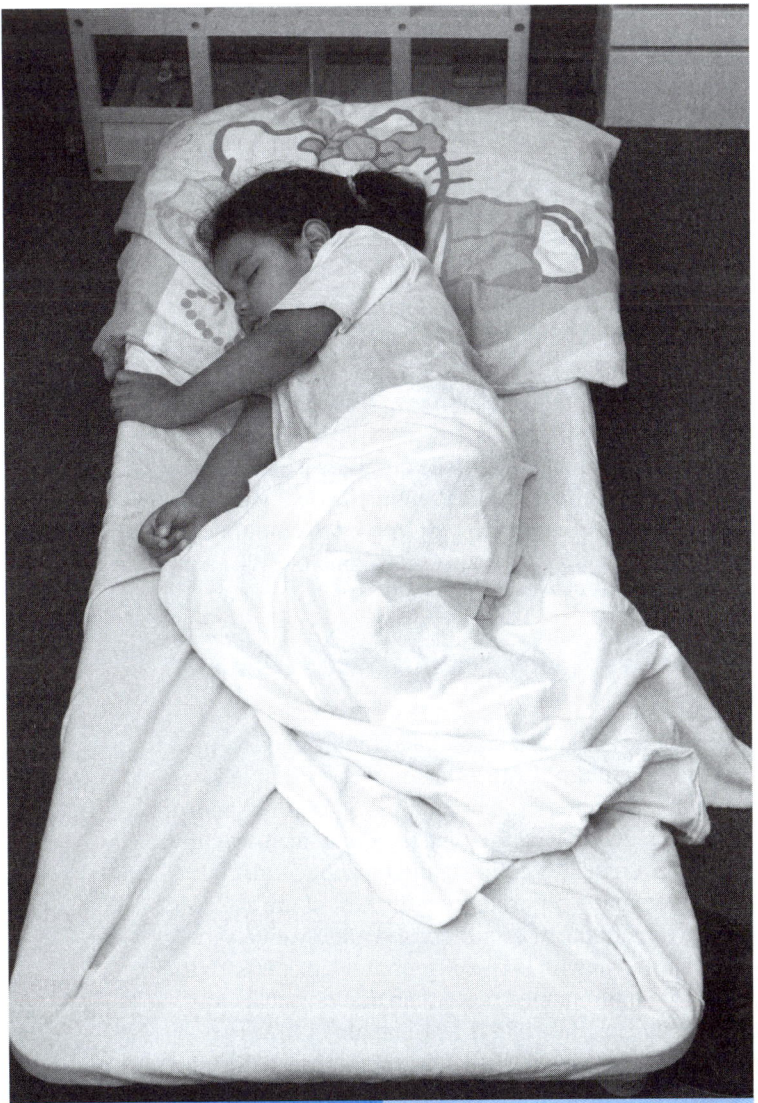

© Ellen B. Senisi

Families must navigate their options, and they often experience considerable stress while doing it.

Setting policies for care of ill children

A facility may care for ill children if it is approved by the licensing authority and has written plans regarding admissible conditions and symptoms, as well as procedures for daily care of ill children. These plans should be reviewed annually by the child care health consultant and the local health authority.

Know what to do when a child appears ill

The program's written policies and procedures should detail the actions to take when a child becomes seriously ill or is injured. Some conditions require calling the emergency medical services number (usually 911). Other situations require bringing the child to a source of medical care within an hour. Still others require consulting a health professional about what to do. Health professional advice could be provided in a telephone conversation, or the recommendation might be for the family to take the child to an appointment at a clinical facility. Personnel must have sufficient training to recognize when a child requires prompt medical attention. The conditions that require medical care right away are outlined in Figure A.14 in Appendix A.

Each child's family should identify at least two emergency contact people who are usually available to take the child home if the parent cannot be reached or is not available. Ensure that contact information for these two individuals is in the child's record, and test their telephone numbers occasionally to be sure they are current. Testing telephone numbers is most easily incorporated into the office routine if you divide the number of children in the program by the number of working days in six months (approximately 120) and test that number of telephone contacts every day.

Temporary care for children with common minor illnesses

Every program and each enrolled family needs a plan to care for ill children. If the child must be excluded from care, at a minimum, the program's plan should address care provided during the time the child must wait until pickup occurs. The child should be kept comfortable in a quiet space separate from the rest of the children where the child can be supervised and receive care from someone who is competent and familiar with the child. Ill children need more than just physical care. During illness, the child is learning about how to cope with being sick. Be sure to share staff observations about the child's illness with the child's family. If medical advice is needed, the information about how the child was during the day is essential to the health care provider's ability to provide advice.

If a child appears *mildly* ill, take him aside, encourage rest, and assess the situation. Observe the child's symptoms. *Remember, you are not expected to diagnose illness.* Report the symptoms you have observed to the proper person(s)—the family, the program director, the health staff person (if any) or health consultant, and/or the child's health provider. Decide whether the program can continue to care for the child. Report the situation to the family and be sure to document what you observed and did for the child. To know what to do for different symptoms, review the current recommendations for care of common symptoms with your program's child care health consultant. Write up a plan for your setting.

At the end of this chapter, you'll find a brief description of some commonly occurring symptoms and chronic health conditions. A more comprehensive resource for competent guidelines prepared for parents is the current edition of *Caring for Your Baby and Young Child: Birth to Age 5,* published by the AAP. This book is regularly reviewed and updated by a panel of national pediatric experts. It can be purchased from the AAP bookstore at **www.aap.org**. For free and current information about care of mild illnesses, search for the symptom or condition on the AAP's Healthy Children website for parents and caregivers, **www.healthychildren.org**.

Special considerations for programs that do not exclude mildly ill children

When young children become ill they need adequate rest, appropriate diet, medications as ordered, and appropriate physical and emotional support. Working parents should be entitled to family sick leave days to care for their ill children. Professionals and the public generally agree that when a child is seriously ill, or when it is not yet clear that the illness is a mild one, the parent should be able to stay home with the child. At a minimum, working parents should be able to use their own sick or personal days to care for their ill children. However, because children are ill frequently, some families have difficulty making alternative arrangements for the days when the child is not very ill and the parents need to be at work.

Facilities unable to care for ill children should be supportive and helpful to families, giving them suggestions for alternative arrangements. Sometimes, with modified activities, a child can be included in the facility's regular group of children. A center may be able to set up a get-well room where ill children who are not able to participate in their regular group can receive care. Some centers set up small satellite family child care homes for their enrolled children to use when ill. Ideally the program will make sure that the children already know the teacher in the get-well room or in the satellite child care home by having her regularly work at the center with each of the groups. Other alternative care arrangements include 1) a worker sent by a home health agency or from a pool of qualified adults to the child's home, or 2) care in a special pediatric unit of a hospital, a facility adjacent to a pediatric office, or another similar setting.

Some facilities offer care for mildly ill children who would otherwise be excluded from a program because they have contagious infections or require more care than most programs could provide. (See criteria described in Chapter 2.) These facilities should meet more specialized requirements, such as having staff members with the qualifications and training that the program's health consultant thinks necessary to care for the specific types of illnesses that the program will accommodate. Other considerations are

- Child-to-staff ratios
- Space and equipment requirements
- Special services from health consultants
- Administrative procedures that differ from those used by facilities that care for well children only

In some states, facilities that care for ill children must be separately licensed. The standards for such facilities are detailed in Section 3.6.2 of *Caring for Our Children*. Those who are considering providing care for children who are excluded from their usual care arrangement should review and follow these standards.

Health consultants

Appropriate involvement of health consultants is especially important for facilities that care for ill children. Programs should use the expertise of health professionals to design and provide an environment with sufficient staff members and facilities to meet the needs of ill children. The health consultant for facilities that provide more than temporary care for mildly ill children waiting to be picked up should be a health professional with training and experience in pediatric health care. See Chapter 9 for details about child care health consultants, including where to look for someone to fill this role for your program.

Caring for Our Children Standard 3.6.2.7 describes the requirements for health consultation for specialized facilities that care for children who are ill as follows:

> Each special facility that provides care for children who are ill should use the services of a child care health consultant for ongoing consultation on overall operation and development of written policies relating to health care. The child care health consultant should have the knowledge, skills, and preparation as stated in Standard 1.6.0.1.

The facility should involve the child care health consultant in development and/or implementation, review, and sign-off of the written policies and procedures for managing specific illnesses. The facility staff and the child care health consultant should review and update the written policies annually.

The facility should assign the child care health consultant the responsibility for reviewing written policies and procedures for the following:

a. Admission and readmission after illness, including inclusion/exclusion criteria

b. Health evaluation procedures on intake, including physical assessment of the child and other criteria used to determine the appropriateness of a child's attendance

c. Plans for health care and for managing children with infectious diseases

d. Plans for surveillance of illnesses that are admissible and problems that arise in the care of children with illness

e. Plans for staff training and communication with parents/guardians and primary care providers

f. Plans for injury prevention

g. Situations that require medical care within an hour

While making arrangements to have this type of service from a health consultant may be difficult and require additional program expense, having such advice is essential for each special facility that provides care for ill children. If possible, the program should use the same health consultant's services for ongoing consultation on overall operation and development of written policies relating to health care. The facility should involve the consultant in development and/or implementation, review, and approval of the written policies and procedures for managing specific illnesses. The program staff members and the consultant need to review and update the written policies annually. The facility should arrange for the health consultant to take responsibility for reviewing written policies and procedures that have health and safety implications.

Giving medication in a child care program

Almost all children, at one time or another, need medication. Families probably will ask you to give medication for a chronic condition, for a mild illness, or as needed for temporary discomfort. The Americans with Disabilities Act (ADA) may require providers to administer medications to children with chronic conditions or special health needs.

Caring for Our Children Standard 3.6.3.1 defines when medication administration is permissible in child care programs. This standard requires that both prescription and nonprescription (over-the-counter, or OTC) medication must be ordered by the prescribing health care professional for a specific child, with written parental permission for the program to administer the medication. (The exception is that nonprescription sunscreen and insect repellent require parental consent but do not require instructions from the child's health professional.) Written instructions from the health care professional should specify the reason for giving the medication, the name of the medication, the dosage, and how long the medication should continue to be given.

The medication must come to the facility in the original container with a label that includes the child's name, date filled, prescriber's name, pharmacy name and phone number, dosage/instructions, and relevant warnings. Folk or homemade remedies or treatments (those not covered by oversight of the federal Food and Drug Administration or not prescribed by a licensed pediatric health care provider) may not be administered in child care. Written procedures that are followed by the program staff should address documentation of the receipt of the medication from the parent with a safety check of the instructions and the container label; proper storage; administration in a private area away from other children and using appropriate technique; and documentation of the dose, time, and any problems associated with administration. The commonly cited "Five Rights" of medication administration in group settings should be assured: Right Medication, Right Child, Right Dose, Right Method, and Right Time. Some add a sixth right to this list: Right Documentation.

Enlist families' help when children require medication. This might include setting up a schedule for giving medications only at home or consulting with the child's health care provider about prescribing medication in a different form (e.g., liquid, pill, or capsule) and/or varying the number of times a day a medication is required (e.g., morning and bedtime instead of three times a day). You might ask a parent to come during the day to give the medication, but it is burdensome to require families to do this unless a parent works near the facility.

The forms in Appendix AA of *Caring for Our Children* make up a Medication Administration Packet. The forms include an authorization for program staff members to give medication, a checklist for teachers to follow when receiving medication from the parent, a Medication Log to document medication that is given, and a Medication Incident Report. In addition, the packet includes a checklist to give to families to ensure that they are aware of and support the steps necessary for the facility to give medication to their child. Giving this checklist to parents and reminding them to use it when requesting medication administration during program hours may help everyone to limit inappropriate requests and make appropriate requests easier to handle.

Check state regulations for requirements related to administering medication to children in your care. Errors in medication administration occur easily; reactions and side effects are common. It is essential that only personnel with appropriate training and demonstrated skills perform this task; therefore, all teachers who give medication to children should receive training about how to safely administer it. Training should include skill and competency assessment in medication administration. Curricula concerning both medication administration and managing infectious diseases, with manuals and videos for instructors and participants, are posted at **www.healthychildcare.org/HealthyFutures.html**. A licensed health professional may teach a course using these curriculum materials.

It is best to have a health professional observe staff members administering medication at the program site after training is complete, and periodically thereafter. Try to arrange for a pharmacist or nurse to do this observation at least once a year. For a checklist that the health professional can use during the skills check observation, see Figure A.15 in the Appendix.

Practical guidelines for administering medication

- Only staff members who have demonstrated the knowledge and skills required to administer medication in group care settings should administer medicine.

- Have the family ask the pharmacist to give them an extra *labeled* bottle to bring to the program so that one can be kept at home.

- Be sure to have the prescribing health professional give very specific instructions about how the medicine should be given (e.g., before or after meals, with a full glass of water, by tilting the head). Some prescription labels and accompanying information sheets provided by the pharmacy have this information.

- Learn the possible side effects of the medication and inform the family immediately if you observe any. Do not give more medication without the approval of the child's parent or physician.

- Always read what the label says about storage. Most medications should not be stored in warm, wet, or lighted places.

- Always read the label carefully before you give any medicine; bottles often look the same.

- Observe the "Five Rights." Give the right medication to the right child; give the right dose by the right method at the right time. Ensure that the child's name is on the bottle as several children may be taking the same medicine. As an extra precaution, put medication in a bag labeled with the child's name in large letters. Double-check the name of the child, dose, time, and method of administration.

- Never leave medicine in a place where children can get to it. If you must answer the telephone or leave the room while medication is out, put it away first or take it with you. A child can take an overdose in seconds.

- Never refer to medicine as candy or something else children like. They may try to get more of it than is prescribed.

Common illnesses and chronic health conditions

The following short descriptions of some short-term (acute) illnesses and ongoing or recurrent (chronic) health conditions are intended to illustrate the types of health needs that are common among young children and the adults who care for them. Use *Managing Chronic Health Needs in Child Care and Schools* and the AAP Healthy Child Care website to search for and learn more about these and other acute illnesses and chronic health conditions.

Fever

Fever is an elevation of the normal body temperature. It is a common symptom in young children; it is not a disease. Many families (and the public in general) have unrealistic fears about fevers. Fevers are rarely harmful, and treatment is not always necessary. An above-average body temperature can be due to a number of factors, including strenuous exercise, time of day (temperature rises in late afternoon), environment (e.g., a hot room, a hot day, or being bundled up), or individual variation. It can be the result of an infection, an illness that causes inflammation but is not an infection, or a reaction to a medicine.

What is considered a significant fever varies by age and whether there is a simple explanation such as having received a vaccine in an expected interval before the fever occurred. Oral temperatures above 101° F (38.3° C), rectal temperatures above 102° F (38.9° C), or axillary (armpit) temperatures above 100° F (37.8° C) usually are considered to be above normal in children. Infants younger than 4 months with fever should be evaluated by a medical professional on the same day. Any infant younger than 2 months with fever should get medical attention immediately—within an hour if possible. The fever is not harmful; however, the illness causing it may be serious in this age group.

Some young children (usually younger than 4 years of age) with fevers may have a brief seizure (lasting less than five minutes). Although these seizures are harmless, the first time it happens, children should be evaluated by a health professional. Seizures caused by

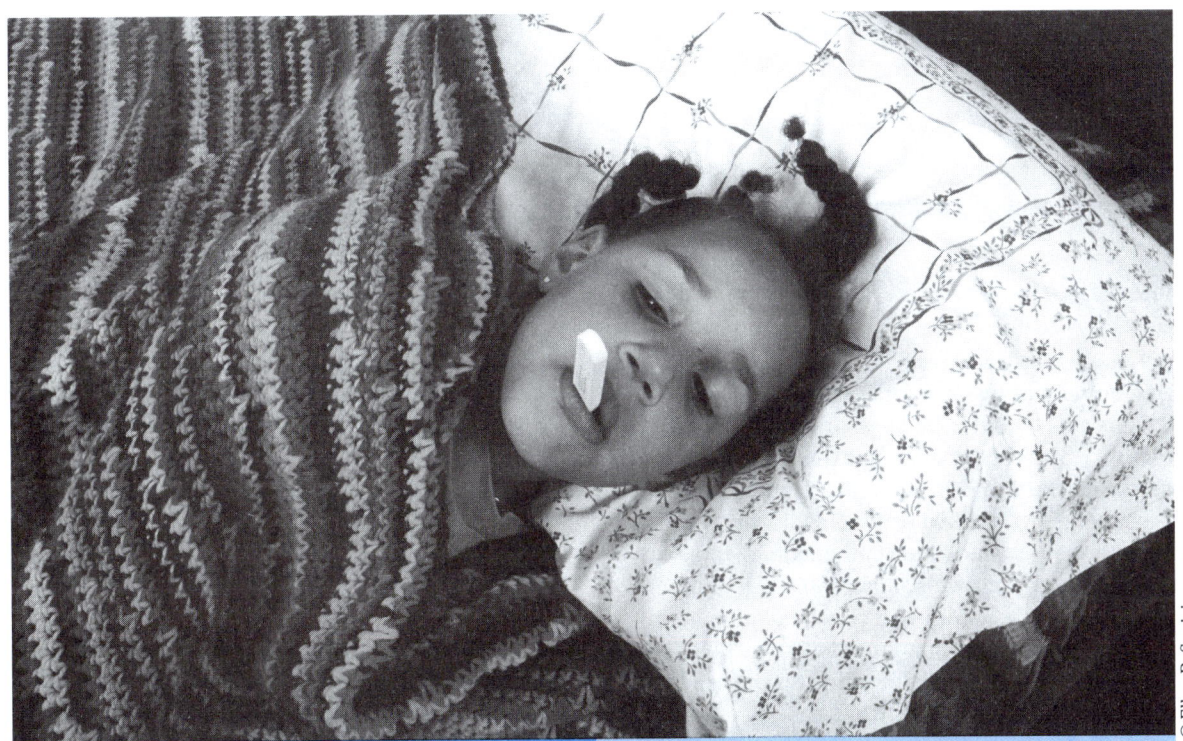

Figure 11.2.

How to Take a Child's Temperature

Perform hand hygiene before and after taking a child's temperature.

Use a digital thermometer.

Armpit Temperatures

- Make sure the armpit is dry and then put the tip of an oral thermometer in an armpit.
- Close the armpit by holding the elbow against the chest until the thermometer signals it has a reading. (Use one that beeps when it is ready to be read.) This usually takes about five minutes. The tip of the thermometer must be covered by skin the whole time. If you do not get a reading, try to take the temperature again.
- This method is not very accurate after a few months of age. However, it will give you an indication of whether the child's temperature is or is not elevated if the child feels warm to you.

Oral Temperatures

- Be sure the child has not had a cold or warm drink in the last 15–30 minutes.
- Put the tip of the thermometer under one side of the tongue and toward the back. Be sure it is under the tongue and not just against the child's cheek.
- Hold the thermometer in place and ask the child to hold it with his lips and fingers (not teeth) until the thermometer signals it has a reading. (Use one that beeps when it is ready to be read.) Keep the lips sealed. Digital thermometers usually give a reading in less than a minute.

Digital Electronic Pacifier Temperature

- Have the child suck on the pacifier until you hear a beep that indicates it has a reading. This may take three to four minutes.

Ear Temperature

- This type of thermometer reads the infrared heat waves released by the eardrum. Very young children (under 1 year of age) have very small and angled ear canals that make it difficult to get an accurate reading with an ear thermometer.
- To straighten the ear canal, grasp the middle of the ear and pull it backward and upward.
- Put the tip of the ear probe into the ear canal until you hear the signal that a reading is ready. The ear probe should not make the child uncomfortable if it is placed correctly. (Read the instructions that come with the device for details about this technique.) Usually this type of thermometer gives a reading in a few seconds.
- If the ear canal is packed with ear wax, the probe may not get an accurate reading.

Temporal Artery Temperature

- This type of thermometer senses the infrared heat waves from the temporal artery, which runs across the forehead. It is the warmth from this artery that your grandmother used to tell if her children had an elevated temperature by putting her hand or cheek on their foreheads.
- Place the sensor part of the thermometer at the center of the forehead, midway between the eyebrow and the hairline.
- Follow the instructions that come with the device to get a reading.

---

fever are hard to prevent as they may occur as the body temperature is rising.

Fevers do not harm the child unless they are caused by overheating from some external cause. A fever that is associated with illness does not usually go above 105° F and does not harm the child. Children with fevers do need to drink more fluids, but there is no need to cool the child down or give medication for fever unless the fever is making the child uncomfortable or is exceptionally high—above 106° F. Such a high temperature is a medical emergency that requires immediate health professional care. Up to that level, the height of the temperature is not a reliable indicator of the severity of illness causing it.

Caring for Our Children Standard 3.6.1.3 reviews the types of thermometers that are appropriate for taking children's temperature. Only digital thermometers should be used. Do not use glass or mercury thermometers. An ear thermometer is an acceptable tool for taking temperatures of children older than 4 months of age. It needs to be positioned correctly to obtain an accurate reading from the child's eardrum and not from the ear canal. Rectal temperatures should be taken only by parents or staff members who have been trained to do so by a health professional. Generally, it is best for staff members to avoid taking rectal temperatures because of the potential for allegations of sexual abuse. By 4 years of age most children can hold an oral thermometer under their tongues long enough to get a reliable oral temperature. Under-the-arm temperatures are less accurate but may be used with infants and young children for whom oral temperature taking is not possible. Thermometers that read temperature from the forehead and temple area are not reliable. Thermometers placed in the mouth or rectum should have a plastic sheath and be cleaned and sanitized after each use according to the manufacturer's directions. For correct interpretation of the temperature reading, document the site at which the temperature was taken, the type of thermometer, the time the temperature was taken, and the thermometer reading. Do not adjust the temperature reading based on where it was measured; just say where it was measured and the reading. (For more details on taking children's temperatures, see Figure 11.2)

Children with fevers do not need to be excluded from care unless the fever is associated with a behavior change or other sign of illness. To learn more about temperature taking and fevers, go to **www.healthy children.org** and search for "temperature."

Teething

When children's teeth work their way through the gums starting at around 4 months of age, they can cause irritation of gum tissue through which they must pass. The area around where the tooth is coming up can become slightly swollen and tender. Teething can make children drool and want to chew or rub their gums on objects. Teething does not usually cause fever. However, the objects teething children chew on can have disease-causing germs on them. Teething occurs at the time that the antibodies transferred to the baby before birth are nearly gone, so infants may get infections easily in the second half of their first year. Firm rubber teething toys are helpful when the baby can hold on to and use them. If they are dropped or handled by other children, they should be cleaned before giving them back to the teething child.

Upper respiratory infections (colds)

Everyone has more colds than any other illness. Infants have 6–10 in that first year, and then gradually have fewer as their experience with different viruses teaches their immune system how to fend off these infections. Even without complications, most colds last at least 7–10 days. Many infants will just be getting over one cold when they come down with the next one. By 3–5 years of age, most children have the same number as the average adult, about four colds a year. Having close contact with other children in a family with siblings or in a child care group slightly increases the number of colds the child will have. If the infant is breastfed, there will be fewer episodes and each one will not last as long.

Most children with colds get better without any special treatment. The course of a cold is familiar to most of us. First you start feeling like you are "coming down with something," and then your nose gets stuffy and starts to run. Sneezing and mild fever, cough, and difficulty swallowing are common. Because infants must breathe through their nose to nurse or drink from a bottle, they have a tough time feeding. Older children can breathe between swallows of fluid from a cup. Offering fluids frequently gets more down than trying to get a child with a cold to drink a lot at once.

No medicine cures a cold. Antibiotics don't treat the viruses that cause colds. Over-the-counter cold medicines should not be used. They don't help children who are younger than 6 years of age and may cause side effects. Doing what is necessary to help the child drink enough fluid helps. The fluid makes it easier for the body to bring infection-fighting cells to the tissues infected by the cold and to keep nasal discharge thin enough to drain properly. Saline nose drops and cool mist humidifiers may help thin the mucus in the nose and shrink swollen nasal membranes so the mucus can drain into the throat where the baby will swallow it. Swallowed mucus ends up in a bowel movement where it is harmless. If the child's cold symptoms are getting worse or do not improve after a week, the family should consult the child's health care provider.

Vomiting and nausea

A child vomits when the stomach is irritated by infection, by a toxic substance the child swallowed or a food that was spoiled and toxic, by hard coughing, or by some condition that stimulates the nerves that make the muscles of the stomach contract and empty the contents. Vomiting is very unpleasant. The main concern with vomiting is that the fluid being lost fairly rapidly causes dehydration. If the child is not voiding as often as usual, and the urine is becoming a darker yellow than usual, you know the child is starting to become dehydrated.

Vomiting is managed by letting the stomach rest for half an hour and then giving three to four teaspoons of water every 15 minutes, or an even smaller amount if the three to four teaspoons do not stay down. After an hour with fluid staying down, double the amount offered every 15 minutes. If the condition doesn't get better with this approach, the family should contact the child's health care provider. Most will recommend special rehydrating fluids that contain water and the minerals that the child loses with vomiting if the symptom lasts more than a few hours.

Diarrhea

Diarrhea is a condition in which the bowel movements are more watery, unformed, and frequent than usual for that person. Infants who are breastfed normally have loose, frequent bowel movements. Changes in diet, an infection, some medications, and anything else that irritates the bowel can cause diarrhea. When the bowel is irritated or normal bacteria that help with digestion are killed by antibiotics, food moves through the bowel too quickly for enough water to be transferred from it into the body. When the bowel has passed stool quickly during an illness, it may take some time for the bowel lining to heal well enough to absorb the food and water properly. So bowel movements may remain looser and more frequent for a while. As with vomiting, the main concern is dehydration. Watching the frequency and color of the urine is a good indicator of whether dehydration is occurring.

Manage diarrhea by avoiding fluids with a large amount of sugar in them. Except for breast milk, milk and milk-based foods can make diarrhea worse. Offer water and foods like rice, noodles, oatmeal, dry cereal, mashed banana, and unsweetened applesauce.

Allergies

An allergy is a condition in which the body's immune system is responding too vigorously to a substance. Normally the immune system recognizes when something enters the body that doesn't belong there. This reaction helps remove harmful substances. However, too much reaction causes symptoms. Allergic reactions can vary from mild to life-threatening. Some allergic reactions give cold-like symptoms. Others cause rashes like eczema, breathing trouble with wheezing, swelling body tissues, or stomach cramps and vomiting.

Common causes of allergy include exposure to pollens, mold, dust mites, animal dander, medications, insects (e.g., cockroaches) and insect stings, and foods. Allergies are the most common type of chronic (long-lasting and/or recurrent) health condition.

Allergic skin conditions include eczema, hives, and contact dermatitis—a reaction to something that touched the skin. Many young children have these conditions. These are treated with medications, moisturizers, antihistamines, and avoiding drying out the skin. Children with these skin problems need to avoid whatever gives them symptoms. Sometimes it is a food, soap, another chemical, an animal, or a fabric. As with many skin conditions, itching can lead to scratching. The scratching opens the skin to bacterial infection. Helpful measures include using cool compresses on itchy areas or cool baths followed immediately (within two to three minutes) by application of a lotion, cream, or ointment to hold the moisture in the skin.

In child care settings, everyone who might care for the child needs to know about a child who has an allergy. They must make sure that the child is protected from contact with the substance to which the child is allergic and know what to do if the child has a reaction. This may require posting the child's allergy, what to do if the child has an allergic reaction, and the child's photo in all parts of the facility that the child uses. Without taking such measures, not only staff and substitutes but also another child's parent or a visitor might inadvertently expose the child to whatever causes a reaction for the child. Parents must be asked to give consent for such open communication, but they are usually grateful for the protection this measure offers. If the child moves around in the facility or goes on a field trip, it may be wise to have the child wear a badge that announces the allergy. Bracelets with this information are available, but they may not be practical for young children. All children who have a chronic condition should have a care plan that identifies the condition and what the child care providers should do about it on a day-to-day basis and in an emergency.

Asthma

When the airways become swollen and blocked with mucus and the muscles around the airways constrict in reaction to some irritation, the person cannot move air through these tubes well. The person starts to cough, wheeze, and work harder to breathe. You will hear the sound of the air being forced through the narrowed tube. This sound is called wheezing. In very young children, the large air tubes are not very big. They are called bronchioles, and when the child grows and has bigger air tubes, they are called bronchi. So when a young child wheezes, the child's health care provider may say the child has bronchiolitis. When an adult wheezes from an infection of the large airways, the health care provider may say the person has bronchitis. Asthma is a condition in which someone wheezes. Since many young children who have a bout of bronchiolitis don't go on to have asthma when they are older, their health care provider may not use the term asthma to describe their wheezing.

Asthma is a very common chronic disease. Around 7 percent of all children have asthma. The symptoms can be triggered by a respiratory infection; by exposure to smoke, dust, mold, and other substances to which the person is allergic; or by exposure to tobacco smoke or very dry or very cold air. The goal in managing asthma is to allow the child to do everything children without asthma can do. The child may use inhaled medications with a spacing device and a mask or mouthpiece or a nebulizer. Some medications prevent symptoms and others control symptoms when an asthma episode occurs. Some children may take oral medications. As is true for children with allergies, children with asthma should have a specialized care plan that includes a list of what triggers the child's symptoms, what to do every day, and what to do if an asthma episode occurs.

Suggested activities

- Review the standards in *Caring for Our Children* Section 3.6.2 about setting up care for children who: 1) would be excluded because they cannot participate in their usual early education program; 2) require more care from their teachers than those adults can provide while competently caring for other children in the group; or 3) have a condition that poses a threat of spread of infection. Is a care facility such as this available in your community? What are the arrangements to use it? What does it cost? If families needed to use this service, what would be the experience from the child's point of view and from the parents' point of view? Would you recommend using such arrangements?

- Recall the illnesses you have had over the past 12 months. For how many days did these illnesses restrict you to staying at home? How many days did you go to work or school with some symptoms? How did you decide whether to limit your activity? What measures did you take to hasten recovery?

- Recall a childhood illness that kept you home from school. What do you remember about it? What gave you comfort? Why do you remember particular aspects of the illness experience?

- Have you given medication or seen someone else administer medication in an early education setting? Did the person giving the medication have special training in how to do it in such a setting? Did the administration procedure meet the standards for providing such care outlined in *Caring for Our Children*? How could the individual's performance be improved?

- Locate an early education program in your community that provides care for its enrolled children whether they are well or mildly ill. (Nearly all programs care for children who have colds.) Do they meet the standards for providing such care outlined in *Caring for Our Children*? How could their performance be improved? Do they use procedures and documents that have the same items found in the Medication Administration Packet? What is missing?

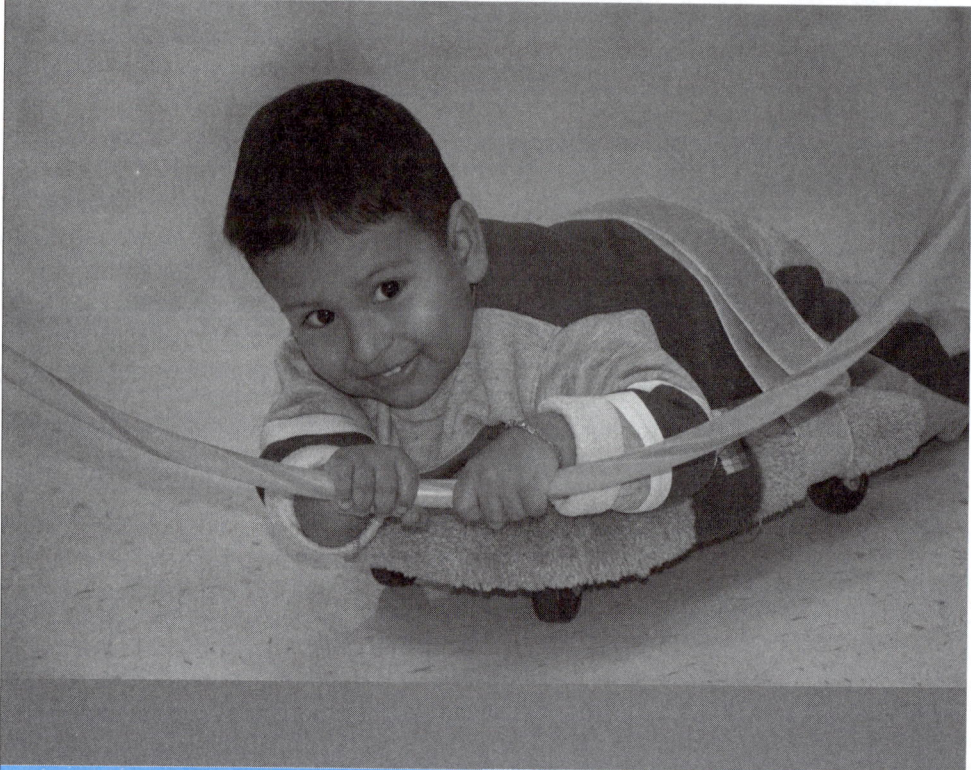

By Peg Callaghan / © NAEYC

Inclusion of Children with Special Needs

MAJOR CONCEPTS

- The broad definition of children with special health needs includes children with medical and developmental/learning issues, as well as those with conditions considered disabilities. A child may have different types of special needs.

- Inclusion of children with special needs enriches the program for typically developing children. This inclusion brings diversity, opportunities to learn how to identify strengths as well as needs for special support, and contacts with specialists who broaden understanding about how to foster optimum development of all children.

- Public and private funding pays for some services that federal and state laws indicate are rights that must be met for children with developmental disabilities and those with chronic health conditions. Teachers have a special duty to make sure children with special needs receive and benefit from the services and resources available to them.

- Children with chronic conditions have varying severity of health conditions that require planning by teachers. Most of these conditions cause only mild or intermittent problems.

- Caring for children with chronic conditions requires closer coordination among the child's health care providers, family members, and the program's staff members than for typically developing children.

Children with a wide range of special needs or disabilities (e.g., speech and language delays, chronic medical conditions, developmental delays, or physical impairments) can benefit from being in group situations with children who do not have special needs. The lives of other children and staff members can be greatly enriched by including children with special needs in early care and education programs.

In 1998, a widely quoted article in *Pediatrics* (McPherson et al.) provided a now commonly used definition of children with special health care needs: "Those who have or are at increased risk for a chronic physical, developmental, behavioral or emotional condition and who also require health and related services of a type or amount beyond that required by children generally" (138). This definition broadly covers all children with special needs or disabilities, not just those with conditions that are conventionally thought to require medical management.

Inclusive care

Inclusion, as a value, supports the right of all children—regardless of their diverse abilities—to participate actively in natural settings with their peers within their communities. A natural setting is one in which children would spend time if they did not have a disability. Such settings include but are not limited to home and family, play groups, child care programs, nursery schools, Head Start programs, kindergartens, and neighborhood school classrooms. Support for inclusion requires help for young children and their families to access and receive health, social service, education, and other supports and services that promote full participation in community life.

Most of the time children with special needs can participate in the normal routines of child care. Some children with special needs require extensive individual program planning, and some need extra services. Others need staff members to help them in minor ways or for a limited period of time. Many chronic health conditions are associated with mild or intermittent symptoms, so children with one or more of these conditions need special care only at those times.

Staff members must be attentive to the needs and reactions of the child who has a disability or special health care need, as well as to those of the other children, families, and staff members. Everyone must be flexible in planning and conducting program activities. At the time of the enrollment decision and thereafter, each program needs to be realistic about what it can and should do to safely and appropriately meet a child's special needs. In many instances, staff members' concerns can be addressed by representatives of other programs who can arrange to provide special services that enable children with special needs to be included in early care settings that serve typically developing children.

Early childhood programs cannot deny care simply because a child has a disability. The Americans with Disabilities Act (ADA), which went into effect in 1992, states that people with disabilities are entitled to equal rights and protections in employment, in receipt of state and local public services, and in access to public accommodations such as preschools, child care centers, and family child care homes. Section 504 of the 1975 Rehabilitation Act includes very similar requirements for any program that receives federal assistance, including those programs administered by religious institutions. The official source for interpretation of ADA is the U.S. Department of Justice, which provides information online at **www.ada.gov**. Search the ADA website for "child care" to identify helpful documents and phone numbers to call with questions about how to handle specific situations. (See Figure 12.1 for a list of examples of information available about child care on the ADA website.)

Meeting the child's and family's needs while caring for other children may seem overwhelming to those working in already short-staffed and inadequately financed programs. Federal law uses some key terms (here italicized) to guide decisions about providing access to people with disabilities. The law requires that programs must provide services with *reasonable accommodation*. Each child's needs must be *evaluated on an individual basis* to determine whether a program can *reasonably accommodate* the child's needs. Generally, the only acceptable reasons to refuse to enroll a child are that the child poses a *direct threat* to others (that cannot be managed) or that caring for the child would *fundamentally alter the nature of the program*.

Even when few adaptations are required to accommodate children with special needs, many programs are reluctant to enroll them. Some try to discourage families from enrolling their children by suggesting they may not be able to receive adequate care. Such actions are illegal under the ADA. While it may be challenging to meet the needs of some children, both typically developing children and those with special needs benefit from shared learning environments that allow them to participate and learn together.

Benefits of inclusion

Focusing on the benefits of including children who have special needs helps to balance the challenges. The following sections briefly highlight the benefits for all children, for families of children with special needs, and for teachers.

Figure 12.1.
Examples of ADA Information Available

The following are examples of information from the richly populated website of the ADA.

Commonly Asked Questions About Child Care Centers and the ADA

A 13-page publication that provides answers to commonly asked questions about how the ADA applies to child care centers.

ADA Questions and Answers

A 32-page booklet in easy-to-use question-and-answer format giving an overview of the ADA's requirements.

Checklist for Readily Achievable Barrier Removal

This document helps identify accessibility problems in small- to medium-sized existing facilities and provides sample solutions for some common architectural barriers.

Tax Credits and Deductions

To assist businesses with complying with the ADA, Section 44 of the IRS Code allows a tax credit for small businesses, and Section 190 of the IRS Code allows a tax deduction for all businesses. These credits and deductions for businesses can be used to cover selected costs of providing access to people with disabilities.

Source: "Child Care Centers and the Americans with Disabilities Act," U.S. Department of Justice, Civil Rights Division, Disability Rights Section. Online: www.ada.gov/chcaflyr.htm.

Inclusion helps all children

Children with special needs who are given the opportunity to play and learn with other children in the classroom learn more about themselves and practice important life skills. For example, they learn to cope with the give-and-take of everyday life where people have differing strengths and needs for support from others. Both typically developing children and those with special needs have opportunities to model and practice new skills every day. This helps all the children take key steps to developing responsibility and independence.

The techniques used to care for children with disabilities foster richer programming for typically developing children also. Inclusion helps children without disabilities to accept and be comfortable with individual differences. Children's attitudes toward peers with special needs can become more positive when they have the opportunity to play together regularly and when teachers support and encourage these interactions. They learn that children with special needs are more like them than they are different. Children with special needs can do some things better than they can do others. They need to eat, play, receive affection, and learn new things. Inclusion allows all children the opportunity to make friends with many different individuals. Often, typically developing children can take part in, enjoy, and benefit from special activities planned to accommodate a child with special needs.

Inclusion helps the families of children with special needs

Children with special needs typically spend more of their hours in the child care setting than in clinics or special treatment programs. As with typically developing children, quality child care gives families both time and support to meet the challenges in their lives, including those that are not directly related to caring for their children. For nearly all families, parents must be able to go to work, perform well on the job, and earn a living to meet their financial responsibilities. Frequently, costs of living are higher for families whose children have a disability or chronic health condition. For all families, but especially for those whose children have disabilities or special health conditions, child care provides some respite and partnership in caring for their children. Inclusive care provides social support from a wider circle of adults who carry on family life and adult responsibilities than parents of children with special needs would have otherwise.

When program staff members and specialists share the responsibility for teaching children, parents feel less isolated. They learn new ways to help their child not only from professionals, but also from one another. Watching their child progress and interact with other children helps parents to think about their child realistically. They will see that some of the behaviors that concern them are typical of all young children, not just their child. For children with developmental disabilities, parents may see that their children are progressing along a path modeled by other children, albeit more slowly.

Inclusion helps teachers

Many of the most effective teaching techniques were first developed for children with disabilities, such as Maria Montessori's methods. Working with children with special needs is a chance for teachers to broaden both teaching and personal experience. Teachers have opportunities to implement therapies and make observations that can be instrumental in meeting children's medical and rehabilitative service needs. Some of the techniques are the same as a teacher would use for a younger child. For example, teachers who help young children learn how to hold their cups by themselves or modulate their behavior appropriately are accommodating the child's developmental level. This type of accommodation is generally what is needed for children with a developmental delay who are functioning as if they are younger than their chronological age.

How is inclusion carried out?

Inclusion can be carried out in a variety of ways. The decisions about the best ways to include a particular child depend on the child's strengths and needs. Every child is an individual, with different abilities and characteristics. All children display a broad range of behavior and abilities. Children with special needs generally have some abilities and behaviors within the range of typical development, and some that are outside of it. The most inclusive setting should be *individually* determined for a *particular* child at a *particular* time and reassessed *regularly*.

Inclusion involves the efforts of many people working as a team. This team includes teachers, the child's family, and specialists providing consultation and direct services on a full- or part-time basis from agencies serving young children with special needs and from the public schools. Planning should involve families and staff members from the child care program and community service agencies. Coordination of efforts is both a challenge and a critical requirement for meeting the needs of a child with a chronic illness or disability.

Staff members' feelings about and attitudes toward children with special needs

Most staff members in early care and education programs did not choose special education as a career and may feel unprepared to work with children with special needs. Each staff member has different attitudes and experiences different feelings, usually both positive and negative, toward children with special needs in the program. Different types of needs may evoke different emotions and responses. Staff members may feel sympathy for the family, acceptance of the child's needs, concern about their ability to meet the child's needs, frustration in not getting needed support, anxiety about doing the right thing, and/or enthusiasm for new challenges and opportunities. Each of these feelings may affect a teacher's responses to a child with a special need.

Feeling sorry for a child or wishing to make tasks easier often leads to an overly protective attitude. Teachers may try to shelter the child from experiences that are part of daily life. This may prevent a teacher from seeing the child's strengths and expecting the most from her. Staff members may feel frustration or resent the extra responsibility or work required to accommodate a child with special needs. They may experience fear and insecurity—natural responses to inadequate information about a child's condition. Feelings of acceptance and caring may surface immediately or may develop over time.

Sharing feelings with other staff members may help. Also, teachers often find that working closely on a daily basis with children who have special needs eases their anxiety and fear. Teachers must see the children as children first and discover their abilities and needs as individuals. The emphasis should be on the whole child rather than on the child's limitations. Teachers of typically developing children and children with special needs find they succeed by adapting their approaches to respond to the individual child's need for adult help and support.

Inclusive education: The Individuals with Disabilities Education Act

Under the federal Individual with Disabilities Education Act (IDEA), state or local school systems are responsible for providing services to children with specific types of special needs.

As explained in Section 8.1 of *Caring for Our Children*,

> The Individuals with Disabilities Education Act (IDEA), a federal law most recently amended in 2004, affords caregivers/teachers a unique opportunity to support children with disabilities that might affect their educational success and to improve services for both the children and families in the child care setting. The purpose of the law is to provide "free appropriate public education" for all "eligible" children, from birth to twenty-one years, in a natural or least restrictive environment. Eligible children under IDEA include those with developmental delays or those with physical or mental conditions that may result in a developmental delay. Part B, Section 619 of this statute supports the needs of eligible preschool-age children through the local school district. Part C provides for a comprehensive system to serve the needs of eligible infants and toddlers between the ages of birth and three years and their families. Child care programs can play a significant role in supporting the developmental needs of children with special health care needs and disabilities in the child care setting.

The purpose of Part B of the law is to provide "free appropriate public education" regardless of disability or chronic illness to eligible children ages 3 through 21, in the least restrictive environment appropriate to the child. Under Part C of IDEA, state agencies are responsible for providing services to infants and toddlers from birth through 3 years with disabilities. Federal funds subsidize the cost of providing these services. Medicaid and private health insurance, including the state- and federally-subsidized Child Health Insurance Program (CHIP), pay some but usually not all of the expenses of daily care for children who have chronic health issues. Federal tax credits and deductions are available to for-profit child care programs to help defray some types of costs associated with serving children with special needs. Early care and education programs can play a significant role in maximizing children's development by making sure that families whose children are eligible for subsidized services apply and receive them as laws require.

Part C of IDEA—Infants and toddlers

Part C makes federal funds available for states to implement an interagency system of early intervention services for eligible infants and toddlers and their families. The state governor selects the lead agency that is responsible for the administration of the program. The intent of Part C is to enhance development and provide other needed services for infants and toddlers who have developmental delays or specific types of diagnosed conditions. A further intent is to support the capacity of families to enhance the development of their children in the home and community and to transition children to appropriate, effective preschool services.

The focus of services provided to the child and family under Part C is the achievement of two related goals:

- Enhance and support the development of young children with disabilities and minimize their need for special education and related services when they enter the public school system.
- Maximize the potential for infants and toddlers with disabilities to enjoy the benefits of their communities and grow into adults capable of living independently, pursuing vocations, and participating in the benefits their communities offer all citizens.

Although a lead agency is responsible for implementation, the program is designed to be a coordinated, collaborative effort among a variety of state agencies. These agencies' activities include screening, assessment, service coordination, and development of an Individualized Family Service Plan (IFSP) for every eligible infant or toddler and family. The IFSP describes the child's developmental, therapeutic, and health needs; summarizes assessments that have been done; describes early intervention services and family support that will be provided; and lists the expected functional outcomes of services.

The process usually begins with screening by a worker who talks with the parent by telephone to determine whether the child is likely to have a problem that qualifies for early intervention services. If so, the child is scheduled for an assessment. Families of children whose screening results do not meet the criteria of the early intervention system for assessment usually receive counseling about what to watch for in their child's development. They are encouraged to make contact with the early intervention system again if the child doesn't meet recognized milestones of development.

Among the more important aspects of the interagency model is the belief that children and their families should be viewed from the perspective of their abilities rather than their deficits. The IFSP and all service providers emphasize the family's and child's strengths and capabilities rather than perceived weaknesses. Service providers strive for progress by enhancing and supporting the family's strengths, focusing on their resources, priorities, and concerns about the child rather than on correcting "deficiencies."

Part C of IDEA requires delivery of services in natural environments to the maximum extent appropriate to the child. These are defined as settings that are "natural or normal for the child's peers who have no disabilities." These natural environments include the child's home, the neighborhood, community programs, child care centers, parks, recreation centers, stores, malls, museums, and so on. The family and providers incorporate elements of the child's regular environment—such as furniture, toys, schedule, siblings, care providers, and extended family—in the planning and delivery of services and supports. In this way they can best discover the child's talents and gifts and use them as a foundation on which to build the child's progress in the normal course of play, relationships, and caregiving. Learning about and understanding the child's routines and using real-life opportunities and activities, such as eating, playing, and interacting with others, greatly enhances adults' ability to work on the child's developmental skills. This approach helps the child achieve the functional outcomes identified in the IFSP.

For these reasons, it is critical to have a representative from the child care program provide input and be available to the team who develops or revises the IFSP. Written informed consent must be obtained from the family before confidential information (written or verbal) can be shared. With consent, appropriate child care staff members can join the IFSP team by providing vital information about the child's current status and the feasibility of implementing whatever is being considered for a child's IFSP. In addition, the child care staff members must understand both the role the child care program is to play and the resources available through the IFSP to support the child's family and the work of the child care staff.

Part B, Section 619 of IDEA—Children 3–5 years of age

Children 3–5 years of age who are eligible for services under Part B of IDEA are generally served through a written Individualized Education Program (IEP). (In some states and communities the IFSP may still be used for preschoolers.) The IEP is developed by a team with the local education agency. The local school system or the agency to which the school delegates this responsibility arranges for implementation of the IEP in either a public or a private preschool. Local education agencies may make arrangements to contract with private providers for preschool services or to provide educationally related services identified in the IEP (e.g., speech and language therapy) in any recognized child care setting. Teachers should become familiar with, and when possible provide input to, the preschooler's IEP. The teacher may be able to participate, with prior informed written parental/guardian consent, in the IEP review meetings to share valuable insight and information regarding the child's needs in the child care setting.

The standards in Chapter 8 of *Caring for Our Children* detail the opportunities and responsibilities that child care programs share with other agencies to serve a child with special needs, with an emphasis on children who have an IFSP or IEP. However, some children with special health needs who do not have a developmental delay are not eligible for these education-based services. The procedures outlined in the standards should be used to guide their care, too. The steps described in the standards include the following:

- Planning for inclusion, including delineating the tasks to be accomplished before enrollment, such as
  - Assessment of the child's special needs
  - Developing a service plan that specifies the type and frequency of special services the child requires
  - Formulating an action plan
- Identifying a staff member to coordinate the child's care in the program and specifying that person's role
- Arranging for contracted services and reimbursements
- Developing measurable objectives and providing documentation in written reports to all those involved in the child's care
- Conducting periodic reevaluation of the child and of the facility's performance in meeting the objectives
- Conducting individualized planning and support to help the child meet learning standards that apply to all children

Children with chronic conditions but no developmental delay

IDEA recognizes children with chronic illness as well as those with developmental disabilities as eligible for funded services *if* the condition might adversely impact their educational success. Usually, children who have chronic medical or behavioral issues but who are not developmentally delayed do not receive services via the process specified in the law to develop IFSPs and IEPs. For children who cannot receive services under IDEA, teachers should seek services from the child's usual source of medical care. Such services may be paid for by health insurance, fees the family can afford, funding from philanthropic organizations, or publicly funded programs such as maternal and child health services subsidized by Title V of the Social Security Act.

Preparing to care for children with special needs

During enrollment, but before a child actually participates in the program, staff members should request detailed information from the family about the child's health issues and special needs. Ask specific questions about how an illness or a special need will affect the child's ability to participate in the program and what services staff members will be expected to provide that differ from those provided for typically developing children. Identify the professionals involved with the child's care. To receive information directly from these professionals about recommendations for the child's accommodation and any measures that might be needed in an emergency, obtain and have parents complete the Health Insurance Portability and Accountability Act (HIPAA) forms their health professionals use to document parent consent for sharing information with appropriate program staff members.

To care for children with special physical, mental, behavioral, or developmental needs, teachers need to be part of a professional team. Children with disabilities and special health care needs should have a multidisciplinary, interdisciplinary, or transdisciplinary assessment by appropriately qualified professionals. The following components should be included in a comprehensive assessment of a child (see *Caring for Our Children* Standard 8.3.0.1):

- A care plan developed by the child's health care providers, preferably those in the child's medical home
- Results of medical and developmental examinations
- Assessments of the child's behavior, cognitive functioning, and current overall adaptive functioning; other evaluations that may have been done
- Evaluations of the family's needs, cultural and linguistic differences, concerns, and priorities

Teachers need as much information as possible about the daily and emergency needs of all children. Any child who has a condition or a special need that may require special attention from teachers should have a care plan. A care plan informs staff members about special training they may need, what procedures they might need to follow, and any modifications to the program's usual routines. The care plan may be very simple or complex depending on the child's needs. It might include contact information for families and doctors, including important subspecialists; medical conditions; allergies; medication(s); medical procedure(s); special diet; special instructions for classroom accommodations, naps, toileting, outdoor activity, or transportation; and special equipment or supplies.

The child's health care provider should complete those parts of the care plan that he or she thinks the child care program needs to know to take care of the child. Some children will have more than one medical and educational specialist, each of whom should contribute information to a care plan. The teacher may need to compile separate information and instructions from the specialists on a single care plan form. The composite care plan should include relevant information from the IFSP or IEP and instructions specific to the child's condition (e.g., asthma, diabetes, seizures). If there are conflicting instructions, the teacher will need to contact the parties involved or engage the help of the program's child care health consultant to resolve the areas that seem to be incompatible. (For sample care plan forms, see Figure A.16 in Appendix A of this book and Appendix O of *Caring for Our Children*.)

The information in the care plan should be reviewed collaboratively by the program's child care health consultant and staff members to plan and provide training for necessary accommodations. Each time the child receives care from a health care professional or from other specialists, the care plan should be reviewed again and updated.

Caring for Our Children Standard 3.5.0.1, after citing the definition of children with special health care needs published in *Pediatrics* in 1998, explains the recommended content of a care plan for such children:

> Any child who meets these criteria should have a Routine and Emergent Care Plan completed by their primary care provider in their medical home. In addition to the information specified in Standard 9.4.2.4 for the Health Report, there should be
>
> a. A list of the child's diagnosis/diagnoses
>
> b. Contact information for the primary care provider and any relevant subspecialists (i.e., endocrinologists, oncologists, etc.)
>
> c. Medications to be administered on a scheduled basis
>
> d. Medications to be administered on an emergent basis with clearly stated parameters, signs, and symptoms that warrant giving the medication written in lay language
>
> e. Procedures to be performed
>
> f. Allergies
>
> g. Dietary modifications required for the health of the child
>
> h. Activity modifications
>
> i. Environmental modifications
>
> j. Stimulus that initiates or precipitates a reaction or series of reactions (triggers) to avoid
>
> k. Symptoms for caregiver/teachers to observe
>
> l. Behavioral modifications
>
> m. Emergency response plans—both if the child has a medical emergency and special factors to consider in programmatic emergency, like a fire
>
> n. Suggested special skills training and education for staff

Modifying an early education program to accommodate children with special needs

Modifications or adaptations in a program's policies, practices, equipment, or routine may be needed to facilitate the active participation of children with special needs. The primary goal of inclusion is to enable all children to participate actively to maximize their development and to allow them to be as independent as possible. A program that enrolls children with special needs should meet these objectives:

- Adapt the program to ensure children's successful participation
- Develop all children's feelings of competence
- Promote peer acceptance
- Avoid overprotection
- Strengthen the teamwork among family, teachers, and other specialists

Adapt the program

Selecting and adapting materials and activities for children with special needs sometimes requires problem solving and creativity. Special materials may be required, many of which can be used by typically developing children as well. Examples of such materials are

- Eating utensils with special grips or edges
- Puzzles with large pieces and/or knobs for children with fine motor needs
- Books with large pictures for children with visual impairments
- Hypoallergenic art materials
- Foods that do not have ingredients that present a problem for children with allergies, food intolerance, or other nutrition issues

In many cases, staff members can adapt materials already available. For example, they can

- Apply masking tape to thicken brush handles and crayons to give children a firmer grip

- Slit a small rubber ball and slide the paintbrush or crayon through it so the children can grab it better
- Paste fabric on a storybook to make it more tactile
- Lower an easel or coat hooks
- Use more visuals to accompany classroom discussions for children with impaired hearing, or use more listening activities for those with visual difficulties
- Use a wedge, standing table, or bolster, or adapt other equipment to help support children physically
- Remove pets or plants from the room or center if they aggravate a child's asthma or allergies

Necessary adaptations depend on the type and severity of a child's needs. For example, to accommodate a child who uses a wheelchair, staff members can

- Measure pathways to ensure that the child can maneuver from one area to another
- Check the height of tables to ensure that the arms of the wheelchair fit under them, add blocks to slightly increase the height, or find an alternate seating arrangement
- Explore the use of a scooter board instead of a wheelchair, if appropriate, for mobility around the classroom
- Ensure ready access to and from the building, adding ramps instead of, or in addition to, steps
- Position an activity table so the child can reach it

Figure A.17 in Appendix A provides a list of adaptive equipment for children with special needs and includes many materials that may already be available in a facility serving typically developing children. Reviewing this list may help reassure staff members when considering enrolling a child who has a disability.

Develop feelings of competency in children

All children need to feel a sense of competence. For some children, learning, adapting to changes in their environment, and relating to other children and unfamiliar adults take more time and effort. To ensure successful experiences for all children, staff members should

- Observe children closely to see what interests them
- Talk with children about themselves, their families, pets, and experiences
- Break tasks into a sequence of smaller units
- Allow sufficient time for children to learn and use new skills before moving on to something else
- Offer a variety of materials and activities suited to different levels of ability
- Provide an emotionally safe classroom by respecting all children
- Focus on the *process* of learning rather than the end result
- Accept different answers from different children
- Set clear, realistic goals for each child

Promote peer acceptance

Children must be provided with positive role models so they can learn to interact with others in a kind, accepting way. When given opportunities to watch adults relating comfortably to children with special needs, typically developing children take the first

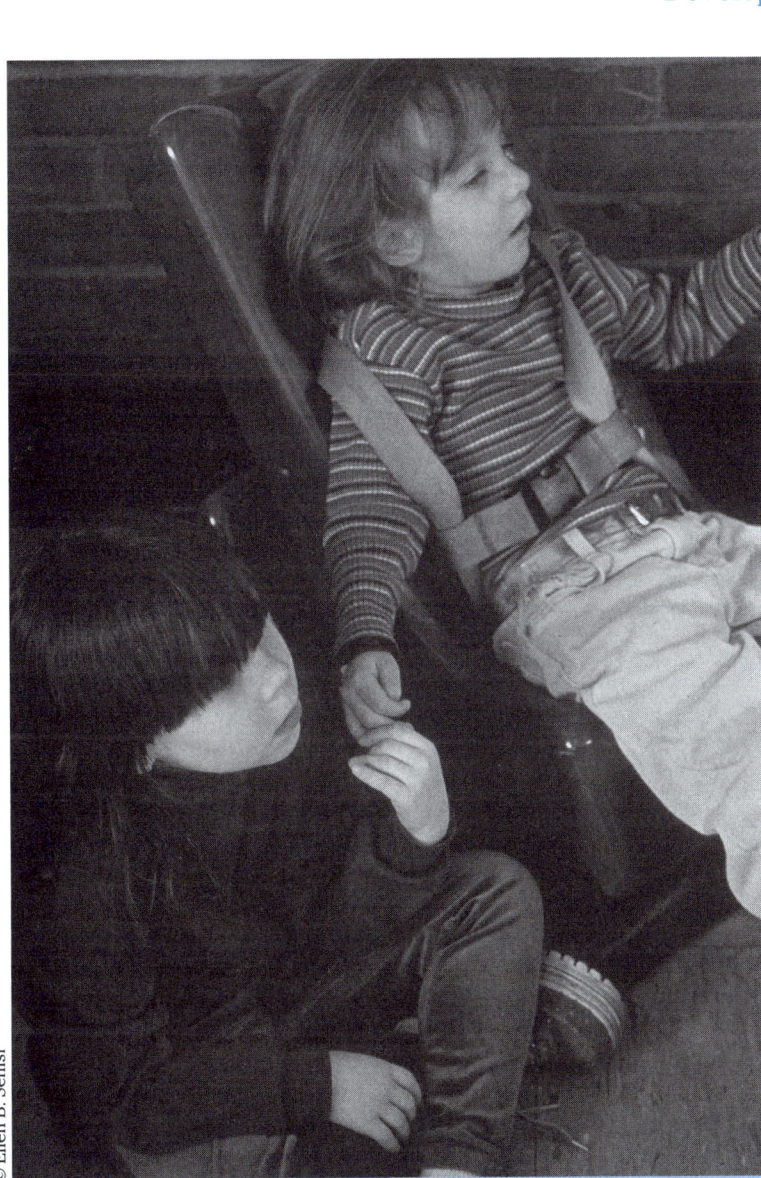
© Ellen B. Senisi

step toward learning peer acceptance. Children should be given factual information about disabilities to dispel misunderstandings and diminish fear. Staff members can encourage the acceptance of a child with special needs in the following ways:

- Always answer children's questions accurately, using language they can easily understand.
- Reassure children that they cannot "catch" a disability.
- Plan activities that allow the other children to see the child with a special need in a successful role.
- Have materials that reflect diversity routinely available. For example, include books about children with special needs in the reading area, and include dolls or puppets with disabilities.
- Invite adults with disabilities into the classroom to participate in activities.
- Focus on a variety of similarities and differences among people.
- Operate from a viewpoint of competence and adaptation rather than from a deficit model that emphasizes weakness.

Avoid overprotection

Overprotection limits a child's opportunities to grow to full potential. Both pity and fear may make a teacher reluctant to allow a child with special needs to take risks, have the opportunity to respond to limits before the teacher intercedes, engage in conflict, and experience *real* success and failure. Staff members can avoid overprotection by remembering to do the following:

- Set limits that apply to *all* children (e.g., all children must wait for a turn on the slide).
- Provide many classroom options and activities for children that they can do without needing to wait for adult guidance or assistance.
- Encourage all children to try new activities if they do not choose to do them on their own.
- Communicate a positive attitude and sincere feelings to the children. Children see their teachers as important role models.

Strengthen teamwork

Including a child with special needs in the program makes teamwork an even greater necessity. Parents, teachers, and administrators must communicate closely and regularly. With family consent, periodic communications with the child's source of health care and any specialists who provide special care or services is essential, too. Collaboration on the following tasks is especially important:

- Identifying the child's strengths and needs
- Planning and implementing a program responsive to the child's needs, including transitional activities when the child moves on to the next source of care
- Noting any changes in the child's condition
- Talking or meeting with other specialists providing therapeutic services
- Sharing information, observations, concerns, and the child's progress
- Obtaining special materials and resources to help work with the child
- Promoting and tracking the connection of the child to a medical home (see Chapter 8 for the definition and discussion of the concept of a medical home)

Focusing on providing a child and family with a supportive, caring environment can often eliminate feelings of possessiveness, inferiority, or superiority among staff members. This focus helps team members see one another's contributions as essential to helping children and families achieve their goals.

Medical procedures

Caring for Our Children Standard 3.5.0.2 provides guidance for accommodating the growing number of children who require some medical procedure during their usual day. Some children require tube feedings, suctioning of their airway, supplemental oxygen, postural drainage, catheterization to release their urine, checking of blood sugar, injections, or other special medical procedures to be performed routinely every day or urgently for a specific circumstance. Some children with these needs, especially school-age children, know how to do certain procedures (e.g., catheterization, blood testing, or injections) on their own.

For all children who require medical procedures while in the early education facility, providers should obtain a written report from the health care provider who prescribed the special treatment (e.g., a urologist for catheterization). The report should include any special preparation needed to perform urgent procedures that are unique to the child with special needs. The clinician's report should include instructions for performing the procedure, how to receive training in performing the procedure, and what to do and who to notify if complications occur.

The skills required to implement special medical procedures are not traditionally taught to teachers as part of their academic or practical experience. Even so, very few children's needs are so complex that they require specialized facilities with health personnel as teachers. Child care staff can learn the same skills that parents learn to carry out the procedures a child might need.

Remember that reasonable accommodation is legally required by the ADA. Therefore, teachers must do their best to make the accommodations required to enroll and ensure the safe care of the child who requires one or more medical procedures. Some state laws require that certain procedures be done only by family members or by a licensed health professional who follows written medical orders for what is required. Adding a licensed health professional if one is not already part of the staff can be costly. Sometimes the expense is covered by health insurance or payments covered by funds from IDEA identified in the IFSP or IEP. Under ADA, the child care program cannot charge the family for the costs involved in reasonable accommodations to meet their child's special needs. The legal definition of "reasonable accommodation" is usually interpreted to mean that accommodation is required unless doing so would put the facility out of business. In other states, medical procedures may be performed by teachers who receive training in the procedures and have the oversight/supervision of a licensed health professional. Check with your state board of medicine and nursing for its requirements. Then work with the family and the child's health care provider to comply with these requirements.

Families are responsible for providing the required equipment for procedures. Training for staff members should be provided by a qualified health care professional and should include opportunities for staff members to demonstrate competence in performing the procedures. Arranging for such training is the responsibility of all concerned—families, clinicians, and teachers—and must be satisfactorily completed before the child enrolls. The training for child care staff to perform these procedures is sometimes paid for by the child's health insurance or is included and paid for in the IFSP or IEP for a child who has developmental disabilities. Creative arrangements may be required to be sure everyone involved has appropriate training. For example, have the medical equipment company deliver the equipment to the child care facility so that the teacher and parent can receive instruction from the company's instructor at the same time.

The facility should allow sufficient time for staff to carry out the necessary procedures. Caring for children who require intermittent catheterization is not as demanding as it first sounds, but it must be done competently and takes a bit more time than taking a child to use the toilet.

Before enrolling a child who will need medical procedures, teachers can request and review fact sheets, instructions, and training. Often the child's parents or clinicians have these materials and know where training is available. When the specifics are known, teachers can make a more responsible decision about what would be required to serve the child.

Emergency planning considerations for children with special needs

To prepare for emergency episodes with a child with a chronic illness, ask the family to describe a situation that required such action in the past. Find out what may cause an urgent or emergency situation and how often it may occur. Ask how the child may behave before, during, and after such an episode and how long the episode usually lasts. Ask the child's parent(s) and doctor to describe and, as appropriate, demonstrate what to do during and following such an episode. Ask if these actions are something you can reasonably be expected to perform alone or if you will need someone else's help.

Since few health professionals have firsthand knowledge about the operation of a child care setting, prepare a list of typical classroom activities for them. Ask the child's health care professional to check off activities that must be avoided and to describe modifications needed for other activities so the child can participate. For more complex conditions, ask the physician to arrange for a knowledgeable health professional to visit the facility and work with the staff members to prepare for competent care of the child.

In conjunction with the federal Maternal and Child Health Bureau of the Health Resources and Services Administration, the American College of Emergency Physicians and the American Academy of Pediatrics (AAP) developed a tool called the Emergency Information Form for Children with Special Needs. This form provides the key information that EMS and emergency room personnel need for treating a child, including current medications and doses, usual baseline findings on physical examination, and rapid treatment options that may be appropriate for the child. This form should be kept up-to-date and always physically available with a child who has special medical needs that might require emergency medical service personnel. To locate this form, search the website of the American College of Emergency Physicians (**www.acep.org**) or the AAP (**www.aap.org**). The form also appears in Appendix BB of *Caring for Our Children*.

Prepare other children in the group for possible health crises by giving them a simple explanation as part of discussing other types of emergencies. Assure children that staff members can handle all such situations. If an event occurs, matter-of-factly review with the children what happened. Allow them to play out what they experienced, draw pictures, and tell stories related to the event until their interest wanes, indicating that they have become comfortable with it.

Resources to plan care for children with special needs

Teachers are not expected to be experts in special education or nursing procedures. Usually, the child's parents have a wealth of information to share about what works and what doesn't work for their child. Teachers can visit other programs where children with similar special needs receive educational services. Specialists, particularly those who have evaluated or worked with the child, usually have valuable suggestions and may be able to offer training and other resources.

If the child is under 3 years of age and eligible for early intervention services under Part C of IDEA, early intervention staff will be a valuable resource. Ideally the child care staff should be ongoing members of the team who plan for the child in the formal process involved in establishing and updating the IFSP and informally, on an ongoing basis. Remember to obtain required permission forms signed by the parent or legal guardian to communicate with the child's health care provider and others working with the child. Don't let paperwork barriers prevent coordination of program goals, activities, and evaluations among all the members of the child's team.

Training sessions, conferences, or workshops can provide background information about chronic illnesses, disabilities, and inclusion. National associations and professional organizations have brochures, internet postings, and sometimes a help line to call for information describing a specific disability. Be aware that some authoritative-sounding organizations may offer distorted and misleading information. Check with the child's health care providers for credible resources for parents. Local hospitals, colleges, clinics, or other community agencies may be able to provide additional information and assistance. The ADA also has useful resources to offer. (See Figure 12.1 for some examples.)

Extensive study of the implications of the ADA by the Child Care Law Center has helped clarify the issues for early education programs. The Child Care Law Center has publications that are nationally relevant, in addition to resources specific to its home state of California. To learn more about what programs are required to do to reasonably accommodate the needs of a particular child, refer to online publications at **www.childcarelaw.org**. Several other chapters in this manual provide helpful information to guide a program's thinking about inclusion. The sections on specific types of special needs, chronic illnesses and disabilities, transportation, and emergency preparedness should be particularly useful when thinking about inclusive care.

The AAP has a quick reference guide called *Managing Chronic Health Problems in Child Care and Schools* to help education professionals understand and address the chronic conditions of children who are seeking to enroll or are already enrolled in their facilities. This book uses the broad definition of special health needs that includes developmental disabilities. For example, the Quick Reference Sheets include topics such as allergies, asthma, attention-deficit/hyperactivity disorder, autism spectrum disorders, Down syndrome, and visual impairments. These one- to two-page Quick Reference Sheets describe a condition, how common it is, the characteristics of children with the condition, professionals who make up the treatment team for this condition, adaptations needed, considerations in an emergency, types of program policies needed, and resources that provide more information about the specific condition. The book also includes useful documents and forms, a glossary of terms that specialists use, and many references and links to additional resources. It is available for purchase from the NAEYC bookstore at **www.naeyc.org** and from the AAP bookstore at **www.aap.org**.

The National Dissemination Center for Children with Disabilities (**www.nichcy.org**) offers publications that discuss evaluation procedures and special education services. The NICHCY website has links to state resource sheets that list state agencies, state chapters of disability organizations, and related parent groups. The work of NICHCY is funded by the Office of Special Education Programs (OSEP), U.S. Department of Education. For more information from OSEP, go to **www2.ed.gov/about/offices/list/osers/osep/index.html**. For general information about disabilities and chronic health care conditions that children or staff members and family members of enrolled children may have, go to **www.cdc.gov/ncbddd**—the National Center on Birth Defects and Developmental Disabilities. This website has some information about each condition and then directs visitors to credentialed organizations that focus on a particular type of health condition. Use the A to Z links to find the condition you want to learn more about.

To provide competent care, be sure to review all of the relevant standards in *Caring for Our Children*. The standards in Chapter 8 of that publication address inclusion, the process to use prior to enrollment, developing a service plan, coordination and documentation, periodic reevaluation, and facility requirements. In addition, Section 8.8 lists the applicable standards found in other chapters that address staff-to-child ratios, staff qualifications, training and continuing education, care plans, medical procedures, feeding plans, care for children with food allergies, facility accommodations and space for therapy services, special equipment, first aid, transportation, transition to new services, information exchange, contents of records, and written policies.

Suggested activities

- Think about people you know who have a chronic illness or disability. What are their abilities? What limitations do they have that could be overcome by some accommodation? How do you know when they are not feeling well? What happens when they have more difficulty than usual with their condition? How does their special need affect them and the people around them? What would happen if these individuals were denied the opportunity to do what brings them in contact with others?

- What experience have you had with inclusion of a child with a special need in an early care and education program? What accommodations did that child require? Was it difficult to meet the child's needs and the needs of the other children at the same time? What would have made it easier?

- Contact your local school district and ask the following:
    - Who is eligible for the development of an IFSP?
    - Who determines whether a child is eligible for services provided under an IFSP? How is a child's eligibility for IDEA services determined? What is the procedure?
    - How long is the waiting time for an assessment of a child who is referred to the early intervention agency because the child is suspected to be developmentally delayed?
    - What services are offered to children with complex medical conditions either with or without a developmental delay?

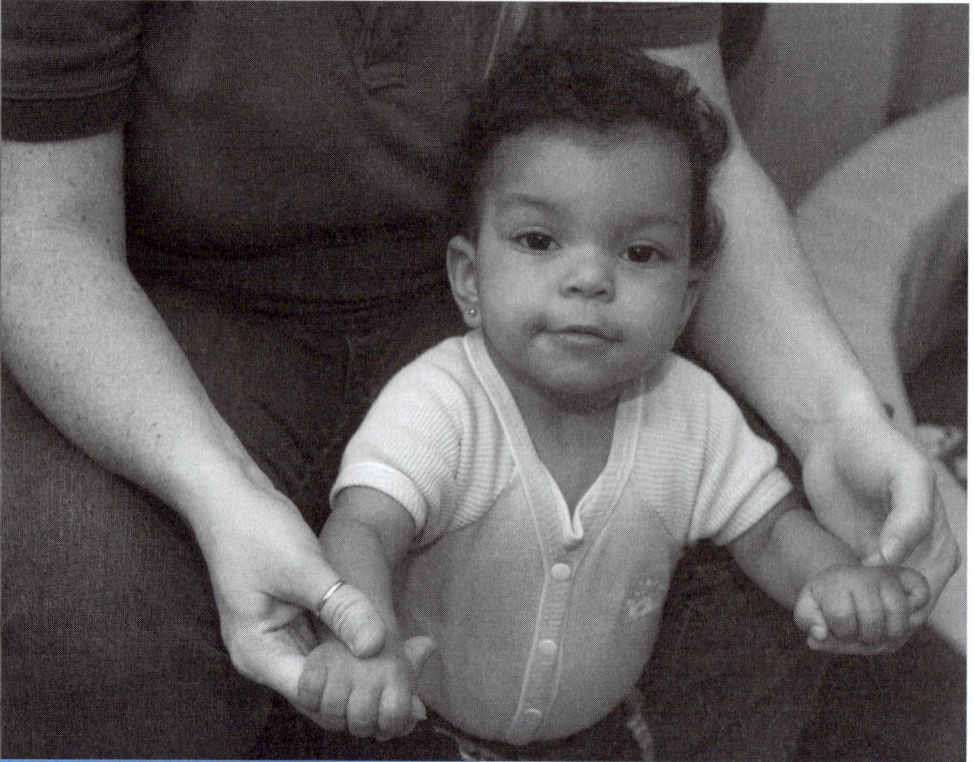

Child Maltreatment (Abuse and Neglect) and Administration of the Health Component

MAJOR CONCEPTS

- Child maltreatment is the currently recommended term professionals in the field use to describe what most state laws call child abuse and neglect.
- Most child maltreatment is perpetrated by family members or individuals living with the family, not by child care personnel.
- Early care and education providers are required by law to report child abuse and neglect.
- The child care program can provide a therapeutic environment for families under stress, and thus play a key role in preventing child abuse and neglect.
- Denial of privacy to children and adults in child care settings can help prevent child maltreatment and the suspicion of child maltreatment.
- Implementing safe, healthy early care and education requires competent administration and evaluation of the program's health component.

The preceding chapters discussed many of the facility and function requirements for operating a safe, healthy child care program. Two special issues remain to be addressed: child maltreatment and the administration of the health component in an early care and education program.

Child maltreatment (abuse and neglect)

In addition to children who have special needs because of medical or developmental health problems, some children have special needs because their families or other caregivers are under unusual stress and cannot provide appropriate care, or because the child's characteristics overwhelm the ability of parents or other caregivers to meet the child's needs. These and other contributing factors can combine to lead to child maltreatment. The many and varied contributions to the maltreatment of children make its identification, treatment, and prevention complex. There are several types of child maltreatment. Each leaves a permanent (physical and/or psychological) mark on the victim.

No standard definition of child maltreatment is used by all professionals who deal with it. Every state has one or more legal definitions that are used to establish official reporting procedures. However, most states recognize four types of maltreatment: neglect, physical abuse, sexual abuse, and emotional abuse. (For definitions and explanations of terminology used by states, see Figure 13.1.) The federal law known as the Child Abuse Prevention and Treatment Act (CAPTA) provides for a clearinghouse for information and grants to states to combat child maltreatment. The Child Welfare Information Gateway (**www.childwelfare.gov**) offers information about CAPTA, definitions of child abuse and neglect, a summary of how states treat these types of maltreatment, and a state-by-state list of the elements covered in each state's statutes relating to child maltreatment.

Identification of children who have been abused or neglected

Abuse occurs in all communities—urban, suburban, and rural—regardless of ethnicity, race, religion, or income level. It is impossible to know how many children are abused each year because the definitions of abuse and neglect, as well as reporting practices, vary from state to state. Nevertheless, the estimates are large. The scope of the problem is outlined in a 2009 publication of the U.S. Department of Health and Human Services (HHS), Administration on Children, Youth and Families, *Child Maltreatment 2007*. According to this document, in 2007, Child Protective Services received 3.2 million referrals involving alleged maltreatment of 5.8 million children. In about a quarter of these reports, at least one child was found to be a victim of child abuse or neglect. An estimated 1,760 children died that year of child abuse or neglect. About 75 percent of these children were younger than 4 years of age. Nearly 80 percent of the perpetrators were parents. More than half of the reports (57.7 percent) of suspected child maltreatment were made by someone who had contact with the child because of the individual's work role. Teachers made the largest percentage of reports.

Educators are mandated reporters; that is, they are required to report all suspected cases of abuse and neglect. Every program has a responsibility to inform staff members of appropriate federal, state, local, and program regulations regarding child abuse and neglect. Teachers may feel that they lack the skills required for accurate identification, or they may be concerned about how a report will affect their relationship with the family and other staff members. However, many families receive support and assistance as a result of such reporting. In 2007, 62.1 percent of victims received services; only 20.7 percent were placed in foster care (U.S. Department of Health and Human Services, 2009). To report suspected child maltreatment, use your state's toll-free phone numbers. For crisis counseling and information about where to call or make a report in your state, call the Childhelp National Child Abuse Hotline at 1-800-4-A-CHILD (1-800-422-4453).

Some indicators help identify suspected cases of abuse and neglect in children. Many are signals that the child is *possibly* being abused; however, some indicate other physical, environmental, or emotional problems. Poor growth can be a sign of any type of abuse or neglect in a child. (For signs and symptoms of child abuse and neglect, see Figure A.18 in Appendix A.)

All staff members should be required to participate in education about child maltreatment, both preservice and as part of continuing education. This education should include how teachers can promote protective factors to prevent child maltreatment, identify signs of stress in families, and provide support and referral to resources. As stated in *Caring for Our Children* Standards 1.4.1.1 and 1.4.5.2, ensuring that staff members learn about child maltreatment should also enable them to prevent and identify shaken baby syndrome (abusive traumatic brain injury) and repeated exposure to domestic violence. In addition to preservice and continuing education about child maltreatment, each adult who works in the program must receive a copy of the program's written policies on staff conduct and on reporting procedures for suspected child abuse. Because children with disabilities are at higher risk of being abused, learning how to prevent their maltreatment should receive particular attention.

Figure 13.1.

What Is Child Abuse and Neglect?

Child abuse and neglect are defined by Federal and State laws....At the Federal level, the Child Abuse Prevention and Treatment Act (CAPTA) defines child abuse and neglect as: "Any recent act or failure to act on the part of a parent or caretaker which results in death, serious physical or emotional harm, sexual abuse, or exploitation, or an act or failure to act which presents an imminent risk of serious harm."

The CAPTA definition of sexual abuse includes "the employment, use, persuasion, inducement, enticement, or coercion of any child to engage in, or assist any other person to engage in, any sexually explicit conduct or simulation of such conduct for the purpose of producing a visual depiction of such conduct; or the rape, and in cases of caretaker or interfamilial relationships, statutory rape, molestation, prostitution, or other form of sexual exploitation of children, or incest with children."

Nearly all States, the District of Columbia, American Samoa, Guam, the Northern Mariana Islands, Puerto Rico, and the U.S. Virgin Islands provide civil definitions of child abuse and neglect in statute. States recognize the different types of abuse in their definitions, including physical abuse, neglect, sexual abuse, and emotional abuse. Some States also provide definitions in statute for parental substance abuse and/or for abandonment as child abuse.

Physical Abuse

Physical abuse is generally defined as "any non-accidental physical injury to the child" and can include striking, kicking, burning, or biting the child, or any action that results in a physical impairment of the child. In approximately 38 States and American Samoa, Guam, the Northern Mariana Islands, Puerto Rico, and the Virgin Islands, the definition of abuse also includes acts or circumstances that threaten the child with harm or create a substantial risk of harm to the child's health or welfare.

Neglect

Neglect is frequently defined as the failure of a parent or other person with responsibility for the child to provide needed food, clothing, shelter, medical care, or supervision to the degree that the child's health, safety, and well-being are threatened with harm. Approximately 24 States, the District of Columbia, American Samoa, Puerto Rico, and the Virgin Islands include failure to educate the child as required by law in their definition of neglect. Seven States specifically define medical neglect as failing to provide any special medical treatment or mental health care needed by the child. In addition, four States define medical neglect as the withholding of medical treatment or nutrition from disabled infants with life-threatening conditions.

Sexual Abuse/Exploitation

All States include sexual abuse in their definitions of child abuse. Some States refer in general terms to sexual abuse, while others specify various acts as sexual abuse. Sexual exploitation is an element of the definition of sexual abuse in most jurisdictions. Sexual exploitation includes allowing the child to engage in prostitution or in the production of child pornography.

Emotional Abuse

Almost all States, the District of Columbia, American Samoa, Guam, the Northern Mariana Islands, Puerto Rico, and the Virgin Islands include emotional maltreatment as part of their definitions of abuse or neglect. Approximately 32 States, the District of Columbia, the Northern Mariana Islands, and Puerto Rico provide specific definitions of emotional abuse or mental injury to a child. Typical language used in these definitions is "injury to the psychological capacity or emotional stability of the child as evidenced by an observable or substantial change in behavior, emotional response, or cognition" and injury as evidenced by "anxiety, depression, withdrawal, or aggressive behavior."

Parental Substance Abuse

Parental substance abuse is an element of the definition of child abuse or neglect in some States. Circumstances that are considered abuse or neglect in some States include:

- Prenatal exposure of a child to harm due to the mother's use of an illegal drug or other substance (14 States and the District of Columbia)
- Manufacture of a controlled substance in the presence of a child or on the premises occupied by a child (10 States)
- Allowing a child to be present where the chemicals or equipment for the manufacture of controlled substances are used or stored (three States)
- Selling, distributing, or giving drugs or alcohol to a child (seven States and Guam)
- Use of a controlled substance by a caregiver that impairs the caregiver's ability to adequately care for the child (seven States)

Abandonment

Approximately 17 States and the District of Columbia include abandonment in their definitions of abuse or neglect, generally as a type of neglect. Approximately 18 States, Guam, Puerto Rico, and the Virgin Islands provide definitions for abandonment that are separate from the definition of neglect. In general, it is considered abandonment of the child when the parent's identity or whereabouts are unknown, the child has been left by the parent in circumstances in which the child suffers serious harm, or the parent has failed to maintain contact with the child or to provide reasonable support for a specified period of time.

Source: Reprinted, by permission, from Child Welfare Information Gateway, *Definitions of Child Abuse and Neglect* (Washington, DC: Author, 2011), 1–5. Online: www.childwelfare.gov/systemwide/laws_policies/statutes/define.pdf.

Risk factors related to child abuse or neglect

All adults have the capacity to strike out in anger, fear, pain, or frustration. Even if we know someone well, we cannot assume that person could not abuse a child. Most people have the ability to control violent impulses, but given certain circumstances, abuse can occur. There are numerous risk factors for child abuse or neglect. They can be related to the child, the adult, or social stresses, and they can be triggered by certain situations. Teachers who are familiar with these risk factors can more accurately identify child abuse and potentially abusive situations.

Child abuse often happens when adults

- Are isolated, without support
- Have unmet needs for nurturance and dependence
- Feel that their failures outnumber their successes
- Were abused themselves and lack nurturing childrearing experiences
- Are under stress
- Keep their frustrations inside until they finally boil over or cannot control their emotions
- Are under the influence of alcohol or other drugs that reduce their ability to control impulses
- Have mental health problems

Many of the causes of child abuse also can be traced to societal or personal problems, such as family difficulties, domestic violence, economic problems, unemployment, and the loss of a way to cope with problems. Figure A.19 in Appendix A summarizes some characteristics and risk factors related to child neglect.

How programs can help abused children and stressed families

Early childhood programs are the only places where young children are seen on a daily basis for an extended time by professionals trained to observe their appearance, behavior, and development. A teacher may be the first person to suspect (and to report) child maltreatment. Every program should have a written policy and procedure to address child maltreatment. Teachers should immediately follow these when they suspect that something is amiss.

Often, children who are victims of maltreatment are not able to learn or participate to their full potential. They may carry physical and emotional scars throughout life. Depending on the kind and/or severity of abuse or neglect, long-term effects can include motor impairment, loss of hearing or vision, mental retardation, and/or learning and emotional difficulties. Thus it is essential that teachers take action to interrupt the cycle of abuse and neglect by helping children and parents receive needed treatment. The teacher's trusting relationship with children is a major factor in helping children and families cope with and resolve such difficult situations.

Appendix N: Protective Factors Regarding Child Abuse and Neglect in *Caring for Our Children* describes strategies that early childhood programs can use to help strengthen protective factors and prevent child maltreatment. This information is reproduced from Strengthening Families, a framework developed by the Center for the Study of Social Policy (**www.strengtheningfamilies.net**), and also from the Child Welfare Information Gateway.

The protective factors are

- Parental resilience
- Social connections
- Knowledge of parenting and child development
- Concrete support in times of need
- Children's social and emotional competence

The program strategies that early education programs can use to foster these protective factors include the following:

- Facilitate friendships and mutual support. Provide a place where parents/guardians can have positive social interactions in a child-friendly setting.
- Strengthen parenting skills. Model and teach positive, effective guidance techniques with explanations about appropriate expectations based on child development.
- Link families to services and opportunities. Offer information about fun things to do as a family and where to turn for help when (any type of) services are needed.
- Respond to family crises. Connect stressed families with community resources when needed.
- Facilitate children's social and emotional development. Provide children with a healthy, nurturing environment that encourages trust and attachment.
- Observe and respond to early warning signs of child abuse or neglect.
- Value and support parents. Help parents develop confidence, and link them to community resources, including mental health professionals, as needed.

Legal and ethical issues

Obtain a copy of the state's child abuse reporting statute. Check with a local department of social services, law enforcement agency, or district attorney's office, or your regional Health and Human Services (HHS) office. Ask what happens after a report is made so that you can explain the procedure to the family when you inform them about your responsibility to report a suspicion. While making a report, ask whether, when, and how someone from the agency will give feedback to the person who made the report about the result of their investigation. Usually, only limited information is given by the social service agency to the person who reported the suspected maltreatment. You may learn only whether the investigation confirmed or did not confirm legally defined maltreatment. Indicate to the agency staff that appropriate staff members from the child care program would like to be advised about how the child care program can help the family cope with the experience of having a report filed, whatever the outcome of the investigation.

NAEYC's *Code of Ethical Conduct and Statement of Commitment* (2011), contains principles related to child maltreatment. These state that

> **P-1.1—Above all, we shall not harm children. We shall not participate in practices that are emotionally damaging, physically harmful, disrespectful, degrading, dangerous, exploitative, or intimidating to children. *This principle has precedence over all others in this Code.* . . .**
>
> **P-1.8**—We shall be familiar with the risk factors for and symptoms of child abuse and neglect, including physical, sexual, verbal, and emotional abuse and physical, emotional, educational, and medical neglect. We shall know and follow state laws and community procedures that protect children against abuse and neglect.
>
> **P-1.9**—When we have reasonable cause to suspect child abuse or neglect, we shall report it to the appropriate community agency and follow up to ensure that appropriate action has been taken. When appropriate, parents or guardians will be informed that the referral will be or has been made.
>
> **P-1.10**—When another person tells us of his or her suspicion that a child is being abused or neglected, we shall assist that person in taking appropriate action in order to protect the child.
>
> **P-1.11**—When we become aware of a practice or situation that endangers the health, safety, or well-being of children, we have an ethical responsibility to protect children or inform parents and/or others who can. . . .
>
> **P-2.13**—We shall maintain confidentiality and shall respect the family's right to privacy, refraining from disclosure of confidential information and intrusion into family life. However, when we have reason to believe that a child's welfare is at risk, it is permissible to share confidential information with agencies, as well as with individuals who have legal responsibility for intervening in the child's interest. . . .
>
> **P-2.15**—We shall be familiar with and appropriately refer families to community resources and professional support services. After a referral has been made, we shall follow up to ensure that services have been appropriately provided. . . .
>
> **P-3B.4**—If we have concerns about a colleague's behavior, and children's well-being is not at risk, we may address the concern with that individual. If children are at risk or the situation does not improve after it has been brought to the colleague's attention, we shall report the colleague's unethical or incompetent behavior to an appropriate authority. . . .
>
> **P-4.6**—We shall be familiar with laws and regulations that serve to protect the children in our programs and be vigilant in ensuring that these laws and regulations are followed.

Common problems with reporting child abuse or neglect

Staff members may have mixed feelings about reporting suspected maltreatment. They may not want to become involved, or they may feel that families have the right to discipline their child in their own way. Teachers also may be reluctant to face the fact that someone known to them may be abusive. These are natural feelings, but they must be overcome for the child's sake.

Some teachers have had previous negative experiences in reporting suspected abuse and neglect and are reluctant to become involved again. Maybe a social worker discouraged reporting, was unresponsive, or did not adequately handle the case. Perhaps someone knows of cases where nothing was done and the abuse continued or escalated. Although these concerns may be valid, a previous bad experience does not mean that the next case will not be handled better. In most states, the law requires filing a report regardless of previous experiences, with no exceptions. Children cannot be protected from maltreatment unless they are first identified and the situation is reported.

Teachers may worry about endangering their relationship with the child's family by reporting a suspicion. Although the identity of the reporter of child abuse is supposed to remain anonymous, families will suspect who reported them by the nature of the information contained in the report. Abusive adults need help, and some are grateful when they receive it. In other situations, parents are unaware that their child is being abused by another adult. Each case requires individual handling. Some parents may be irate at first, or even act in a threatening manner. Be sure to inform the social service agency and the police if these things happen. In general, it is best to advise the parent that an abuse/neglect report is being filed, as required by law, and that help is available for the family. Even if the person adamantly denies any abuse or neglect, or knowledge of abuse by others, filing of suspected abuse or neglect is required so child protective services can investigate and initiate action if appropriate.

Sometimes it is difficult to tell a parent beforehand about making a report. If a child is in imminent danger and the parent may disappear with the child, call the appropriate agency immediately and do not tell the parent. However, most often, the child's teacher will know and care about the parent, and the situation may be such that the child will not be in imminent danger. Staff members may worry that telling the parent will evoke hostility and anger that may result in removal of the child from the program. However, failure to inform families about making a report may lead them to feel betrayed or deceived. As a general rule, it is better to inform the family of a decision to make a report. Start by explaining that educators are *required* by law to report all instances of suspected child abuse. It is the job of the investigators to determine whether there is actual abuse. Although parents may be very angry, showing concern for the child may help them see that there was no choice in the matter.

Preventing maltreatment in programs for young children

Every program should implement the following essential precautions to prevent maltreatment of children in their care. These measures also help to protect the program from being wrongly suspected of allowing maltreatment to occur. Devastating turmoil usually results when someone who works in a child care program is accused of being involved in maltreatment of a child, whether the accusation turns out to be false or true.

Background checks

Directors of centers and providers of family child care should conduct careful background checks of all adults who will come into contact with children in the program. Such checks should be part of licensing in states where licensing or registration of individual caregivers is required. In family child care homes, all children over the age of 10 and other adults present should also be screened, whether or not these individuals are involved in providing care to the children in the home.

Check with local law enforcement and social service agencies about how to access and document the following elements of background screening (adapted from *Caring for Our Children* Standard 1.2.0.2):

- Verification of name and address, Social Security number, and education
- Employment history
- Licensing by any state agencies (e.g., foster care, mental health, nursing homes)
- Driving history documented by state records
- Verification of legitimacy and reliability of information given by references
- Search for alias
- Mention in court records
- Fingerprints on file
- State and national criminal history
- Mention in public registries of child abuse and neglect or sex offenses

All of the specific elements listed above should be included in background screening before allowing anyone to work in the program in any capacity. The prospective employee must give consent for the background screening and should not be considered eligible for the job without it. The first step is to verify the usual identifying information of a potential employee, such

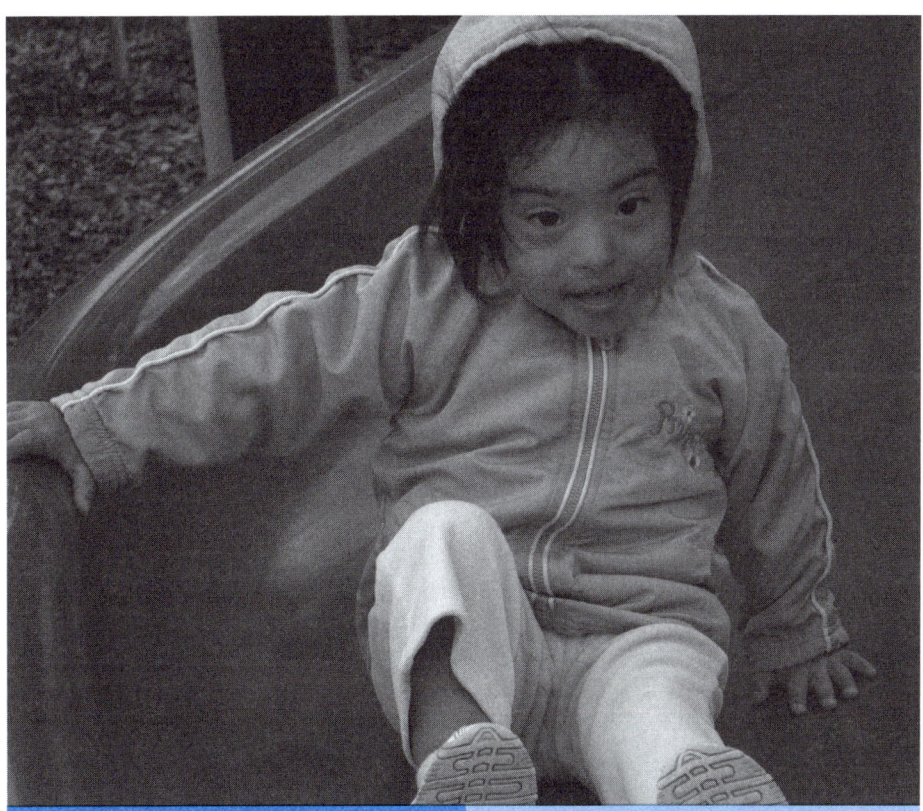

as name, address, Social Security number, education, employment history, and references. Then, if the results suggest the person might be suitable, the other items should be checked. The inquiry should include whether there have been any convictions, arrests, investigation findings, or court cases related to child maltreatment. Drug tests may be required. The screening should be done again if any concerns arise after someone is working in the program. States that do this checking as a function of a credentialing system for employees in programs that care for children reduce the burden on an individual program. However, vigilance is best whenever there is any concern.

Do not hire anyone with a record of prior child abuse of any type or allow anyone to work or volunteer with children if they acknowledge being sexually attracted to children or abusing them. Check all records before allowing an adult to have contact with children. If the person is needed immediately, before all the screening steps are complete, arrange to have another adult present to observe and intercede at all times.

Many abusive adults have not been reported and entered into child abuse registries. While these adults are unlikely to admit their past or current abuse to another person, employment applications should include the question about previous experience with hitting, shouting, losing control, or sexual misconduct. These questions may discourage some potentially abusive individuals from seeking employment in the program. In addition, asking these questions alerts potential staff members about behaviors that are unacceptable. Failure of a prospective employee or a current staff member to disclose previous convictions of child abuse is grounds for not hiring that individual or for dismissal if already on staff.

Other ways to learn about an individual include observation of the candidate performing the job for which she is applying and a probation (trial) period for new employees and volunteers. During the probation period, observe and discuss the person's performance with co-workers and families. Everyone in any way involved with the children in that person's group should be encouraged to drop in and observe too.

The most important measure program directors can take to prevent child maltreatment is to ensure that there is adequate daily supervision of all staff members. Children should not be taken to any area of the facility where they cannot be easily viewed by other adults. The physical layout of the facility should reduce the likelihood of isolation or privacy of individual teachers with children, especially where children may be undressed or have their private parts exposed. Provide windows and mirrors, and remove doors on toilet stalls and toileting rooms for children who need assistance with toileting, so that all adult-child interactions can be seen.

Set up the facility and program operations to prevent maltreatment

Denial of privacy to adults and the increased possibility of observation by another adult are strong deterrents to abuse or accusations of abuse. Where teachers must work in isolation, such as in early or late care or in family child care homes, in addition to screening the teacher and adults who will be in the building when children are in care, members of children's families and regulatory specialists should make unannounced visits as often as possible.

Early attention and intervention by early educators can save a child from harm and help strengthen the family's ability to appropriately nurture the child. Build a trusting, sharing relationship with families. Become aware of, and let parents know about, community agencies that provide support services, such as respite care, counseling, temporary shelter, drug treatment, and food stamps. Share child development and childrearing techniques. Let families know when the staff members recognize signs of stress in their children. Share concerns with families and listen as they share their concerns. Any teacher, volunteer, or parent who suspects someone is maltreating a child should not wait to report it. Report the concern to the appropriate staff member with administrative or supervisory authority and to the agency responsible for taking such reports.

Another part of prevention is educating young children, particularly in the area of sexual abuse. Adults are responsible for keeping children safe. Children cannot be expected to recognize and resist inappropriate touching. However, children can learn about their right to say no to something that does not seem right and about how to tell a trusted adult about the experience. They should know that they will not be blamed if something happens that was not right but that they didn't recognize at first was not right. Be aware that the concept of teaching children about "good touches" and "bad touches" is not appropriate. Care must be taken not to teach children that genital touching or fondling is *bad*. Doctors must check children's genitals on occasion, touching will eventually become a normal and good part of *mature* sexual practice, and masturbation is commonplace among preschoolers. Children can be taught that doctors must check their private parts but that, otherwise, if someone wants to check or touch their private parts, or do something else they think is not right, they should say no and find another grown-up they trust to tell about it.

Teachers may be concerned that touching children in any manner might be mistaken for maltreatment. However, positive touch is essential for comfort, assistance, and nurturing. Parents should be advised about the physical contact the staff members usually have with the children and be encouraged to discuss any concerns about such touching. The best way to handle a situation that might cause concern, such as a male teacher having children sit on his lap or assisting children in the toilet room, is to let parents know in advance that these activities are part of the curriculum and are always observed for appropriateness by another staff member. If a child gets a new bruise while in child care, discuss it with a supervisor and inform the parent about what happened. Seeing a bruise on a child that is unexplained can lead to suspicion about maltreatment. For additional information on how to address issues related to child abuse, and to access a large library of resource materials on the topic, visit **www.childwelfare.gov**.

Discipline

All child care programs should have a philosophy and policy that provide developmentally appropriate guidelines for disciplining children. This must be effectively communicated to staff members and families. *Corporal punishment is not acceptable under any circumstances.* Effective guidance/classroom management techniques teach the child how to behave, rather than focusing on punishment for misbehavior. As noted in *Caring for Our Children* Standard 2.2.0.6,

> The word *discipline* means to teach and guide. Discipline is not punishment. The discipline standard therefore reflects an approach that focuses on preventing behavior problems by supporting children in learning appropriate social skills and emotional responses.

Natural consequences of misbehavior are reasonable: the child who hits is not allowed to be in close proximity to other children while being given opportunities to express frustration and anger in more acceptable ways. Natural consequences are the loss of participation or the opportunity to do something, but they do not include denial of daily functions of living, such as eating, sleeping, and toileting.

Use sound child development principles to set expectations and realistic limits for children. For example, not many 3-year-old children will sit still and be attentive for longer than 15 minutes, even if the activity they were watching (e.g., a puppet show) was interesting to them at the start. A 2-year-old child wants to have opportunities to control his actions. The child will often refuse something the adult deems desirable if offered only one option but will more readily choose it when offered two acceptable alternatives. Children should be taught positive and appropriate words, actions, and ways of relating to other children and adults. Modeling positive patterns of interaction and communication with all children and families is one of the most effective ways to teach.

Injury

If a child arrives with an injury requiring immediate medical attention, arrange for a visit to a doctor or to an emergency room for treatment. If you notice bruises, cuts, burns, or other injuries on a child, ask the parent how the injury occurred, what treatment was provided, and what care or precautions must be taken. As a routine practice, the program should keep careful records about every child, noting all injuries that children have when they arrive at the program and any injuries that happen while the child is at the program. Include a description of the injury, date, time, place it happened, and how it occurred, statements by parent or child, and treatment the child received. Always notify parents immediately if any injury or illness occurs while the child is participating in the program. (See Figure A.6 in Appendix A.) There are certain types of injuries that strongly suggest abuse. These include burns on the skin; hand prints on the child's body; striped bruises that suggest the child was hit with a cord or stick; other types of imprints of objects on the child's body; or a swelling, bruise, or cut on a body part that the child tells you happened as the result of deliberate injury. Shaken baby syndrome, described in Chapter 3, is traumatic brain injury from rapid acceleration/deceleration of the child's head from shaking or being tossed in the air, or another activity.

Reporting procedures

What and when to report. *No state requires that the reporter have proof that abuse or neglect has occurred.* The law may specify that you need only to have a suspicion or a "reason to believe." Child abuse and neglect must be reported *as soon as it is suspected* because delay may expose the child to significant harm.

Where to report. Report the concern to the child abuse reporting hotline, department of social services, child protective services, or police as required by your state and local laws. Phone numbers and the reporting system requirements should be posted clearly where staff members can access them easily. Many states have information sheets and forms that can be given to all staff members. Staff members need to know they will not be disciplined or fired for making the report. Parents/guardians should be informed at enrollment of the legal obligation of staff members to report any suspected maltreatment. The previously mentioned Childhelp National Child Abuse Hotline at 1-800-4-A-CHILD (1-800-422-4453) provides 24-hour-a-day, 7-day-a-week access to information on where and how to file a report. Note that the hotline cannot take a report of abuse directly; staffers can counsel you about the need to make a report, refer you to the appropriate reporting agency, and assist you in making the call if you wish.

How to report. Reporting forms and the contents of reports of suspected child abuse and neglect vary from state to state. All states require that a verbal or written report (or both) be made to the specified agency. Obtain copies of your state's reporting form so you can be prepared to give all the information during a telephone report.

Elements to include in a child maltreatment policy

Every early education program's written policy on child abuse and neglect should include the following:

- Requirements for staff members to receive training about preventing and reporting suspected child abuse and neglect

- Procedures for reporting suspected maltreatment (e.g., who must be informed; who makes the report; who communicates with the other families, the staff, and the press)

- A code of conduct for staff members relating to their behavior with children, including permissible methods of guidance/classroom management techniques and prohibition of unobservable interaction of adults with children in the facility—especially in situations in which children receive assistance with dressing, undressing, and toileting

- Program commitment to providing stress management when needed and breaks for teachers of no less than 15 minutes every four hours and at least a 30-minute break for lunch; paid time off

- A method for teachers to signal for and receive immediate relief by a substitute when they feel they cannot continue to provide safe and nurturing care

- Procedures for investigating job applicants and volunteers prior to hiring and whenever suspicion is raised concerning a staff member

- Approaches to management of children who have been victims of maltreatment, including special training for staff members by experts in behavior management of child abuse victims

Administration of the health component

Competent administration is required to implement all aspects of the health component in the program. For all hours of operation, the delegation of authority should be documented in writing and explicit so it is clear to all who are involved with the program. The staff members who are in charge of individual children should be explicitly designated as well.

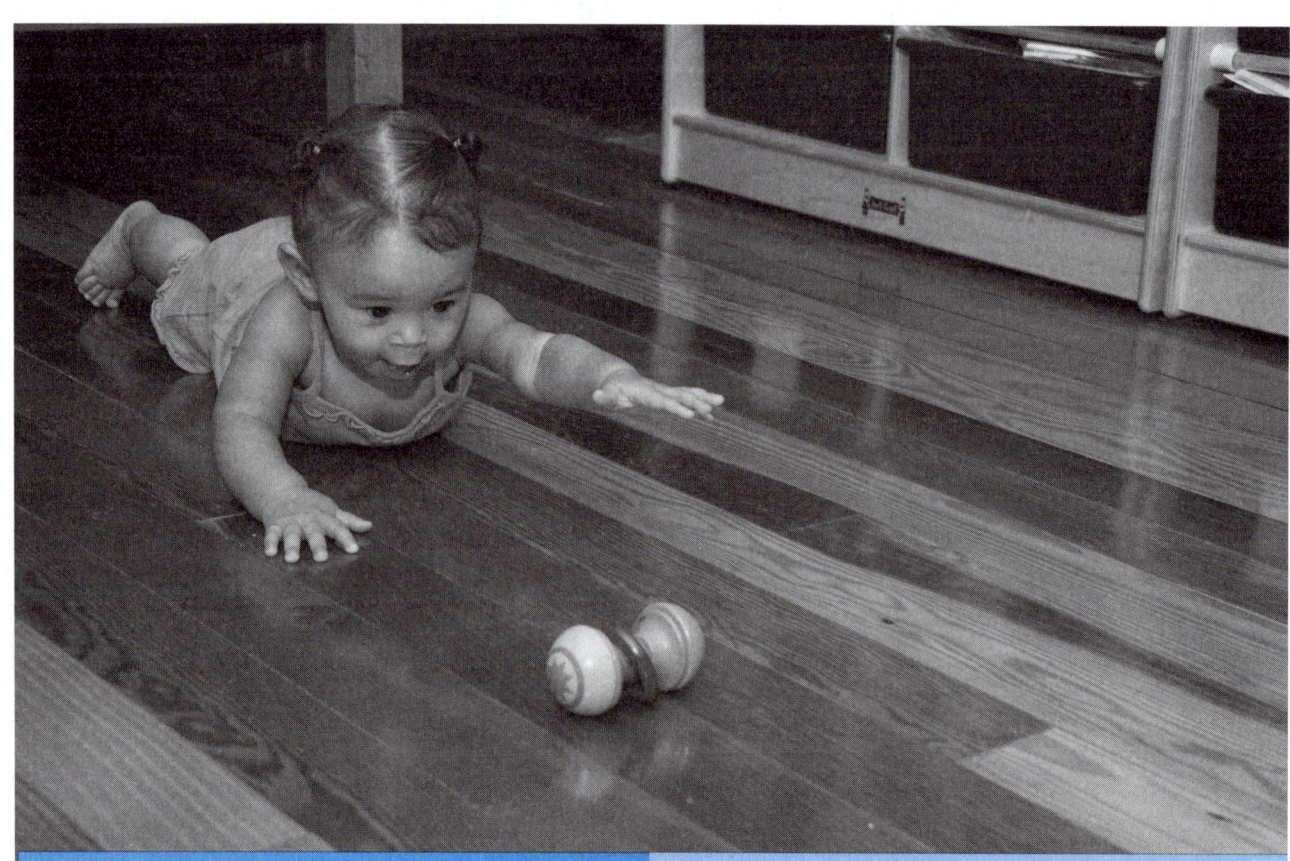

Role of the governing body and the administrator

The governing body of a center should appoint an administrator whose duties related to health and safety include

- Ensuring compliance with all applicable health and safety rules, regulations, facility policies, and procedures
- Developing, implementing, and updating the facility's health and safety policies and informing all families, employees, and volunteers about them
- Hiring, supervising, assigning duties and responsibilities to, evaluating, and firing or excusing adults who work in the facility, especially as the performance of these adults relates to health and safety (e.g., physical health, mental health, oral health, and nutrition)
- Providing or ensuring that all adults and children receive appropriate education about health and safety issues, including preservice training and continuing education for staff members and volunteers
- Providing for continuous supervision of visitors and all non-facility personnel
- Ensuring and following up on the findings of routine safety and maintenance checks by 1) planning for corrective action and 2) assigning a specific person to arrange for or provide repair and maintenance
- Recommending an annual budget and managing finances to support the operation of the facility in a safe and healthy way
- Maintaining required records for staff members, volunteers, and children to ensure confidentiality; appropriately using the data to prevent injury and infection and plan for children's care and regulatory oversight
- Providing for parent involvement and education; offering opportunities for activities that foster interaction among families to encourage mutual support
- Providing oversight of any research studies or activities of students from institutions of higher education who are using the facility or working with children as part of a practice experience
- Reporting to the governing body on a regular basis about all facets of the operation of the program

Of course, family child care providers often fill multiple roles and may perform all duties that a center administrator would handle.

Facility health policies

The facility should have written policies that specify the ages and abilities of the children who are served in the program, how children's individual and special needs will be addressed, the services provided, the management of administrative functions, and all other procedures. Including explicit procedures for implementing each policy will make the work of developing the policies worthwhile. A child care health consultant, the administrator, the staff members, and representatives of the families should be included in the development, annual review, and updates of the policies and procedures. The written policies should be provided electronically or in hard copy to all staff members and parents in a language they can understand and at least two weeks before any new policies go into effect. All who receive a copy of the policies should indicate in writing that they have received, read (or had the policies read to them), and understand them. *Caring for Our Children* Chapter 9 (and other chapters of this manual) provides additional details for the following topics to be covered by the policies:

- Admission criteria and enrollment procedures; preadmission agreement, preadmission enrollment information for each child
- Pick-up/drop off, sign-in/sign-out routines; persons authorized to pick up a child; safe passenger and pedestrian practices; notice of nonattendance, arrangements when late or no pick-up occurs
- Payment of fees, deposits, and refunds
- Written description of the program based on a statement of principles
- Methods and schedules of communications between parents and staff members on a daily basis—for periodic reviews of the child's progress, for illness or injury, in a facility emergency, and when anything unusual occurs
- Supervision indoors and outside
- Accepted guidance/classroom management techniques
- Inclusion of children with special needs; sharing of information about therapies and treatments the child requires
- Nondiscrimination
- Termination of enrollment; transitions to other programs
- Staffing, including specific assigned responsibilities to teachers, substitutes, and volunteers (by role and, where appropriate, by name)
- Child health services, including health assessments with screenings and immunizations
- Plans for health promotion and prevention, including identification of the child's medical home, information exchange and tracking related to routine preventive health services, health consultation, health education for children/staff members/families, oral health, sun safety, environmental quality measures to avoid noxious and toxic exposures (e.g., to pesti-

cides, poisons), safety surveillance, and preventing obesity

- Food and nutrition, including food handling, human milk, feeding and food brought from home, as well as a daily schedule of meals and snacks; nutrition service records (e.g., budget, expenditures for food, menus, inspection reports, nutrition education, and recipes)
- Confidentiality of records
- Physical activity both outdoors and when children are physically active indoors, play areas, screen time, and frequency/location/type of outdoor play
- Sleep areas and equipment; safe sleep practices
- Sanitation and hygiene
- Care of acutely ill children, exclusion and alternate care for ill children whom staff members decide may not remain in their usual care arrangement, records of illness/symptoms/absence from the facility and reporting notifiable diseases to the health department, review of documented illness to detect patterns amenable to prevention, and sharing of information about family health that might affect the child's well-being
- Medication administration
- Handling of urgent medical care
- Handling of outbreaks of disease
- Documentation of immunizations, including exemptions and plans for exclusion of children who lack age-appropriate immunizations
- Documentation of injuries occurring at the facility and periodic review (at least semiannually) to detect patterns amenable to prevention
- Presence and care of any animals on the premises
- Evening and night care plan
- Prohibited substances (e.g., smoking, tobacco, alcohol, illegal drugs, and firearms)
- Human resources management—staff health and maintenance; content of staff and volunteer records, professional development records, and attendance records for those involved in caring for the children and all other staff members; benefits; and performance evaluation
- Facility records related to insurance coverage, maintenance of records, and availability of records for inspection by licensing and other authorized personnel; records and documents available to parents/guardians (e.g., license or operating certificate, reports of violations and corrections related to inspections, and accreditation or other quality status awards)
- Maintenance of the facility and equipment, including play areas, safety checks, equipment audits, recall checks, requirements for manufacturers/installers' warrantees, and requirements for contractors' compliance with facility policies
- Prevention and reporting of child maltreatment
- Handling of threatening incidents and security
- Plans for management of disasters, emergencies, drills, evacuation, alternative shelter arrangements
- Use of consultants (e.g., child care health, mental health, and early education), including frequency of planned visits and documentation of visits and electronic consultation (including name of consultant, date and time for visit, recipient of services, reason, service provided, recommendations, follow-up)
- Transportation and field trips
- Review and revision of policies, plans, and procedures

Administrators should use the standards in Chapter 9 of *Caring for Our Children* to set objectives for the program. While the scope of what could be done is vast, getting started and working to improve over time will make a big difference in the quality of care. Health policies should be a living document used to orient new staff members and families, evaluate the performance of seasoned staff members, and annually reassess the intention expressed in the policies. In addition to using health policies as a tool for improvement, the administrator should ensure that there is a comprehensive written plan of daily activities. This plan should be based on developmentally appropriate practice that integrates health and safety practices.

Keeping health records up-to-date is important, but the value lies in using the data to ensure that children receive the services they need both within the program and from their regular sources of medical and oral health care. Health records should be confidential, but families need to understand the benefits of granting access to those records to the people who can use the information to help their children. The family, the teachers, and the child's health professionals should be able to share information to effectively coordinate supportive care, and the administrator must be the one to establish this three-way communication.

Every child care program, large or small, needs a health consultant who is more just than a name and phone number. The health consultant should visit the facility and be guided by the staff members' priorities and the health consultant's observations of significant risks to provide the most meaningful services. For a large center, observations need to be extensive. Formal instruction and follow-up is necessary to see whether training has been effective. Communication requires willingness on the part of the consultant and the program's staff members to learn each other's approaches and support working together toward common goals.

Every program should establish a community resource file that is updated at least annually and is available to share with parents as needed. To the extent possible, information should be provided in the languages spoken by parents. This file will grow as staff members identify additional family needs and resources to meet those needs. A copy of the file should be accessible, and families and staff members should be encouraged to contribute to it.

Administration is not an end; it is a process that leads to desired outcomes, and it is most successful when those outcomes are clearly defined. With clearly defined common objectives, administrators can harness the efforts of families, staff members, consultants, and community resources to make early care and education a truly safe and healthy place that supports the well-being of children and families.

Suggested activities

- Inquire of the child welfare agency serving your area how child abuse and neglect reports are handled. How does your state define abuse and neglect? What type of professional help is available to stressed families who are at risk of abuse or have already abused their children?

- If possible, ask to speak to a child welfare worker about whether there have been any instances in which a child abuse report was made by an early educator as a mandated reporter. Acknowledging the need to avoid mention of anyone's name, ask whether such reports by early education staff members have led to providing help for a child and the child's family.

- Ask several providers to share a copy of their written health policies. Which of the items listed in this chapter are covered; which are not? If you were a new staff member at each of these facilities, would you know from what you read what you were expected to do about health and safety practice in that setting?

Appendices

Appendix A. Forms and Checklists   196

Appendix B. Acronyms Used in This Book   230

Appendix C. Links to Internet Resources in This Book   231

**Appendix D. Crosswalk of *Healthy Young Children* and NAEYC   233
Early Childhood Accreditation Criteria**

Figure A.1.

DIAPERING

This poster is based on *Caring for Our Children, 3rd Edition*, a publication of the American Academy of Pediatrics, American Public Health Association, and the NRC for Health and Safety in Child Care and Early Education. It was created by CCA Global with guidance from the PA Chapter of the AAP.

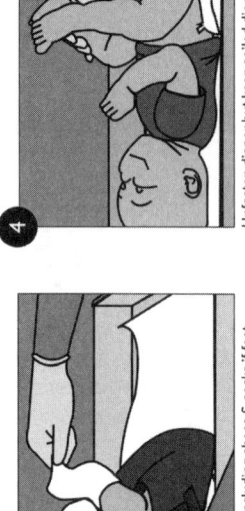

1. Cover surface with disposable paper. Remove from containers & place on diapering surface **away from child's reach**: Wipes • Clean diaper • Dab of diapering cream on facial tissue • Plastic bag for soiled clothes • [Put on gloves if using]

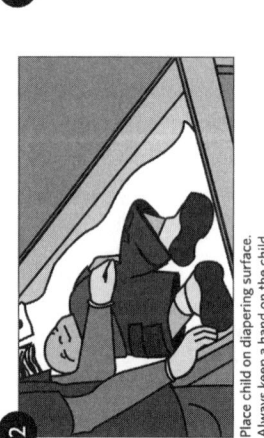

2. Place child on diapering surface. Always keep a hand on the child.

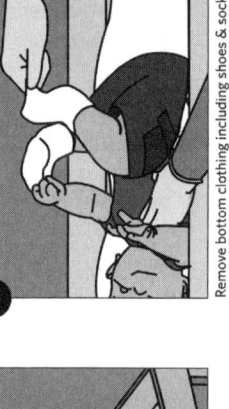

3. Remove bottom clothing including shoes & socks if feet cannot be kept from contacting soiled skin or surfaces. [If clothing is soiled, remove and place in plastic bag.]

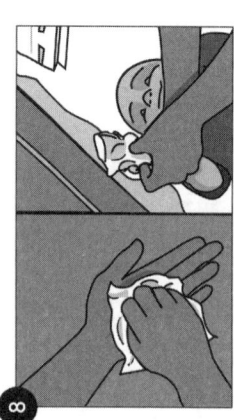

4. Unfasten diaper but keep soiled diaper under child's bottom.

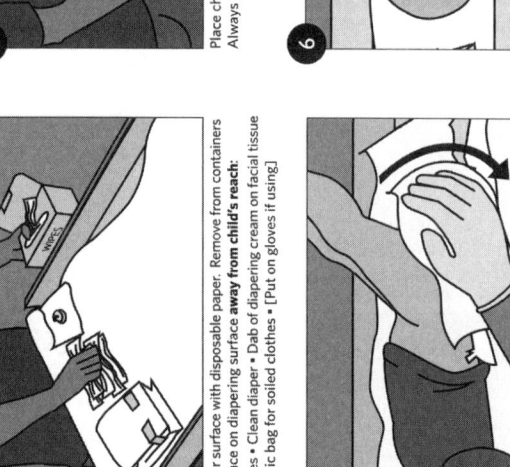

5. Lift child's legs and clean bottom from front to back. Use fresh wipe each time.

6. Put soiled wipes in soiled diaper. Then remove diaper and dispose in plastic-lined hands-free covered can.

7. Remove gloves. Dispose in hands-free can.

8. Use separate fresh wipe on adult's and child's hands. Dispose in hands-free can.

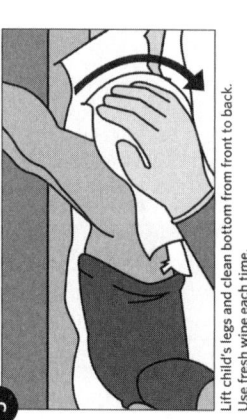

9. If paper is soiled, fold clean side of paper back under child's bottom.

10. Put clean diaper under child's bottom. [If using diaper cream, apply with facial tissue.]

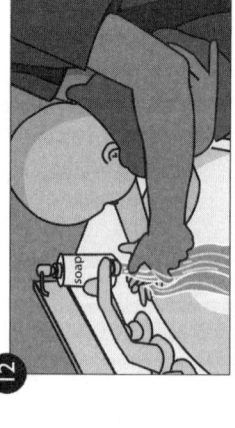

11. Fasten diaper and dress child.

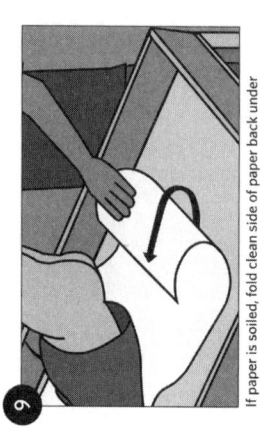

12. Wash child's hands at sink.*

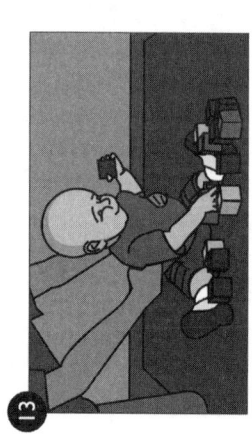

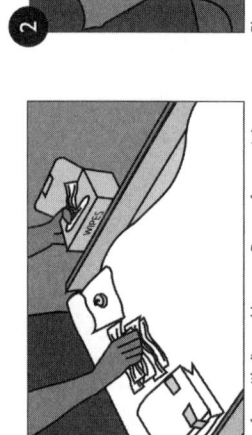

13. Return child to supervised area.

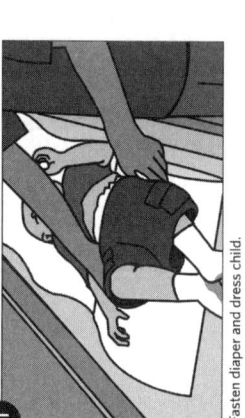

14. Clean and Disinfect — Wash | Rinse | Disinfect (Soap + Water | Water | Bleach Water)

A. Dispose of changing table paper.
B. If diapering surfaces are visibly soiled:
 • Wash surfaces with detergent, water & paper towels.
 • Rinse surfaces with water.
C. Wet all diapering surfaces with disinfectant solution.
D. Leave solution on for required contact time.

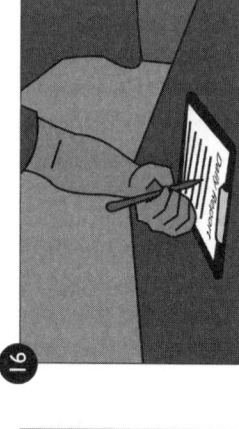

15. E. WASH HANDS: *Use of an alcohol-based hand sanitizer is OK for adults and children over 24 months.
F. If diapering surface is wet after required contact time, dry with clean paper towel before next change.

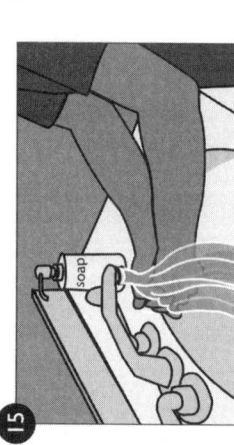

16. Record in Daily Report form for family
 • Time of diaper change
 • Diaper contents
 • Any problems such as loose stool, skin irritation, etc.

© 2012 CCA Global Partners, Inc. This poster is based on *Caring for Our Children*, 3rd edition, a publication of the American Academy of Pediatrics, American Public Health Association, and the NRC for Health and Safety in Child Care and Early Education; created by CCA Global with guidance from the PA Chapter of the AAP. Reprinted by permission from CCA Global.

Figure A.2.

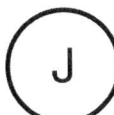

Selecting an Appropriate Sanitizer or Disinfectant

One of the most important steps in reducing the spread of infectious diseases in child care settings is cleaning, sanitizing, and disinfecting surfaces that could possibly pose a risk to children or staff. Routine cleaning with detergent and water is the most useful method for removing germs from surfaces in the child care setting. However, some items and surfaces require an additional step after cleaning to further reduce the number of germs on a surface to a level that is unlikely to transmit disease.

What is the difference between sanitizing and disinfecting?

Sometimes these terms are used as if they mean the same thing, but they are not the same.

Sanitizer is a product that reduces germs on inanimate surfaces to levels considered safe by public health codes or regulations. A sanitizer may be appropriate to use on food contact surfaces (dishes, utensils, cutting boards, high chair trays), toys that children may place in their mouths, and pacifiers.

Disinfectant is a product that destroys or inactivates germs on an inanimate object. A disinfectant may be appropriate to use on non-porous surfaces such as diaper change tables, counter tops, door and cabinet handles, and toilets and other bathroom surfaces.

The U.S. Environmental Protection Agency (EPA) recommends that EPA-registered products be used whenever possible. Only a sanitizer or disinfectant product with an EPA registration number on the label can make public health claims that they are effective in inactivating germs. Major manufacturers of chlorine bleach and hydrogen peroxide products offer products that are EPA-registered and sold either in retail stores or commercial janitorial supply stores.

Always follow the manufacturer's instructions when using EPA-registered products described as sanitizers or disinfectants. This includes pre-cleaning, how long the product needs to remain wet on the surface or item, whether or not the product should be diluted or used as is, and if rinsing is needed. Please note that the label instructions on most disinfectants indicate that the surface must be pre-cleaned before applying the disinfectant.

Are there alternatives to chlorine bleach?

If a product that is not chlorine bleach is registered with the EPA and described as a sanitizer or as a disinfectant and is used according to the manufacturer's instructions, it can be used in child care settings. Check the label to see how long you need to leave the sanitizer or disinfectant in contact with the surface you are treating, whether you need to rinse it off before contact by children, and for any precautions when handling.

Some child care settings are using products with hydrogen peroxide as the active ingredient instead of chlorine bleach. Hydrogen peroxide breaks down into water and oxygen.

Check to see if the product has an EPA registration number and follow the manufacturer's instructions for use and safe handling. Remember that EPA-registered products will also have available a Material Safety Data Sheet (MSDS) that will provide instructions for the safe use of the product and guidance for first aid response to inadvertent exposure to the chemical.

If you are looking for environmentally friendly products, one EPA-registered product is a botanical-based disinfectant whose active ingredient is thymol which requires a ten minute contact time and, if applied to toys or food contact surfaces, a water rinse is required before use.

In addition, some manufacturers of sanitizer and disinfectant products are working towards developing "green cleaning products" that can attain EPA registration. As new environmentally friendly cleaning products appear in the market, check to see if they are EPA-registered.

Household Bleach and Water

If purchasing an EPA-registered product for sanitizing or disinfecting is not an option, then household bleach diluted with water is a practical alternative. It is economical, convenient, and readily available. It is effective if the proportional amount of bleach to water is appropriate for the task. Using too little bleach may make the mixture ineffective. However, using too much bleach may create a potential health hazard.

When purchasing chlorine bleach, make sure that the bleach concentration is for household use, and not for industrial applications. Household chlorine bleach is typically sold in retail stores as 5-10% hypochlorite solution (regular strength). Use only unscented bleach.

Some chlorine bleach products sold in retail stores may be EPA-registered and described as a sanitizer or disinfectant. Check the label to see if the product has an EPA registration number and follow the manufacturer's instructions

If the chlorine bleach product is for household use and does not have an EPA registration number, here are two recipes that you can use. Which recipe you choose will depend on whether you need to sanitize or disinfect a surface.

To safely prepare bleach solutions:
- Dilute bleach with cool water and do not use more than the recommended amount of bleach.
- Select a bottle made of opaque material.
- Make a fresh bleach dilution daily; label the bottle with contents and the date mixed.
- Wear gloves and eye protection when diluting bleach.
- Use a funnel.
- Add bleach to the water rather than the water to bleach to reduce fumes.
- Make sure the room is well ventilated.
- Never mix or store ammonia with bleach or products that contain bleach.

Appendix J

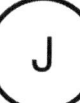

Purpose	Recipe
Sanitizer For food contact surface sanitizing (dishes, utensils, cutting boards, high chair trays), toys that children may place in their mouths, and pacifiers.	1 tablespoon of bleach + 1 gallon of cool water Let stand for 2 minutes or air dry.
Disinfectant For use on non-porous surfaces such as diaper change tables, counter tops, door and cabinet handles, toilets.	¼**- ¾ cup of bleach + 1 gallon of cool water (or 1 to 3 tablespoons of bleach + 1 quart of cool water) applied as a spray or poured fresh solution, not by dipping into a container with a cloth that has been in contact with a contaminated surface Let stand for 2 minutes or air dry.

To safely use bleach solutions:
- Apply the bleach dilution after cleaning the surface with soap or detergent and rinsing with water.
- If using a spray bottle, adjust the setting to produce a heavy spray instead of a fine mist.
- Allow for a two minute contact time or air dry.
- Apply when children are not present in the area.
- Ventilate the area by allowing fresh air to circulate and allow the surfaces to completely air dry or wipe dry after two minutes of contact with the surface before allowing children back into the area.
- Store all chemicals securely, out of reach of children and in a way that they will not tip and spill.

Adapted from: California Childcare Health Program. 2009. Sanitize safely and effectively: Bleach and alternatives in child care programs. *Health and Safety Notes* (July).

A Final Note

Remember that any cleaning, sanitizing, or disinfecting product must always be safely stored and out of reach of children. Always follow the manufacturer's instruction for safe handling to protect yourselves and those in your care.

References:
1. California Childcare Health Program. 2009. Sanitize safely and effectively: Bleach and alternatives in child care programs. *Health and Safety Notes* (July). http://www.ucsfchildcarehealth.org/pdfs/healthandsafety/SanitizeSafely_En0709.pdf.
2. U.S. Environmental Protection Agency. 2008. What are antimicrobial pesticides? Pesticides Website. http://www.epa.gov/oppad001/ad_info.htm.
3. U.S. Environmental Protection Agency. 2009. Selected EPA-registered disinfectants. Pesticides Website. www.epa.gov/oppad001/chemregindex.htm.
4. Grenier, D., D. Leduc, eds. 2008. *Well beings: A guide to health in child care.* 3rd ed. Ottawa: Canadian Paediatric Society.
5. Rutala, W. A., D. J. Weber, the Healthcare Infection Control Practices Advisory Committee (HICPAC). 2008. *Guideline for disinfection and sterilization in healthcare facilities, 2008.* Atlanta, GA: Centers for Disease Control and Prevention, National Center for Preparedness, Detection, and Control of Infectious Diseases, Division of Healthcare Quality Promotion. http://www.cdc.gov/hicpac/pdf/guidelines/Disinfection_Nov_2008.pdf.
6. U.S. Department of Health and Human Services, Public Health Service, Food and Drug Administration. 2009. Food code. College Park, MD: Food and Drug Administration. http://www.fda.gov/Food/FoodSafety/RetailFoodProtection/FoodCode/FoodCode2009/default.htm.

** Corrected to "1/4" from "1/2" in second printing, August 2011.

Source: Appendix J, *Caring for Our Children.* Reprinted with permission.

Figure A.3.

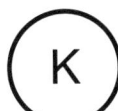

Routine Schedule** for Cleaning, Sanitizing, and Disinfecting

Areas	Before Each Use	After Each Use	Daily (At the End of the Day)	Weekly	Monthly	Comments
Food Areas						
• Food preparation surfaces	Clean, Sanitize	Clean, Sanitize				Use a sanitizer safe for food contact
• Eating utensils & dishes		Clean, Sanitize				If washing the dishes and utensils by hand, use a sanitizer safe for food contact as the final step in the process; Use of an automated dishwasher will sanitize
• Tables & highchair trays	Clean, Sanitize	Clean, Sanitize				
• Countertops		Clean	Clean, Sanitize			Use a sanitizer safe for food contact
• Food preparation appliances		Clean	Clean, Sanitize			
• Mixed use tables	Clean, Sanitize					Before serving food
• Refrigerator					Clean	
Child Care Areas						
• Plastic mouthed toys		Clean	Clean, Sanitize			
• Pacifiers		Clean	Clean, Sanitize			Reserve for use by only one child; Use dishwasher or boil for one minute
• Hats			Clean			Clean after each use if head lice present
• Door & cabinet handles			Clean, Disinfect			

**Corrected to "Routine Schedule" from "Guide" in second printing, August 2011.

• Floors			Clean		Sweep or vacuum, then damp mop, (consider micro fiber damp mop to pick up most particles)
• Machine washable cloth toys				Clean	Launder
• Dress-up clothes				Clean	Launder
• Play activity centers				Clean	
• Drinking Fountains			Clean, Disinfect		
• Computer keyboards		Clean, Sanitize			Use sanitizing wipes, do not use spray
• Phone receivers			Clean		
Toilet & Diapering Areas					
• Changing tables		Clean, Disinfect			Clean with detergent, rinse, disinfect
• Potty chairs		Clean, Disinfect			
• Handwashing sinks & faucets			Clean, Disinfect		
• Countertops			Clean, Disinfect		
• Toilets			Clean, Disinfect		
• Diaper pails			Clean, Disinfect		
• Floors			Clean, Disinfect		Damp mop with a floor cleaner/ disinfectant
Sleeping Areas					
• Bed sheets & pillow cases				Clean	Clean before use by another child
• Cribs, cots, & mats				Clean	Clean before use by another child
• Blankets					Clean

Source: Appendix K, *Caring for Our Children.* Reprinted with permission.

Figure A.4.

Sample Letter to Families about Exposure to Communicable Disease

Name of Child Care Program:_____

Address of Child Care Program:_____

Telephone Number of Child Care Program:_____

Date: _____

Dear Parent or Legal Guardian:

A child in our program has or is suspected of having:_____

Information about this disease:

The disease is spread by:_____
_____

The symptoms are:_____
_____
_____

The disease can be prevented by:_____
_____
_____
_____

What the program is doing:_____
_____
_____
_____

What you can do at home:_____
_____
_____
_____

If your child has any symptoms of this disease, call your doctor to find out what to do. Be sure to tell your doctor about this notice. If you do not have a regular doctor to care for your child, contact your local health department for instructions on how to find a doctor, or ask other parents for names of their children's doctors. If you have any questions, please contact:

_____   at (____)_____
(Caregiver's name)   (Telephone number)

Source: Appendix K, *Model Child Care Health Policies*, 2002.

Figure A.5.

Safety Checklist for Active Play Areas

The following checklist is based primarily on the recommendations of the US Consumer Product Safety Commission (CPSC) as specified in the *Public Playground Safety Handbook*. Not every recommendation is included in this checklist; please refer to the most current guidelines in the Public Playground Safety Handbook, included in this module and available at www.cpsc.gov. Playground equipment should also meet the most current ASTM Standards F1487 for children ages 2-12 years of age and F2373 for children less than 2 years of age. Information on the current edition of these standards is available at www.astm.org. Portable equipment does **not** meet the ASTM standard for public play equipment and therefore should not be used on early learning programs' playgrounds. Early learning programs with indoor play areas should refer to ASTM F2373-*Standard Consumer Safety Performance Specification for Public Use Play Equipment for Children 6 Months Through 23 Months*, for more guidance on areas unique to their facilities.

Successfully completing this checklist will help you make your play area safer.

By checking "Yes" below, you confirm that the recommendation has been met or that a hazard is **NOT** present. When you check "No," be sure to add it to your corrective action plan on the last page of this checklist.

Please note: You will need a yardstick and/or measuring tape to complete this checklist.

There are three age groups referred to in this checklist:

- Toddlers: children aged 6 months through 2 years of age;
- Preschool-age: children aged 2 years through 5 years; and
- School-age: children aged 5 years through 12 years.

The Early Childhood Education Linkage System (ECELS) of the PA Chapter, American Academy of Pediatrics does not accept any liability associated with the assessment of your play area.

Surfacing

Measure the highest point on every piece of play equipment. For swings, the highest point is from the pivot point where the swing is suspended down to the ground. For elevated platforms the highest point is the height of the platform down to the ground. For all other structures, height is measured from the highest point of the structure down to the ground.

Yes No

☐ ☐ Surfaces underneath play equipment that allow children to get off the ground are covered with impact-absorbing material according to the recommendations for critical height (Table below from CPSC *Public Playground Safety Handbook*, April, 2008).

Table 2. Minimum compressed loose-fill surfacing depths			
Inches	Of (Loose-Fill Material)	Protects to	Fall Height (feet)
9	Shredded/recycled rubber		10
9	Sand		4
9	Pea Gravel		5
9	Wood mulch (non-CCA)		7
9	Wood chips		10

Surfacing cont.

Yes No

- ☐ ☐ Unitary rubber surfacing like rubber pads and poured-in-place rubber surfacing meets the ASTM F1292 Standard for the highest point of the play equipment.
- ☐ ☐ The following surfacing materials are not in use underneath play equipment that children can climb: asphalt, concrete, soil or hard-packed dirt, grass, turf, linoleum, or carpeting.
- ☐ ☐ The dirt in the play area has been tested and found free of toxic materials, including lead.
- ☐ ☐ There are no toys or objects with a diameter less than 1 1/4 inch accessible to children who are still placing objects in their mouths.
- ☐ ☐ Loose fill should be avoided for playgrounds intended for Toddlers.
- ☐ ☐ Children do not play on dark colored surfacing that is exposed to intense sun.
- ☐ ☐ Children do not play on frozen safety surfacing.

Use Zones

Yes No

- ☐ ☐ Use zone, the area under and around the equipment where impact absorbing surfacing is required, is a minimum of 3 feet for Toddler play areas in early learning programs.
- ☐ ☐ Use zone is a minimum of 6 feet for Preschool-age and School-age children.
- ☐ ☐ If two pieces of equipment, side by side, are lower than 30" high the use zone between them is six feet or more.
- ☐ ☐ If two pieces of equipment are side by side and one or both is higher than 30" the use zone between them is nine feet or more.
- ☐ ☐ Use zones for moving equipment such as swings and merry-go-rounds do not overlap.
- ☐ ☐ For to-fro swings: the impact-absorbing surfacing material extends twice the height of the pivot point to the ground in front and twice the height of the pivot point to the ground in back of the swings.
- ☐ ☐ For full bucket swings: The impact-absorbing surfacing material extends twice the height from the bottom of the seat to the pivot point in front and twice the height of the bottom of the seat to the pivot point in back.
- ☐ ☐ For tire swings: The impact attenuating surface extends the height from the top of the tire to the pivot point plus 6 feet.
- ☐ ☐ For slides: The impact-absorbing surfacing material extends at least 6 feet from the end of the slide chute—or a distance that equals the height of the slide platform. The impact absorbing surface never needs to extend more than 8 feet.
- ☐ ☐ For slides: No use zone overlaps the use zone at the exit of a slide.

Protrusion & Entanglement

Yes No

- ☐ ☐ All metal edges are rolled.
- ☐ ☐ There are no small pieces of the equipment (like hardware and small bars) that stick out from the equipment that could puncture a child or that could catch clothing.
- ☐ ☐ There are no strings or loose items on children's clothing or around children's necks that could get caught on play equipment.
- ☐ ☐ Any exposed bolts do not protrude more than two threads beyond the face of the nut; exposed bolts have no burrs or sharp edges.
- ☐ ☐ There are no open "S" hooks.
- ☐ ☐ There is a warning sign posted near or on slides or other equipment where potential strangulation may occur.

Entrapment

Yes **No**

☐ ☐ There are no openings in any pieces of play equipment for Preschool-age and School-age 3 ½ and 9 inches that could cause head entrapment.

☐ ☐ There are no head entrapment openings 3 inches to 9 inches for Toddlers.

Equipment Placement

Yes **No**

☐ ☐ Equipment that moves such as swings and merry-go-rounds are placed on the outside edge of the playground.

☐ ☐ Traffic patterns are designed to prevent children from bumping into each other.

Trip Hazards

Yes **No**

☐ ☐ All anchoring devices, such as footings and bars at the bottom of climbers, are below the playing surface.

☐ ☐ There are no exposed tree or plant roots.

☐ ☐ Changes in elevation are made obvious by the use of brightly colored visual or other barriers.

Appropriate Activities & Equipment

Yes **No**

☐ ☐ Age-specific play areas are separated by distance or a physical barrier.

☐ ☐ Equipment is warranted by the manufacturer as suitable for the age of the users (2–5 years and 5–12 years) according to ASTM Standard F1487 and Toddlers according to the ASTM Standard F2373.

Crush & Shearing Points

Yes **No**

☐ ☐ All openings are too big or too small to entrap a child's finger in a moving part.

☐ ☐ All wooden parts are smooth and without splinters.

☐ ☐ All corners are rounded, especially at exit ends and sides along a slide bed.

☐ ☐ Exposed ends of tubing have caps that cannot be removed without tools. There are no openings in the equipment where insects can build nests.

Guardrails, Handrails, and Safety Barriers

Yes **No**

☐ ☐ Guardrails or protective barriers are provided to prevent unintentional or deliberate falls off elevated platforms.

☐ ☐ For Preschool-age children: Elevated surfaces more than 20 inches high have a guardrail or protective barrier; those more than 30 inches high have a protective barrier (an enclosing device that is intended to prevent both unintentional and deliberate attempts to pass through the barrier).

☐ ☐ For Toddlers, elevated surfaces more than 18 inches high have protective barriers.

☐ ☐ For School-age children: Elevated surfaces more than 30 inches high have a guardrail or protective barrier; those more than 48 inches high have a protective barrier.

☐ ☐ Handrails are between 1 inch and 1 ½ inches and are at waist to shoulder height of (22 inches–38 inches) for Preschool-age and School-age. Handrails are between 0.6 inches and 1.20 inches and are at waist to shoulder height (15 inches–20 inches) for Toddlers.

☐ ☐ Boundaries such as painted lines or dividers separate play equipment from walking areas.

☐ ☐ Bike or trike riding areas are separate from other areas.

☐ ☐ Playgrounds are fenced in.

Unsafe Equipment

Yes	No	
☐	☐	There are no heavy swings or swings made out of wood, metal, or other rigid materials.
☐	☐	There are no animal figure swings.
☐	☐	There are no multiple-use occupancy swings (swings used by more than one child at a time) other than tire swings.
☐	☐	There are no swing sets with more than 2 swings per bay.
☐	☐	There are no rope swings; all ropes are anchored at both ends.
☐	☐	There are no trapeze bars or free swinging rings (exception: rings with chains less than 7 inches long).
☐	☐	Any see-saws present have a spring centering device for children 2-5 years of age. If see-saws are used, for older children there must be a shock-absorbing material required to cushion seat impact on the surface and the maximum height of the seat above the protective surfacing must not exceed 5 feet.
☐	☐	There are no trampolines.
☐	☐	There are no swinging gates.
☐	☐	If possible, after installation and before use, the equipment has been thoroughly inspected by a Certified Playground Safety Inspector (CPSI). Request that the CPSI provide a copy of their **current** National Recreation and Park Association's certification.

Maintenance

Yes	No	
☐	☐	Daily checks include: broken glass, animal waste, trash, toxic plants or plant debris, damage by vandals, displaced surfacing, broken equipment, chipping paint, puddles of water, insect hazards, need for lubrication of moving parts.
☐	☐	All hardware fasteners, permanent coverings, or connecting devices are tight and cannot be removed without tools.
☐	☐	All surfaces are intact.
☐	☐	All structures are sturdy enough that they will not move or tip over when the weight of an adult is put against them.
☐	☐	There is no peeling paint (lead in peeling paint on play equipment is a common hazard). Play equipment manufactured prior to 1978 is likely to contain leaded paint.
☐	☐	All ropes are tight, secured at both ends and strands cannot be pulled apart.

Supervision

Yes	No	
☐	☐	All areas where children can play are in view of an adult at all times.
☐	☐	The same child:staff ratio is maintained during active play indoors and outdoors.
☐	☐	Every child is accounted for at all times by a supervising adult. Some method of assuring that no child is hidden or missing from the group must be used.
☐	☐	When children must leave the play area to use the toilet, to get first aid, or for any other reason, supervision of the child who leaves and the children who remain in the play area is secure and consistent.
☐	☐	Children are prevented from playing in a way that challenges them beyond their abilities or that puts others at risk of significant injury.
☐	☐	Practitioners understand the basics of playground safety.
☐	☐	Practitioners understand the signs of traumatic brain injury and can give recommended first aid.

Slides

Yes   No

☐   ☐   Slides for Toddlers are no taller than 32 inches high and have side rims at least 4 inches high.

☐   ☐   Slides for Preschool-age and School-age are no taller than 6 ½ feet and have side rims at least 4 inches high.

☐   ☐   There should be a bar or other means to channel the user into a seated position to go down the slide.

☐   ☐   Slide ladders have flat steps and a handrail on each side. For Preschool-age and School-age, steps are ≤ 9 inches apart. Rungs are ≤ 12 inches apart. (If steps are ≤ 9 inches apart, check for entrapment). Slide ladders for Toddlers steps are less than or equal to 7 inches apart and all risers are closed.

☐   ☐   Slide beds for Toddlers are sloped no greater than 24 degrees.

☐   ☐   Slide beds for Preschool-age and School-age have a flat surface at the bottom to slow children down and are sloped at no greater than a 30 degree angle overall.

☐   ☐   Check the surface temperature of all slides before use to prevent burns. Slides with metal beds are shaded to prevent overheating.

☐   ☐   There are no full spiral slides, only short spiral slides (one 360° turn or less), are accessible to Toddlers or Preschool-age.

Sand

Yes   No

☐   ☐   Sand digging areas are in the shade.

☐   ☐   Sand digging areas are contained by smooth frames.

☐   ☐   Sand is covered when not in use to prevent infectious disease and injury risk when animals and insects get into it.

Swings

Yes   No

☐   ☐   Swings are not attached to any other type of equipment.

☐   ☐   Swing footings are stable and buried below the ground and covered by protective surfacing.

☐   ☐   There is no corrosion evident on hooks or chains.

☐   ☐   There are no "A" frames with horizontal cross bars present.

☐   ☐   Full bucket swings are in a separate bay from the other swings.

☐   ☐   Swing hangers are spaced wider than the seats, not less than 20 inches.

☐   ☐   There is a minimum space of 24 inches between seats and 30 inches between the swings and supporting structure for Preschool-age and School-age. There is a minimum of 20 inches between seats and between the swings and the support structure for Toddlers.

☐   ☐   The distance between the bottom of the seat and the protective surface is at least 12 inches.

☐   ☐   The distance between the bottom of the full bucket swing and the protective surface is at least 24 inches.

Multi-Axis Tire Swings

Yes   No

☐   ☐   Tire swings are not attached to any other type of play equipment.

☐   ☐   Tire swings do not share a bay with any other type of swing and are not mounted on any structure with other play components.

☐   ☐   There are no exposed steel belts in steel-belted radial tire swings.

☐   ☐   There are drain holes in tire swing tires.

☐   ☐   The minimum clearance between the extended tire and support structure is 30 inches.

☐   ☐   The tire swing itself weighs less than 35 pounds.

☐ ☐ There are no tire swings used by Toddlers.

Climbers

Yes No

☐ ☐ Climbers have a safe way off for children who cannot complete the activity.

☐ ☐ No places exist where Preschool-age and School-age children can fall more than 18 inches onto any component of the climber. No places exist where Toddlers can fall more than 7 inches onto any component of the climber.

☐ ☐ Connections between ropes, cables, or chains are securely fixed.

☐ ☐ There are no free standing arch climbers, sliding poles, chain walks, and free standing climbers with flexible components or parallel bars accessible to Toddlers or Preschool-age.

☐ ☐ Horizontal ladders and chinning bars are used only by children who are over 4 years of age. There are no overhead rings or track rides accessible to Toddlers or Preschool-age.

☐ ☐ Climbers for Toddlers have a maximum surface for foot support of 32 inches.

Merry-Go-Rounds

Yes No

☐ ☐ The platform is continuous, approximately circular.

☐ ☐ There are no components, including handgrips, that extend beyond the perimeter of the platform.

☐ ☐ Unless the merry-go-round is tub shaped, there are 1–1 ½ inch handgrips available.

☐ ☐ There are no accessible shearing or crush points.

☐ ☐ The peripheral speed of rotation is limited to 13 feet/second and verified by the manufacturer.

☐ ☐ Merry-go-rounds should not be used on playgrounds intended for Toddlers.

Spring Rocking Equipment

Yes No

☐ ☐ The seat accommodates only the intended number of users at one time.

☐ ☐ There are hand grips and foot rests for each seating position.

☐ ☐ Handgrips for Preschool-age and School-age are between 1–1 ½ inches in diameter; minimum length 3 inches for one hand, and 6 inches for two hands. Handgrips for Toddlers are between 0.60 and 1.20 inches.

☐ ☐ Foot rests are a minimum width of 3 ½ inches.

☐ ☐ Seats for Preschool-age and School-age are not less than 14 inches nor more than 28 inches above platform surface. Seats for Toddlers are not less than 12 inches and not greater than 16 inches.

☐ ☐ There are no log rolls accessible to Toddlers or Preschool-age.

Other Hazards

Yes No

☐ ☐ There are no litter or animal feces in the play area that may attract insects, hide hazards, and harbor infectious disease agents.

☐ ☐ There are no attractive climbing hazards (such a trees) that are accessible from an object placed underneath them.

☐ ☐ There are no plants present that are toxic, thorny, attract bees or have seeds or berries that could cause a choking hazard.

☐ ☐ There is a fence that encloses the play area.

☐ ☐ Shade is provided on the playground. There is a warning sign that states that equipment and surfacing exposed to intense sun can burn.

☐ ☐ Proper site selection and drainage is provided to prevent wash out of loose fill safety surfacing.

Please explain your plan to fix or take out of play any hazardous items or items checked "No."

Hazard to be Fixed	Person Responsible	Action Needed	Date to be Completed	Date Completed
Example: Loose fill (wood mulch) displaced from slide exit zone	staff	Rake loose fill back to original location	immediately	today (or insert date)

Please print legibly.

Name _____ Director's Name _____

Program's Name _____ Program's Phone number _____

Adapted, by permission, from ECELS-Heatlhy Child Care PA, PA Chapter, American Academy of Pediatrics.

Figure A.6.

Incident Report Form

Fill in all blanks and boxes that apply.

Name of Facility: _____ Phone: _____

Address of Facility: _____

Child's Name: _____ Sex: M F Birthdate: ___/___/___

Incident Date: ___/___/___ Time of Incident: ___:___ am/pm Witnesses: _____

Name of Legal Guardian/Parent Notified: _____ Notified by: _____ Time Notified: ___:___ am/pm

☐ EMS Not Notified ☐ EMS (911) or Other Medical Professional Notified: _____ Time Notified: ___:___ am/pm

Location where incident occurred: ☐Playground ☐Classroom ☐Bathroom ☐Hall ☐Kitchen ☐Doorway
  ☐Gym ☐Office ☐Dining Room ☐Stairway ☐Unknown ☐Other (specify)_____

Any Equipment / Product involved: ☐Climber ☐Slide ☐Swing ☐Playground Surface ☐Sandbox ☐Trike/Bike
  ☐Hand toy (specify): _____ ☐Other Equipment (specify): _____

If injury occurred, cause of Injury (describe) or indicate no injury occurred:

_____

  ☐Fall to surface; estimated height of fall _____ feet; Type of surface: _____
  ☐Fall from running or tripping ☐Bitten by child ☐Motor vehicle ☐Hit or pushed by child ☐Injured by object
  ☐Eating or choking ☐Insect sting/bite ☐Animal bite ☐Exposure to cold ☐Exposure to heat
    ☐Other (specify):_____

  Parts of body injured: ☐Eye ☐Ear ☐Nose ☐Mouth ☐Tooth ☐Part of face ☐Part of head ☐Neck
  ☐Arm/Wrist/Hand ☐Leg/Ankle/Foot ☐Trunk ☐Other (specify): _____

  First aid given at the facility ☐Comfort ☐Pressure ☐Elevation ☐Cold pack ☐Rinse with water ☐Bandage ☐Rest
  ☐Other (specify) _____

_____

  Treatment Provided by (Name): _____ Phone:_____
  ☐EMS
  ☐No doctor's or dentist's treatment required
  ☐Treated as an outpatient (e.g. office or emergency room)
  ☐Hospitalized (overnight) # of days: _____

  Number of days of limited activity from this incident: _____ Follow-up plan for care of the child: _____

_____

Corrective action needed to prevent reoccurrence: _____

_____

Name of Supervisor Notified: _____

Name of Official/Agency Notified: _____

Signature of Staff Member Completing Form: _____ Date: _____

Signature of Legal Guardian/Parent:_____ Date: _____

Copies 1) child's folder 2) parent 3) injury log

The original version of this form appeared in *Model Child Care Health Policies*, a publication of the Early Childhood Education Linkage System (ECELS), a program of the PA Chapter, American Academy of Pediatrics. This revision is as of 1/10/2012, © PA AAP

Figure A.7.

Emergency Telephone List

EMERGENCY NUMBERS (include area codes)
_____

Emergency medical system (EMS)_____

Poison Control Center—call 1-800-222-1222.
   The national number automatically connects your
   call to your Regional Poison Control Center.

Police_____

Fire_____

Health consultant_____

Hospital_____

Nearest emergency facility_____

Local health department_____

State department of health_____

Child abuse reporting_____

Rape crisis center_____

Women's shelter_____

Suicide prevention hotline_____

Gas company_____

Water company_____

Heating equipment service_____

Electric company_____

Plumber_____

Taxi_____

Parents Anonymous_____

Alcoholics Anonymous_____

PROGRAM INFORMATION

This telephone is located at_____

Telephone number_____

Program name_____

Description of building_____

Directions for reaching this location from a major road_____

ALWAYS PROVIDE THIS INFORMATION WHEN CALLLING FOR EMERGENCY HELP:

1. Name of the caller; name of the facility

2. Nature of emergency

3. Telephone number

4. Address

5. Easy directions

6. Exact location of injured person(s) (e.g., backyard behind parking lot)

7. Number and age(s) of person(s) involved

8. Condition(s) of person(s) involved

Optional information:

9. Help already given

10. Ways to make it easier to find the building (e.g., a staff member standing out front, waving red flag)

DO NOT HANG UP BEFORE THE OTHER PERSON HANGS UP!

Figure A.8.
Recommended Daily Meal Patterns for Breakfast and Lunch/Supper

TABLE 7-3 Recommended Daily Meal Patterns for Breakfast and Lunch/Supper: Amounts of Food by Age Group, Meal, and Food Group[a]

Food Group[b] (Measure)	1 Year	2–4 Years	5–13 Years
			Breakfast
Fruit or non-starchy vegetables (cup)[c]	¼	½	½
Grain/bread (oz eq)[d]	½	1	1½
			AND
Lean meat or meat alternate (oz eq)[e]	½	1	1
			OR
Grain/bread (oz eq)[d]	1	2	2½
			AND
Lean meat or meat alternate (oz eq)[e]	0	0	0
	(Amounts of grain/bread and meat or meat alternate vary across the week. See footnote e.)		
Milk (cup)	½	½	¾
			Lunch/Supper
Fruit (cup)	¼	½	½
Vegetable (cup)[f]	¼	½	1
Grain/bread (oz eq)[d]	½	1	2
Lean meat or meat alternate (oz eq)[e]	½	1	2
Milk (cup)	½	½	1

NOTE: oz eq = ounce equivalent; svgs = servings; wk = week.

[a]See Table 7-9 and Appendix K for sample menus planned using these patterns.

[b]See Appendix Table H-1 for a listing of foods by food group and subgroup. See Table 7-8 for applicable food specifications to control calories, reduce sodium, and ensure diet quality. Specifications address topics such as the type of milk, forms of fruit, and fat content of meats.

[c]Non-starchy vegetables include all vegetables in Appendix Table H-1 except those listed in the starchy vegetable subgroup.

[d]At least half of the grain/bread must be whole grain-rich. Other grain/bread must be enriched.

[e]Meat/meat alternates should be served 3 days per week at breakfast for all age groups. On each of the days without meat or meat alternates, serve an additional ½ oz eq of bread/grain for children age 1 year and an additional 1 oz eq of bread/grain for all other age groups.

[f]The number of cups indicated represents the total amount of vegetables served at lunch/supper. Offer two different vegetables per meal. With reference to either lunch or supper (or both), serve dark green vegetables at least twice per week, orange vegetables at least twice per week, legumes at least once per week, starchy vegetables no more than twice per week, and other vegetables at least three times per week. *See Appendix Table H-1 for listings of vegetables in each subgroup.* (emphasis added)

Source: Adapted, by permission, from Institute of Medicine, *Child and Adult Care Food Program: Aligning Dietary Guidance for All* (Washington, DC: National Academies Press, 2011), 120. Online: www.fns.usda.gov/ORA/menu/Published/CNP/FILES/cacfpiom.pdf.

Figure A.9.

Weekly Meal Pattern for Regular Snacks

TABLE 7-4 Weekly Meal Pattern for Regular Snacks: Number of Servings from Each Food Group per Week and Amount per Serving, by Age Group[a]

Food Group[b]	1 Year	2–4 Years	5–13 Years
	Number of Servings per Week (Amount/Serving)[c]		
Fruit	2 (½ c)	2 (½ c)	2 (½ c)
Orange vegetable[d]	1 (⅛ c)	1 (¼ c)	1 (½ c)
Non-starchy vegetable[e]	1 (⅛ c)	1 (¼ c)	1 (½ c)
Grain/bread[f]	2 (½ oz eq)	2 (1 oz eq)	2 (1 oz eq)
Lean meat or meat alternate	2 (½ oz eq)	2 (1 oz eq)	2 (1 oz eq)
Milk	2 (½ c)	2 (½ c)	2 (½ c)

NOTE: c = cup; oz eq = ounce equivalent.

[a]See Table 7-9 and Appendix K for sample regular snack menus that follow these patterns.

[b]See Appendix Table H-1 for a listing of foods by MyPyramid food group and subgroup. See Table 7-8 for applicable food specifications to control calories, reduce sodium, and ensure diet quality. Specifications address topics such as the type of milk, forms of fruit, and fat content of meats.

[c]The patterns for each age group show number of servings and amount per serving for either a morning or afternoon snack. If both morning and afternoon snacks are provided daily, the same pattern is to be used for each. Over the course of a 5-day week, a total of 10 servings would be offered for the morning snack and the same number for the afternoon snack (if both were provided); 2 servings would be offered for each daily snack.

[d]See Appendix Table H-1 for a list of orange vegetables.

[e]Non-starchy vegetables include all vegetables in Appendix Table H-1 except those listed in the starchy vegetable subgroup.

[f]At least half of the grain/bread must be whole grain-rich (see specifications in Table 7-8). Other grains must be enriched.

Source: Adapted, by permission, from Institute of Medicine, *Child and Adult Care Food Program: Aligning Dietary Guidance for All* (Washington, DC: National Academies Press, 2011), 121. Online: www.fns.usda.gov/ORA/menu/Published/CNP/FILES/cacfpiom.pdf.

Figure A.10.

Behavioral Data Collection Sheet

This sheet is intended to be used by caregivers to document a child's behavior that is of concern to them. The behavior may warrant evaluation by a health care provider, discussion with parents, and/or consultation with other professionals.

Child's name: _____   Date: _____

1. Describe behavior observed: (See below for some descriptions.)
   _____

2. Behavior noted from: _____ to _____
                         (time)   (time)

3. During that time, how often did the child engage in the behavior? (e.g. once, 2-5 times, 6-10 times, 11-25 times, >25 times, >100 times) _____

4. What activity(ies) was the child involved in when the behavior occurred? (e.g. was the child involved in a task? Was the child alone? Had the child been denied access to a special toy, food, or activity?) _____

5. Where did the behavior occur? _____

6. Who was around the child when the behavior began? List staff, children, parents, others.
   _____

7. Did the behavior seem to occur for no reason? Did it seem affected by changes in the environment?
   _____

8. Did the child sustain any self-injury? Describe. _____

9. Did the child cause property damage or injury to others? Describe. _____
   _____

10. How did caregiver respond to the child's behavior? If others were involved, how did they respond?
    _____

11. What did the child do after caregiver's response? _____

12. Have parents reported any unusual situation or experience the child had since attending child care?

Child Care Facility Name: _____

Name of Caregiver (completing this form): _____

Behaviors can include:
- *repetitive, self-stimulating acts*
- *self-injurious behavior (SIB) such as head banging, self-biting, eye-poking, pica (eating non-food items), pulling out own hair*
- *aggression / injury to others*
- *disruption such as throwing things, banging on walls, stripping*
- *agitation such as screaming, pacing, hyperventilating*
- *refusing to eat / speak; acting detached / withdrawn*
- *others*

Check a child's developmental stage before labeling a behavior a problem. For example, it is not unusual for a 12 month old to eat non-food items, nor is it unusual for an 18 month old to throw things. Also, note how regularly the child exhibits the behavior. An isolated behavior is usually not a problem.

S. Bradley, JD, RN,C - PA Chapter American Academy of Pediatrics
reviewed by J. Hampel, PhD and R. Zager, MD

ECELS-Healthy Child Care PA; PA Chapter, American Academy of Pediatrics 11-04

Source: Reprinted, by permission, from the Pennsylvania Chapter, American Academy of Pediatrics, Early Childhood Linkage System-Healthy Child Care Pennsylvania. Online: www.ecels-healthychildcarepa.org/content/Behavioral%20Data%20Collection%20Sheet%2011-04.pdf.

Figure A.11.

Special Care Plan for a Child with Behavioral Issues

This sheet is intended to be used by health care providers and other professionals to formulate a plan of care for children with severe behavior problems that parents and child care providers can agree upon and follow consistently.

Part A: To be completed by parent/custodian.

Child's name: _____   Date of birth: _____

Parent name(s): _____   _____

Parent emergency numbers: _____   _____

Child care facility/school name: _____   Phone: _____

Health care provider's name: _____   Phone: _____

Other specialist's name/title: _____   Phone: _____

Part B: To be completed by health care provider, pediatric psychiatrist, child psychologist, or other specialist.

1. Identify/describe behavior problem: _____

2. Possible causes/purposes for this type of behavior: (Circle all that apply.)

   - medical condition _____   tension release
           (specify)   developmental disorder
   - attention-getting mechanism   neurochemical imbalance
   - gain access to restricted items/activities   frustration
   - escape performance of task   poor self-regulation skills
   - psychiatric disorder _____   other: _____
           (specify)

3. Accommodations needed by this child: _____
   _____

4. List any precipitating factors known to trigger behavior: _____
   _____

5. How should caregiver react when behavior begins? (Circle all that apply.)

   - ignore behavior   physical guidance (including hand-over-hand)
   - avoid eye contact/conversation   model behavior
   - request desired behavior   use diversion/distraction
   - use helmet*   use substitution
   - use pillow or other device to block self-injurious behavior (SIB)*
   - other: _____
   _____

*directions for use described by health professional in Part D.

S. Bradley, JD, RN, C - PA Chapter American Academy of Pediatrics
reviewed by J. Hampel, PhD and R. Zager, MD
April, 1997

6. List any special equipment this child needs: _____
   _____

7. List any medications this child receives:

   Name of medication: _____   Name of medication: _____
   Dose: _____   Dose: _____
   When to use: _____   When to use: _____
   Side effects: _____   Side effects: _____
   _____   _____
   Special instructions: _____   Special instructions: _____
   _____   _____

8. Training staff need to care for this child: _____
   _____

9. List any other instructions for caregivers: _____
   _____

Part C: Signatures

Date to review/update this plan: _____
Health care provider's signature: _____ Date: _____
Other specialist's signature: _____ Date: _____
Parent signature(s): _____ Date: _____
_____ Date: _____
Child care/school director: _____ Date: _____
Primary caregiver signature: _____ Date: _____

Part D: To be completed by health care provider, pediatric psychiatrist, child psychologist, or other specialist.

Directions for use of helmet, pillow, or other behavior protocol: _____
_____
_____
_____
_____
_____

S. Bradley, JD, RN, C - PA Chapter American Academy of Pediatrics
reviewed by J. Hampel, PhD and R. Zager, MD
April, 1997

Figure A.12.

Developmental Health History

Child's Name_____ Nickname_____
                 (Last)   (First)

Birthdate _____ / _____ / _____

PHYSICAL HEALTH

What health problems has your child had in the past?_____
_____

What health problems does your child have now?_____
_____

Other than what you listed above—
Does your child have any allergies? If so, to what?_____
_____

How severe?_____

Does your child take any medicine regularly? If so, what?_____
_____

Has your child ever been hospitalized? If so, when and why?_____
_____

Does your child have any recurring chronic illness or health problem (such as asthma or frequent earaches)?
_____

Has a disability been diagnosed (such as cerebral palsy, seizure disorder, developmental delay)?
_____

Do you have any other concerns about your child's health?_____
_____

DEVELOPMENT (compared to other children this age)

Does your child have any problems with talking or making sounds? Please explain. _____
_____

Does your child have any problems with walking, running, or moving? Please explain._____
_____

Does your child have any problems seeing? Please explain._____
_____

Does your child have any problems hearing? Please explain._____
_____

Does your child have any problems using her or his hands (such as with puzzles, drawing, small building pieces)? Please explain. _____
_____

Does your child have any problems with mood or behavior? Please explain._____
_____

DAILY LIVING

What is your child's typical eating pattern?_____
_____

Write **N/A** (nonapplicable) if your child is too young for the following questions to apply._____
_____

What foods does your child like?_____
    dislike?_____

How well does your child use table utensils (cup, fork, spoon)?_____

How does your child indicate bathroom needs?_____
Word(s) for *urination:*_____ Word(s) for *bowel movement:*_____

Special words for body parts:_____

What are your child's regular bladder and bowel patterns?_____

Do you want us to follow a particular plan for toileting?

For *toddlers,* please describe use of diapers or toileting equipment (such as potty, toilet seat adapter).
_____

What are your child's regular sleeping patterns?_____

Awakes at_____Naps at_____Goes to bed at_____

What help does your child need to get dressed?_____

SOCIAL RELATIONSHIPS/PLAY

What ages are your child's most frequent playmates?_____

Is your child (circle all that apply) friendly? aggressive? shy? withdrawn?_____

Does your child need extra time/preparation to change from one activity to another?_____

Does your child play well alone? _____ What is your child's favorite toy? _____

Is your child frightened by (circle all that apply) animals? rough children? loud noises? new experiences?
    the dark? storms? anything else?_____

Who does most of the disciplining? _____ What works best when you discipline
your child? _____

With which adults does your child have frequent contact?_____

How do you comfort your child?_____

Does your child use a special comforting item (such as a blanket, stuffed animal, doll)?_____

Parent signature_____ **Date**_____

Figure A.13.

Observation and Symptom Record

Child's name: _____

Date: _____ Observations and symptoms: _____

Describe when the observations were made. When any symptoms or atypical behavior occurred, describe how often, how long, and how intense they seemed: _____
_____

Circle any symptoms the child shows:

runny nose	earache
trouble breathing	vomiting
itching	trouble urinating
sore throat	headache
stiff neck	diarrhea
trouble sleeping	pain
cough	stomachache
rash	wheezing

Other symptoms: _____
_____

Exposure to medications, animals, insects, soaps, new foods: _____

Exposure to other people who were sick (names and what sickness): _____

Child's other problems that might affect this illness (such as allergy, asthma, anemia, diabetes, emotional trauma):
_____

What has been done so far? _____

What the program would like the child's health care provider to share with the child's family and teachers:
_____

Program staff member completing this form: _____

Response from the child's health care provider: _____

Name of child's health care provider completing this form: _____

Source: Adapted, by permission, from S.S. Aronson, ed., *Model Child Care Health Policies*, 5th edition (American Academy of Pediatrics, forthcoming).

Figure A.14.

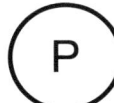

Situations that Require Medical Attention Right Away

In the two boxes below, you will find lists of common medical emergencies or urgent situations you may encounter as a child care provider. To prepare for such situations:
1) Know how to access Emergency Medical Services (EMS) in your area.
2) Know how to reach your Poison Center right away, nationally call 1-800-222-1222.
3) Educate staff on the recognition of an emergency, and when in doubt, call EMS.
4) Know how to contact each child's guardian and primary health care provider. Obtain permission from parents/guardians to speak directly to each child's health care professional.
5) Develop plans for children with special medical needs together with their family and primary care provider.
6) Compile information on when and how to contact public health authorities.

At any time you believe the child's life may be at risk, or you believe there is a risk of permanent injury, seek immediate medical treatment. Do not hesitate, when in doubt, call EMS.

Determine contingency plans for times when there may be power outages, transportation issues etc.

Document what happened and what actions were taken; share verbally and in writing with parents/guardians.

Some children may have urgent situations that do not necessarily require ambulance transport but still need medical attention. The box below lists some of these more common situations. The legal guardian should be informed of the following conditions. If you or the guardian cannot reach the physician within one hour, the child should be brought to a hospital.

Call Emergency Medical Services (EMS) immediately if:

- You believe the child's life is at risk or there is a risk of permanent injury.
- The child is acting strangely, much less alert, or much more withdrawn than usual.
- The child has difficulty breathing, is having an asthma exacerbation, or is unable to speak.
- The child's skin or lips look blue, purple, or gray.
- The child has rhythmic jerking of arms and legs and a loss of consciousness (seizure).
- The child is unconscious.
- The child is less and less responsive.
- The child has any of the following after a head injury: decrease in level of alertness, confusion, headache, vomiting, irritability, or difficulty walking.
- The child has increasing or severe pain anywhere.
- The child has a cut or burn that is large, deep, and/or won't stop bleeding.
- The child is vomiting blood.
- The child has a severe stiff neck, headache, and fever.
- The child is significantly dehydrated: sunken eyes, lethargic, not making tears, not urinating.
- Multiple children affected by injury or serious illness at the same time.
- When in doubt, call EMS.
- After you have called EMS, remember to contact the child's legal guardian.

Get medical attention within one hour for:

- Fever* in any age child who looks more than mildly ill.
- Fever * in a child less than two months (eight weeks) of age.
- A quickly spreading purple or red rash.
- A large volume of blood in the stools.
- A cut that may require stitches.
- Any medical condition specifically outlined in a child's care plan requiring parental notification.

*Fever is defined as a temperature above 101°F (38.3°C) orally, above 102°F (38.9°C) rectally, or 100°F (37.8°C) or higher taken axillary (armpit) or measured by an equivalent method.

References:

1. Aronson, S., ed. 2005. *Pediatric first aid for caregivers and teachers.* Elk Grove Village, IL: American Academy of Pediatrics.

2. Aronson, S., T. R. Shope, eds. 2008. *Managing infectious diseases in child care and schools: A quick reference guide.* Elk Grove Village, IL: American Academy of Pediatrics.

Approved by the AAP Committee on Pediatric Emergency Medicine, January 2009.

Source: Appendix P, *Caring for Our Children.* Reprinted with permission.

Figure A.15.

Medication Administration Skills Checklist

HEALTHY FUTURES MEDICATION ADMINISTRATION SKILLS CHECKLIST

Name of Person Being Observed _____ Date _____

Circle the 'Y' in the "Yes" column, 'P' in the "Partial" column or 'N' in the "No" column to indicate if observed performance matches the details on this *SKILLS CHECKLIST*. Use the "Comments" column to indicate what needs improvement if performance of an item was not fully satisfactory.

Item to Check	Yes	Partial	No	Comments
RECEIVING MEDICATIONS				
Safety Check Person giving medication checks: ☐ Medication received meets criteria (original child-resistant container, label elements) ☐ Child health record on file ☐ Child had previous trial dose ☐ Parent gave information about when last dose was given, child's reaction to medication and medication administration techniques used at home	Y	P	N	
GIVING THE MEDICATION				
Prepare to Administer Medication ☐ Wash hands ☐ Prepare work area (clean/sanitize if needed) ☐ Take out medication (from locked storage) ☐ Relock locked storage if leaving storage area ☐ Check label and forms to see that they match ☐ Gather proper measuring devices ☐ Check that time is right to give dose	Y	P	N	
Prepare the Medication ☐ Select appropriate measuring device ☐ Measure amount noted on the label ☐ Change form of medication ONLY if label says to do so	Y	P	N	
Prepare the Child (states and demonstrates for infant, preschool and school age child)	Y	P	N	
Medication Administration Procedure Check 5 rights: child, medication, dose, time and route ☐ Check right child & note any special instructions in documents & on medication label ☐ Check medication preparation is correct ☐ Re-check child's name, date, time, dose, how medication is to be given (route) on both the medication container and permission slip ☐ Give the medication accurately, not more or less than ordered	Y	P	N	

ECELS-Healthy Child Care PA, PA Chapter, American Academy of Pediatrics   4-13-12

Item to Check	Yes	Partial	No	Comments
☐ Praise the child ☐ Check the label again ☐ Return and lock medication in storage area ☐ Document medication administration right after giving dose ☐ Clean measuring device ☐ Wash hands				
Observe child's response to the medication.	Y	P	N	

DOCUMENTATION				
Documentation Forms are available to capture three types of essential information: ☐ Authorization to give medication ☐ Receiving medication ☐ Medication Log to record details of administered medication	Y	P	N	
Authorization Form to give medication is being used in the program that includes: ☐ Child's information ☐ Prescriber's information ☐ Permission to give medication from parent or guardian	Y	P	N	
Receiving Medication Form is being used that includes documentation that medication met criteria to be accepted: ☐ Presence of readable original prescription or manufacturer's label ☐ Name and strength of medication on label ☐ Date of Rx and expiration date timely ☐ Name of child (first and last) matches intended recipient ☐ Instructions for storage ☐ Instructions for administration	Y	P	N	
Medication Log Form includes: ☐ Name of child ☐ Name of medication ☐ Day, time, dose, route, staff signature ☐ Reported errors or mishaps ☐ Return or disposal of medication ☐ For "as needed" medications, reason medication was given	Y	P	N	

_____ _____
Printed Staff Member Name   Staff Member Signature   Date

_____ _____
Printed Health Professional Name   Health Professional Signature   Date

Source: Reprinted, by permission, from the Pennsylvania Chapter, American Academy of Pediatrics, Early Childhood Linkage System-Healthy Child Care Pennsylvania. Online: http://www.ecels-healthychildcarepa.org/section.cfm?subID=8.

Figure A.16.

Care Plan for a Child With Special Needs in Child Care

Today's Date _____

Full Name of Child	Birth Date	Child's Present Weight
Parent's/Guardian's Name (Please * first person to contact.)	Cell/Home/Work Phone #	Signature for Consent*
Emergency Contact Person (Name/Relationship)	Cell/Home/Work Phone #	*Consent for health care provider to communicate with my child's child care provider to discuss information relating to this care plan.
Primary Health Care Provider	Emergency Phone #	Authorization for Release of Information Form completed? ☐N/A ☐Yes ☐No
Specialty Provider	Emergency Phone #	Emergency Information Form for Children With Special Needs completed? ☐N/A ☐Yes ☐No
Specialty Provider	Emergency Phone #	Specialty Care Plan(s) completed? ☐N/A ☐Yes ☐No

Allergies ☐No ☐Yes If yes, please specify.

Medical Conditions

Needed Accommodations: (Please describe accommodation and why it is necessary.)

Diet/Feeding

Classroom Activities   Toileting

                         Outdoor or Field Trips

Nap/Sleep   Transportation

Recommended Treatment

Medications to be Given at Child Care ☐No ☐Yes Specify medications on Medication Administration Forms.	If yes, Medication Administration Forms completed? ☐Yes ☐No
Medications Given at Home ☐No ☐Yes	If yes, please list in additional information section or attach info.
Special Equipment/Medical Supplies ☐No ☐Yes	If yes, please list in additional information section or attach info.
Special Staff Training Needs ☐No ☐Yes	If yes, please list in additional information section or attach info.
Special Emergency Procedures ☐No ☐Yes	If yes, please list in additional information section or attach info.
Other specialists working with this child ☐No ☐Yes	

Parent Signature Acknowledging Review of Above Information

Additional Information/Comments on Child, Family, or Medical Issues	Additional Information Attached ☐No ☐Yes
Health Care Provider's Signature	Health Care Provider's Name Printed

ECELS-Healthy Child Care PA; PA Chapter, American Academy of Pediatrics 9-2010

Source: Reprinted, by permission, from ECELS-Healthy Child Care Pennsylvania; PA Chapter, American Academy of Pediatrics. Online: www.ecels-healthychildcarepa.org/index.cfm.

Figure A.17.

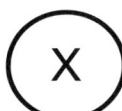

Adaptive Equipment for Children with Special Health Care Needs

Children on a gluten-free diet and those with latex allergies must be protected from ingesting or coming in contact with equipment/materials that may contain these substances. Check manufacturer's specifications and/or labels of all equipment, feeding materials, and toys including art supplies.

Physical Therapy/Occupational Therapy Equipment

Infants, Ages Birth to Two

Equipment
Floor mats, 2 to 3 inches of varying firmness
Therapy balls of varying sizes
Wedges: 4, 6, 8, and 12 inch
Inflatable mattress
Air compressor (for inflatables)
Therapy rolls and half rolls of varying sizes
Nesting benches, varying heights
Wooden weighted pushcart
Toddler swing
Floor mirror
Dycem non-slip matting

Feeding
Bottle straws
Cut-out cups
Bottle holders
Built-up handled utensils
Scoop bowls
Coated spoons

Toys
Books
Mirror
Ring stack
Container toys
Pegboard
Rattles
Squeeze toys
Tracking toys
Toys for pushing, swiping, cause and effect
Adapted switches
Form boards
Large beads
Large crayons

Pre-K, Ages Two to Five

Equipment
Floor mats, 2 to 3 inches of varying firmness
Therapy balls: 16, 20, 24, and 37 inch diameter
Nesting benches
Therapy rolls: 8, 10, and 12 inch diameter
Steps
Floor mirrors
Climbing equipment
Small chair and table
Scooter board
Dycem non-slip matting
Suspended equipment (see also Adaptive Physical Education Equipment, Balance/Gross Motor Coordination)
Walkers, sidelyers, proneboards, adapted chairs
Adapted tricycles

Toys
Easel
Tricycles
Ride-on scooters
Wagon
Wooden push cart
Manipulative toys (puzzles, beads, pegs and pegboard, nesting toys, etc.)
Fastening boards (zippers, snaps, laces, etc.)
Paper, crayons, chalk, markers
Sand/water table
Playdough or clay (consider gluten free and latex free alternatives)
Target activities (beanbags, ring toss)
Playground balls (see under Adaptive Physical Education Equipment, Eye-Hand Coordination)

Speech and Language Development

Infants, Ages Birth to Two

Equipment
Mirrors, wall and hand-held
Assorted spoons, cups, bowls, plates
Mats and sheets
Preston feeding chairs
High chair

Toys
Dolls (soft with large features and feeding bathing and daily living equipment)
Rattles (noisemakers and easy to grasp)
Manipulative toys (for pulling, pushing, shaking, cause and effect)
Assorted picture books (large pictures, one-a-page, photographs, simple plot)
Building blocks
Balls/belts
Telephone
Stacking rings
Shape sorters
Xylophone, Drum

Assessments and Books
Small Wonder Activity Kit

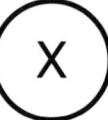

Pre-Feeding Skills by Suzanne Morris
Parent-Infant Communication
Bayley Scales of Infant Development
Communication and Symbolic Behavior Scale
Movement Assessment in Infants by S. Harris and L. Chandler
RIDES
HAWAII HELP
Early Learning Accomplishments Profile and Kit (Kaplan)
Receptive Expressive Emergent Language Test 3
Rosetti Infant/Toddler Language Scale

Pre-K, Ages Two to Five

Equipment
Mirrors, wall and hand-held
Tongue depressors
Penlight
Stopwatch
Tape recorder and tapes
Toothettes
Horns and Whistles

Toys
Dolls (with movable parts and removable clothing)
Manipulative toys (cars and toys for pushing, stacking, cause and effect)
Building blocks
Dollhouse
Pretend play items (dress-up clothes, dishes, sink, food, telephone)
Playdough or clay (consider gluten free and latex free alternatives)
Puzzles (individual pieces or minimal interlocking parts)
Picture cards (nouns, actions, etc.)
Puppets
Animals
Storybooks with simple plot lines (large pictures and few, if any, words)

Assessments and books
Clinical evaluation of Language Fundamentals - Pre-School
Sequenced Inventory of Communication
Test of Auditory Comprehension of Language
Goldman Fristore Test of Articulation
Pre-School Language Assessment Inventory
Assessment of Phonological Processes
Expressive Vocabulary Test-2
Peabody Picture Vocabulary Test-4

Adaptive Physical Education Equipment

Pre-K, Ages Two to Five

Balance/Gross Motor Coordination
Incline mat
Balance beams, 4 and 12 inch wide
Floor mats, 2 inch
Bolsters
Rocking platforms
Scooters (sit-on type)
Tunnel (accordion style)
Training stairs
Hurdles, adjustable height
Pediatric climbing wall

Eye-Hand Coordination
Balls (to hit, throw, and catch)
Beanbags and Target
Hula hoops
Lightweight paddles/rackets
Lightweight bats
Traffic cones
Batting tees
Beachballs

Eye-Foot Coordination
Balls for kicking
Foot placement ladder
Footprints or "stepping stones"
Horizontal ladder

Figure A.18.

Recognizing Child Abuse and Neglect: Signs and Symptoms

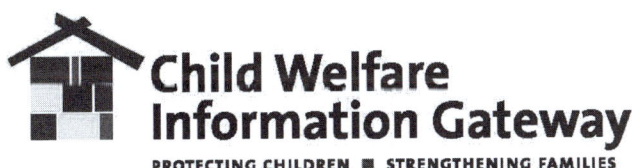

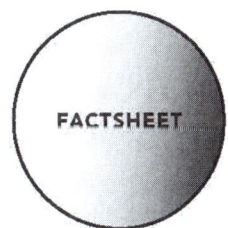

June 2007

Disponible en español
www.childwelfare.gov/pubs/
factsheets/sp_signs.cfm

Recognizing Child Abuse and Neglect: Signs and Symptoms

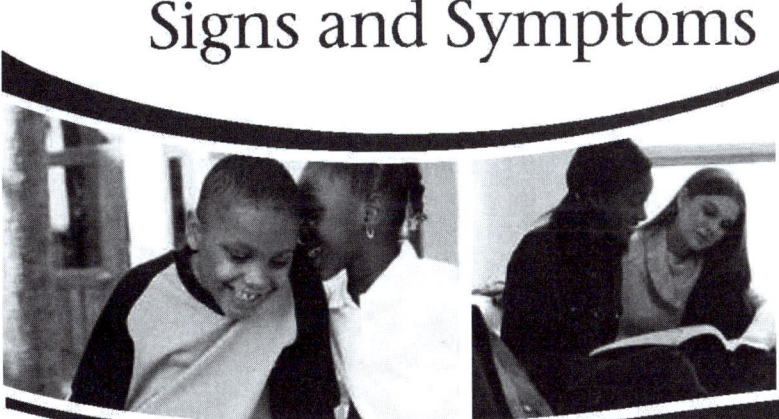

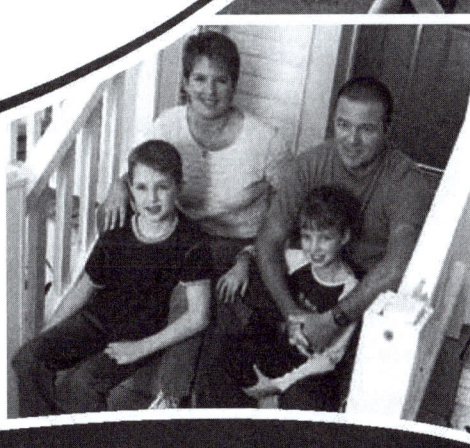

The first step in helping abused or neglected children is learning to recognize the signs of child abuse and neglect. The presence of a single sign does not prove child abuse is occurring in a family, but a closer look at the situation may be warranted when these signs appear repeatedly or in combination.

If you do suspect a child is being harmed, reporting your suspicions may protect the child and get

What's Inside:

- Recognizing child abuse
- Types of abuse
- Signs of physical abuse
- Signs of neglect
- Signs of sexual abuse
- Signs of emotional maltreatment

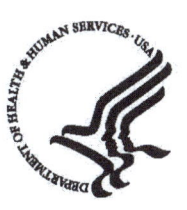

U.S. Department of Health and Human Services
Administration for Children and Families
Administration on Children, Youth and Families
Children's Bureau

Child Welfare Information Gateway
Children's Bureau/ACYF
1250 Maryland Avenue, SW
Eighth Floor
Washington, DC 20024
703.385.7565 or 800.394.3366
Email: info@childwelfare.gov
www.childwelfare.gov

Recognizing Child Abuse and Neglect: Signs and Symptoms   www.childwelfare.gov

help for the family. Any concerned person can report suspicions of child abuse and neglect. Some people (typically certain types of professionals) are required by law to make a report of child maltreatment under specific circumstances—these are called mandatory reporters. For more information, see the Child Welfare Information Gateway publication, *Mandatory Reporters of Child Abuse and Neglect:* www.childwelfare.gov/systemwide/laws_policies/statutes/manda.cfm

For more information about where and how to file a report, contact your local child protective services agency or police department. An additional resource for information and referral is the Childhelp® National Child Abuse Hotline (800.4.A.CHILD).

Recognizing Child Abuse

The following signs may signal the presence of child abuse or neglect.

The Child:

- Shows sudden changes in behavior or school performance
- Has not received help for physical or medical problems brought to the parents' attention
- Has learning problems (or difficulty concentrating) that cannot be attributed to specific physical or psychological causes
- Is always watchful, as though preparing for something bad to happen
- Lacks adult supervision
- Is overly compliant, passive, or withdrawn
- Comes to school or other activities early, stays late, and does not want to go home

The Parent:

- Shows little concern for the child
- Denies the existence of—or blames the child for—the child's problems in school or at home
- Asks teachers or other caregivers to use harsh physical discipline if the child misbehaves
- Sees the child as entirely bad, worthless, or burdensome
- Demands a level of physical or academic performance the child cannot achieve
- Looks primarily to the child for care, attention, and satisfaction of emotional needs

The Parent and Child:

- Rarely touch or look at each other
- Consider their relationship entirely negative
- State that they do not like each other

Types of Abuse

The following are some signs often associated with particular types of child abuse and neglect: physical abuse, neglect, sexual abuse, and emotional abuse. It is important to note, however, that these

---

This material may be freely reproduced and distributed. However, when doing so, please credit Child Welfare Information Gateway. Available online at www.childwelfare.gov/pubs/factsheets/signs.cfm.

Recognizing Child Abuse and Neglect: Signs and Symptoms

types of abuse are more typically found in combination than alone. A physically abused child, for example, is often emotionally abused as well, and a sexually abused child also may be neglected.

Signs of Physical Abuse

Consider the possibility of physical abuse when the **child**:

- Has unexplained burns, bites, bruises, broken bones, or black eyes
- Has fading bruises or other marks noticeable after an absence from school
- Seems frightened of the parents and protests or cries when it is time to go home
- Shrinks at the approach of adults
- Reports injury by a parent or another adult caregiver

Consider the possibility of physical abuse when the **parent or other adult caregiver**:

- Offers conflicting, unconvincing, or no explanation for the child's injury
- Describes the child as "evil," or in some other very negative way
- Uses harsh physical discipline with the child
- Has a history of abuse as a child

Signs of Neglect

Consider the possibility of neglect when the **child**:

- Is frequently absent from school
- Begs or steals food or money
- Lacks needed medical or dental care, immunizations, or glasses
- Is consistently dirty and has severe body odor
- Lacks sufficient clothing for the weather
- Abuses alcohol or other drugs
- States that there is no one at home to provide care

Consider the possibility of neglect when the **parent or other adult caregiver**:

- Appears to be indifferent to the child
- Seems apathetic or depressed
- Behaves irrationally or in a bizarre manner
- Is abusing alcohol or other drugs

Signs of Sexual Abuse

Consider the possibility of sexual abuse when the **child**:

- Has difficulty walking or sitting
- Suddenly refuses to change for gym or to participate in physical activities
- Reports nightmares or bedwetting

This material may be freely reproduced and distributed. However, when doing so, please credit Child Welfare Information Gateway. Available online at www.childwelfare.gov/pubs/factsheets/signs.cfm.

Recognizing Child Abuse and Neglect: Signs and Symptoms

- Experiences a sudden change in appetite
- Demonstrates bizarre, sophisticated, or unusual sexual knowledge or behavior
- Becomes pregnant or contracts a venereal disease, particularly if under age 14
- Runs away
- Reports sexual abuse by a parent or another adult caregiver

Consider the possibility of sexual abuse when the **parent or other adult caregiver:**

- Is unduly protective of the child or severely limits the child's contact with other children, especially of the opposite sex
- Is secretive and isolated
- Is jealous or controlling with family members

Signs of Emotional Maltreatment

Consider the possibility of emotional maltreatment when the **child:**

- Shows extremes in behavior, such as overly compliant or demanding behavior, extreme passivity, or aggression
- Is either inappropriately adult (parenting other children, for example) or inappropriately infantile (frequently rocking or head-banging, for example)
- Is delayed in physical or emotional development
- Has attempted suicide
- Reports a lack of attachment to the parent

Consider the possibility of emotional maltreatment when the **parent or other adult caregiver:**

- Constantly blames, belittles, or berates the child
- Is unconcerned about the child and refuses to consider offers of help for the child's problems
- Overtly rejects the child

RESOURCES ON THE CHILD WELFARE INFORMATION GATEWAY WEBSITE

Child Abuse and Neglect
www.childwelfare.gov/can/index.cfm

Defining Child Abuse and Neglect
www.childwelfare.gov/can/defining/

Preventing Child Abuse and Neglect
www.childwelfare.gov/preventing/

Reporting Child Abuse and Neglect
www.childwelfare.gov/responding/reporting.cfm

This factsheet was adapted, with permission, from *Recognizing Child Abuse: What Parents Should Know*. Prevent Child Abuse America. © 2003.

This material may be freely reproduced and distributed. However, when doing so, please credit Child Welfare Information Gateway. Available online at www.childwelfare.gov/pubs/factsheets/signs.cfm.

Source: Reprinted, by permission, from Child Welfare Information Gateway, *Recognizing Child Abuse and Neglect: Signs and Symptoms* (Washington, DC: Author, 2007). Online: www.childwelfare.gov/pubs/factsheets/signs.pdf.

Appendix A 229

Figure A.19.

Conceptual Model of Child Neglect

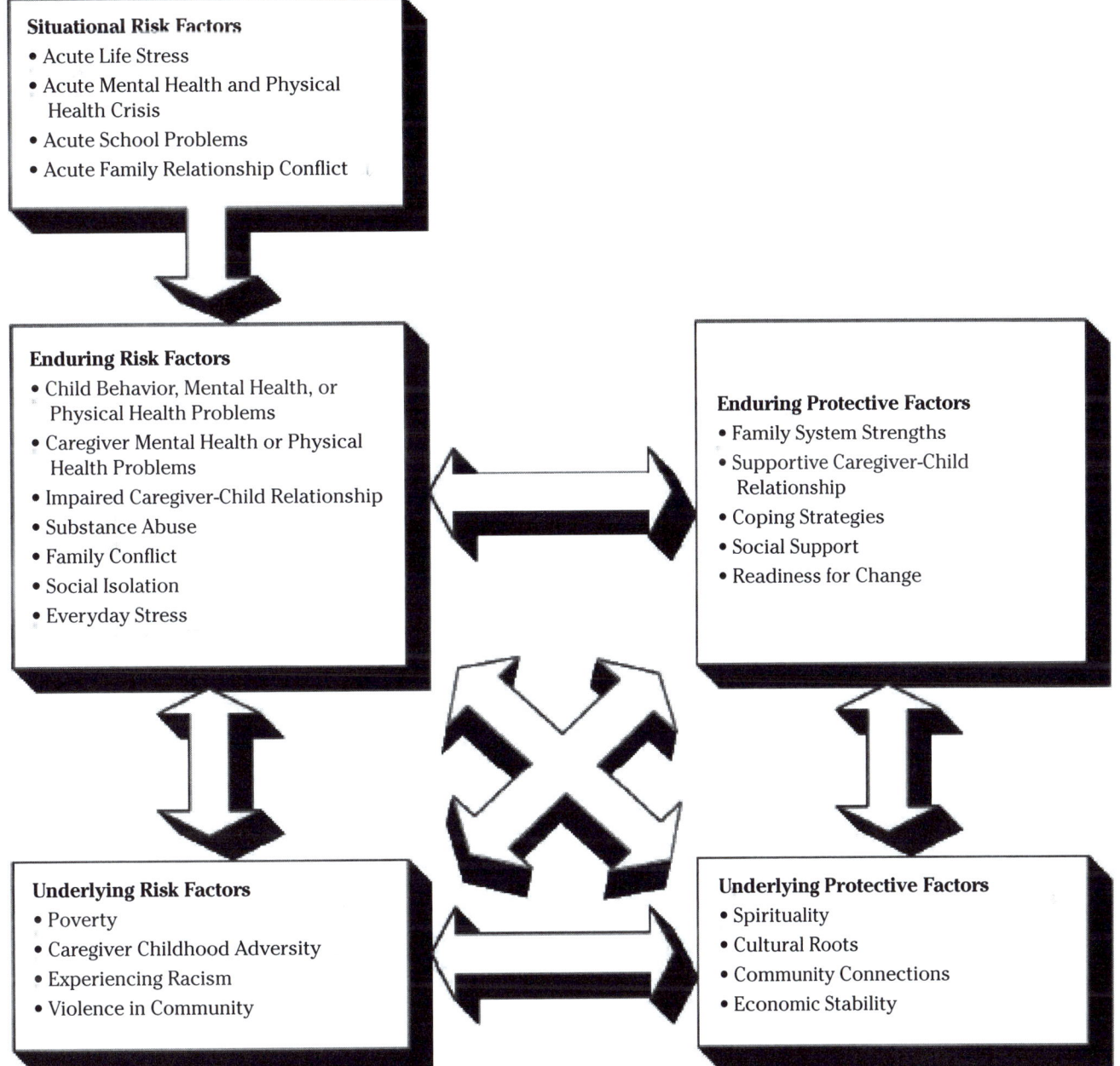

Source: D. DePanfilis, *Child Neglect: A Guide for Prevention, Assessment, and Intervention* (Washington, DC: Children's Bureau, Office on Child Abuse and Neglect, 2006), 30. Online: www.childwelfare.gov/pubs/usermanuals/neglect/neglect.pdf.

Acronyms Used in This Book

AAP: American Academy of Pediatrics
ACIP: Advisory Committee on Immunization Practices (a committee of the CDC)
ACMI: Art and Creative Materials Institute
ADA: Americans with Disabilities Act
AIDS: acquired immune deficiency syndrome
ALA: American Lung Association
ANA: American Nurses Association
ASHRAE: The American Society of Heating, Refrigerating and Air-Conditioning Engineers
ASTM: formerly American Society for Testing and Materials, now ASTM International
BMI: body mass index
CACFP: Child and Adult Care Food Program
CAPTA: Child Abuse Prevention and Treatment Act
CCHC: child care health consultant
CDC: Centers for Disease Control and Prevention
CHIP: Children's Health Insurance Program
CMV: cytomegalovirus
CPR: cardiopulmonary resuscitation
CPS: Child Protective Services
CPSC: Consumer Product Safety Commission
CSEFEL: Center on the Social and Emotional Foundations for Early Learning
EEI: Edison Electric Institute
EMS: emergency medical services
EPA: Environmental Protection Agency
EPSDT: Early Periodic Screening, Diagnosis, and Treatment Program
FAAN: Food Allergy and Anaphylaxis Network
FDA: U.S. Food and Drug Administration
FNS: Food and Nutrition Service (an agency of the USDA)
GFCI: ground-fault circuit interrupter
HIPAA: Health Insurance Portability and Accountability Act
HIV: human immunodeficiency virus
HVAC: heating, ventilation, and air conditioning

IDEA: Individuals with Disabilities Education Act
IEP: Individualized Education Program
IFSP: Individualized Family Service Plan
IOM: Institute of Medicine
IPM: Integrated Pest Management
MSDS: Material Safety Data Sheet
NAEYC: National Association for the Education of Young Children
NAPNAP: National Association of Pediatric Nurse Practitioners
NFPA: National Fire Protection Association
NHTSA: National Highway Traffic Safety Administration
NICHCY: National Dissemination Center for Children with Disabilities
NNii: National Network for Immunization Information
NRPA: National Recreation and Park Association
NSF: National Sanitation Foundation
NTI: National Training Institute for Child Care Health Consultants (housed at the University of North Carolina–Chapel Hill)
OSHA: Occupational Safety and Health Administration
OTC: over-the-counter (medication)
SBA: Safe Building Alliance
SIDS: sudden infant death syndrome
TACSEI: Technical Assistance Center on Social Emotional Intervention
TB: tuberculosis
Tdap: tetanus-diphtheria-acellular pertussis vaccine
TST: tuberculin skin test
UL: Underwriters' Laboratory
USDA: United States Department of Agriculture
USDHHS: United States Department of Health and Human Services
VNA: Visiting Nurse Association
WIC: Special Supplemental Nutrition Program for Woman, Infants, and Children

Links to Internet Resources in This Book

American Academy of Pediatrics, **www.aap.org**

American Association of Poison Control Centers (AAPC), **www.aapcc.org/dnn/default.aspx**

American College of Emergency Physicians (ACEP), **www.acep.org**

Americans with Disabilities Act, **www.ada.gov**

American Heart Association, **www.heart.org**

Art and Creative Materials Institute (ACMI), **www.acminet.org**

ASTM International, **www.astm.org**

Bright Futures, **http://brightfutures.aap.org**
- Periodicity schedule, **http://brightfutures.aap.org/pdfs/Guidelines_PDF/20-Appendices_PeriodicitySchedule.pdf**

California Childcare Health Program, [Integrated Pest Management: A Toolkit for Early Care and Education Programs]; The California Training Institute Curriculum for Child Care Health Advocates, **www.ucsfchildcarehealth.org** (see also **www. cerch.org**)
- Consent for Exchange of Information Form, **http://ucsfchildcarehealth.org/pdfs/forms/CForm_ExchangeofInfo.pdf**

Caring for Our Children, 3rd edition, **www.nrckids.org/CFOC3/**

Center for Early Childhood Mental Health Consultation (CECMHC), **www.ecmhc.org**

Center on the Social and Emotional Foundations for Early Learning (CSEFEL), **http://csefel.vanderbilt.edu**

Centers for Disease Control and Prevention (CDC), **www.cdc.gov**
- Animal-related diseases, **www.cdc.gov/healthypets/**
- BMI calculation, **www.cdc.gov/healthyweight/assessing/bmi/index.html**
- Growth charts, **www.cdc.gov/growthcharts**
- National Center on Birth Defects and Developmental Disabilities (NCBDDD), **www.cdc.gov/ncbddd**
- Overweight and obesity, **www.cdc.gov/obesity/childhood/**
- Recommended vaccines, **www.cdc.gov/vaccines**
- Water safety, **www.cdc.gov**

Child Care Law Center, **www.childcarelaw.org**

Child Welfare Information Gateway, **www.childwelfare.gov**

Color Me Healthy Teacher's Guide, **www.colormehealthy.com**

Dietary Guidelines for Americans, **www.health.gov/dietaryguidelines/**

ECELS-Healthy Child Care Pennsylvania, diapering poster and *MCCHP* Health and Safety checklist, **www.ecels-healthychildcarepa.org**

Environmental Protection Agency (EPA), Integrated Pest Management, **www.epa.gov/pesticides/ipm/**

Equal Employment Opportunity Commission, **www.eeoc.gov**
- Disability laws, **www.eeoc.gov/laws/**
- Employment Tests and Selection Procedures fact sheet, **www.eeoc.gov/policy/docs/factemployment_procedures.html**

The Food Allergy and Anaphylaxis Network (FAAN), **www.foodallergy.org**

Head Start, I Am Moving, I Am Learning, **http://eclkc.ohs.acf.hhs.gov**

Healthy Child Care America, **www.healthychildcare.org**
- Curriculum for Managing Infectious Diseases in Early Education and Child Care Settings; Curriculum for Medication Administration in Early Education and Child Care Settings, **www.healthychildcare.org/HealthyFutures.html**

Healthy Children, AAP parenting information, **www.healthychildren.org**

MyPlate, **www.chooseMyPlate.gov**

National Association for the Education of Young Children (NAEYC), **www.naeyc.org**

National Center on Birth Defects and Developmental Disabilities (NCBDDD), **www.cdc.gov/ncbddd**

National Dissemination Center for Children with Disabilities, **www.nichcy.org**

National Fire Protection Association (NFPA), **www.nfpa.org**

National Heart, Lung, and Blood Institute (NHLBI), body mass index, **www.nhlbisupport.com/bmi/**

National Highway Traffic Safety Administration (NHTSA), **www.nhtsa.gov**

National Program for Playground Safety (NPPS), **www.playgroundsafety.org**

National Recreation and Park Association (NRPA), **www.nrpa.org**

National Training Institute for Child Care Health Consultants (NTI), **http://nti.unc.edu**

Occupational Safety and Health Administration (OSHA) regional offices, **www.osha.gov/html/RAmap.html**

Office of Special Education Programs (OSEP), **www2.ed.gov/about/offices/list/osers/osep/index.html**

Nemours Health and Prevention Services Best Practices for Physical Activity guide, **www.nemours.org/filebox/service/preventive/nhps/paguidelines.pdf**

Pediatric First Aid for Caregivers and Teachers (PedFACTs), **www.pedfactsonline.com**

Poison Control Center at the Children's Hospital of Philadelphia (CHOP), **www.chop.edu/service/poison-control-center/**

Prevent Blindness America, **www.preventblindness.org**

Safe Kids water safety tips, **www.safekids.org**

Strengthening Families, a framework developed by the Center for the Study of Social Policy, **www.strengtheningfamilies.net**

Technical Assistance Center on Social Emotional Intervention (TACSEI), **www.challengingbehavior.org**

U.S. Consumer Product Safety Commission (CPSC), **www.cpsc.gov**
- Crib safety requirements, **www.cpsc.gov/info/cribs/index.html**

U.S. Department of Agriculture (USDA), **www.usda.gov**
- Child and Adult Care Food Program (CACFP), **www.fns.usda.gov/cnd/care/**
- Food and Nutrition Service, **www.fns.usda.gov/fns/**
- Healthy meal portions/patterns, **www.fns.usda.gov/cnd/care/ProgramBasics/Meals/Meal_Patterns.htm**
- Meals Resource System, **http://healthymeals.nal.usda.gov**

U.S. Department of Health and Human Services (HHS), health information, **www.healthfinder.gov**

U.S. Environmental Protection Agency (EPA), **www.epa.gov**
- Design for the Environment (DfE), **www.EPA.gov/dfe**
- Information on UV Index, **www.epa.gov/sunwise/uvindex.html**

U.S. Equal Opportunity Employment Commission, Job Applicants and the Americans with Disabilities Act fact sheet, **www.eeoc.gov/facts/jobapplicant.html**

U.S. Fire Administration (USFA), **www.firesafety.gov/kids**

U.S. Food and Drug Administration (FDA), information on sunscreen, **www.fda.gov/sunscreen**

University of North Carolina at Chapel Hill's Nutrition and Physical Activity Self-Assessment for Child Care (NAP SACC), **www.center-TRT.org**

WellCareTracker™, run by the Pennsylvania chapter of the AAP, **www.wellcaretracker.org**

World Health Organization, guidelines for preparing formula, **http://who.int/foodsafety/publications/micro/pif2007/en/index.html**

Crosswalk of *Healthy Young Children* and NAEYC Early Childhood Accreditation Criteria

NAEYC offers a national, voluntary accreditation system to set professional standards for early childhood education programs, and to help families identify high-quality programs. The NAEYC Accreditation Standards and Criteria are based on research and professional experience, which define program quality. The following table provides a crosswalk of HYC chapter and section titles and NAEYC Accreditation criteria related to health and safety issues.

It is intended to serve as an easy reference guide for programs utilizing the NAEYC Accreditation criteria to guide program improvement efforts. For the most up-to-date information regarding the NAEYC Accreditation Standards and Criteria and their assessment during NAEYC Accreditation site visits, please refer to The Online Resource Center Headquarters to support program quality improvement (TORCH) at www.naeyc.org/torch.

HYC Chapter	HYC Section Title	Page #	Topic Related	NAEYC Criterion
Chapter 2. Preventing Infections	Prevent Infections from Spreading	8	Encourage Breastfeeding	5.B.09
	Prevent Infections from Spreading	9	Spacing of Cots/Cribs/Mats	9.A.01, indicator h
	Prevent Infections from Spreading; Controlling the Spread of Infection Through Cleaning, Sanitizing, and Disinfecting	9; 30	Hand Hygiene	5.A.09
	Prevent Infections from Spreading	10	Animals and Vermin	5.C.05, 9.D.08
	Prevent Infections from Spreading	11	Insect Bites	5.A.07
	Prevent Infections from Spreading	12	Diaper-Changing Procedures	5.A.08
	Require Certain Immunizations and Routine Health Supervision Services; Vaccine-Preventable Diseases	13; 24	Child and Adult Immunizations	5.A.01, 10.D.05, 10.E.0
	Report Some Illnesses; Notification of Exposure to Communicable Diseases	14; 27	Reporting Illness	5.A.04, 5.A.05
	Exclude Some Children and Staff Members for Illness	14	Exclusion/Inclusion Due to Illness	5.A.02, indicator b, indicator g, 5.A.04, 10.B.08, 10.D.01, indicator b
	Diseases Spread by Direct Contact or Contact with Surfaces with Germs on Them; Controlling the Spread of Infection through Cleaning, Sanitizing, and Disinfecting	21; 27	Cleaning, Sanitation, and Disinfecting Frequency	5.C.01, 5.C.03, and 9.C.06
	Infectious Diseases Spread through Blood	22	Standard Precautions	5.C.02
	Notification of Exposure to Communicable Diseases	27	Infectious Disease Policies	10.D.01 indicator a, b, d
	The Role of Ventilation, Temperature, and Humidity in Resistance to Infectious Disease	31	Ventilation, Temperature, and Humidity	9.D.05
	Staff/Child Turnover and Infectious Disease	32	Staff Turnover	10.B.09, 10.B.13, 10.B.15

HYC Chapter	HYC Section Title	Page #	Topic Related	NAEYC Criterion
Chapter 3. Preventing Injuries	Program Planning for Safety inside the Facility	36	Indoor/Outdoor Resilient Surfacing	9.A.06, 9.B.06
	Program Planning for Safety inside the Facility	37	Choking	5.B.14, 9.C.16
	Program Planning for Safety inside the Facility	38	Pediatric First Aid Training, Including Management of a Blocked Airway and Rescue Breathing	5.A.03
	Planning for Safety inside the Facility	40	Plant Safety	9.D.08
	Safety Beyond the Classroom	41	Certified Playground Safety Inspector	9.B.07
	Safety Beyond the Classroom	41	Playground Equipment and Materials	9.B.01-9.B.07
	Safety Beyond the Classroom	45	Sunscreen and Insect Repellant	5.A.07
	Safety Beyond the Classroom	46	Drowning Hazards	9.C.12, 5.A.12
	Safety Beyond the Classroom	47	Weather and Outdoor Play	5.A.06
	Special Safety Tips for Infants and Toddlers	47	Exclusion of Baby Walkers	9.C.08
	Special Safety Tips for Infants and Toddlers	50	Bathroom Barriers for Infants/Toddlers	9.C.17
	Special Safety Tips for Infants and Toddlers	50	Cot/Crib Spacing	9.A.01
	Special Safety Tips for Infants and Toddlers	50	Safe Sleep/SIDS Prevention	5.A.12
	Safety Education and Hazard Checks	51	Classroom Rules and Safety	1.D.02, 2.K.03, 2.K.04, 6.A.02, 9.C.07, 9.C.08
	Supervision	51	Supervision of Children	3.C.01, 3.C.02, 3.C.03, 3.C.04, 3.C.05, 9.A.05, 9.B.03, and 9.C.12
Chapter 4. Ready for Emergencies and Injuries	Prepare for Emergencies	56	Written Emergency Policies and Procedures	10.B.08, 10.D.08, 10.D.09
	Prepare for Emergencies	56	Family Contact Information	5.A.01
	Prepare for Emergencies	56	First Aid/CPR Training	5.A.03
	Prepare for Emergencies	57	First Aid Kit	9.C.10
	Getting Help	57	Medical and Dental Emergencies	10.D.09
	Emergency Evacuation	58	Emergency Evacuation Plan	10.D.08
	Emergency Evacuation	59	Practicing Safety Procedures	2.K.02

HYC Chapter	HYC Section Title	Page #	Topic Related	NAEYC Criterion
Chapter 5. Promoting Health with Good Nutrition	The Nutrition Consultant	65	Health/Nutrition Consultant	5.A.02, 5.B.03
	National Standards and Recommendations for Nutrition in Early Care and Education Programs; Community Nutrition Resources; Running a Food Service	66; 85	Child and Adult Care Food Program (CACFP)	5.B.01, 5.B.02
	General Approaches to Eating	67	Chairs/Tables for Eating	9.A.01
	General Approaches to Eating	67	Family-Style Meals	3.D.07, 3.D.12
	Feeding Infants	69	Feeding on Cue	5.B.12
	Feeding Infants	69	Breastfeeding	5.B.09
	Feeding Infants	70	Storage and Preparation of Human Milk and Formula	5.B.10
	Feeding Infants	73	Juice and Solid Foods	5.B.11
	Feeding Infants	74	Introduction of Cow's Milk	5.B.13
	Basic Nutrition Facts	75	Timing of Meals/Snacks	5.B.16
	Food Habits Are Learned: Nutrition Education	75	Nutrition Curriculum	2.K.01, 2.K.02
	Food Habits Are Learned: Nutrition Education	77	Food as Reward/Punishment	1.B.10
	Food Safety	78	Food Preparation and Storage	5.B.01, 5.B.03
	Food Safety	78	Drinking Water	5.B.06
	Food Safety	78	Food Brought from Home	5.B.02
	Common Nutritional Concerns	80	Fat, Sugar, and Salt	5.A.02
	Common Nutritional Concerns	81	Milk	5.B.13
	Common Nutritional Concerns	82	Special Feeding Needs and Food Allergies	5.B.04, 5.B.05, 5.A.01, 5.C.04
	Running a Food Service	85	Menu Planning	5.A.02, 5.B.15
	Storage of Nonfood Supplies	87	Storage of Toxic Substances	9.D.09
	Insect and Rodent Control in Food Areas	87	Integrated Pest Management (IPM)	9.D.08
Chapter 6. Promoting Health with Physical Activity	National Standards for Physical Activity for Children in Group Care	89	Active Play	2.A.07, 2.A.11
	National Standards for Physical Activity for Children in Group Care	89	Physical Development and Outdoor Materials and Equipment	2.C.01, 2.C.04, 2.K.01, 9.A.04, 9.B.01
	Playing Outdoors	91	Outdoor Play	3.A.03, 5.A.06, 9.B.04
	Playing Outdoors	92	Protection from Sun and Other Hazards	5.A.07, 9.D.08, 5.C.05, 5.A.09, 9.B.05
	Structured Physical Activities	94	Games with Structure	2.C.04

HYC Chapter	HYC Section Title	Page #	Topic Related	NAEYC Criterion
Chapter 7. Promoting Health through Oral Health, Mental Health, and Health Education	Oral Health	97	Toothbrushing and Oral Health Curriculum	5.A.16, 2,K.01, 2.K.05
	Oral Health	97	Sugar	5.A.02, 5.B.11, 5.A.14
	Oral Health	100	Dental Emergencies	10.D.09
	Mental Health	101	Challenging Behavior	1.E.01, 1.E.02, 1.E.03, 1.E.04
	Mental Health	102	Health Consultants and Resources for Children Who Exhibit Challenging Behavior	5.A.02, 7.C.02, 7.C.05, 8.A.01, 8.A.05, 10.B.10
	Mental Health	105	Adult Mental Health	10.D.01
	Health Education For Children, Staff Members, and Families	106	Health Education for Children	2.K.01, 2.K.05
	Health Education For Children, Staff Members, and Families	107	Health Education for Staff Members	6.A.03, 6.A.04
Chapter 8. Medical Care—Clinical Health Services for Children	Health Care	111; 120	Child Health Records	5.A.01
	Tracking and Advocating for Preventive Health Care Records	122	Confidentiality of Child Health	10.B.08, 10.D.05
	Communicating with Families	123	Communication with Families	1.A.01, 1.A.03, 7.A.06, 7.A.09, 7.A.10, 7.A.12, 7.B.01, 7.B.04, 7.B.05, 7.B.06
Chapter 9. Staff Members and Consultants for Safe and Healthy Child Care	Program Responsibilities of All Personnel	127	Personnel Policies	10.E.01
	Health and Safety Concerns in Recruiting, Selecting, and Retaining Staff Members	127	Health Assessment of Staff and Volunteers	10.E.04
	Health and Safety Concerns in Recruiting, Selecting, and Retaining Staff Members	132	Staff Orientation and Training	6.A.03, 6.A.04, 5.A.03
	Health and Safety Concerns in Recruiting, Selecting, and Retaining Staff Members	133	Staff Turnover	10.B.09, 10.B.11, 10.B.13
	Adult Health Needs—Occupational Risks	133	Occupational Health	10.D.01
	Adult Health Needs—Occupational Risks	135	Staff Benefits	10.E.06
	Infectious Disease Risks for Adults	135	Hygiene and Universal Precautions	5.A.09, 5.C.02
	Breaks	138	Staff Breaks	10.E.07
	Child Care Health Consultants	138	Child Care Health Consultants	5.A.02

HYC Chapter	HYC Section Title	Page #	Topic Related	NAEYC Criterion
Chapter 10. Facility Design and Support Services for Safe and Healthy Early Care and Education	Space and Structural Design	145	Amount of Indoor Space/Child	9.C.01
	Space and Structural Design	146	Surfaces	5.C.02, 9.A.01
	Space and Structural Design	146	Outdoor Play Areas	9.B.04, 9.B.07
	Space and Structural Design	146	Indoor Play Areas	5.A.06, 9.A.06
	Equipment and Furnishings	146	Equipment and Furnishings	9.A.01, 9.C.05, 5.A.08, 5.A.09, 9.A.04, 9.B.01, 9.A.03, 9.C.07
	Equipment and Furnishings	147	Communal Water Play	5.A.10
	Air Quality, Ventilation, Heating, and Cooling	147	Indoor Air Quality	9.D.05
	Lighting	147	Natural Light	9.C.04
	Noise Levels	147	Noise Reduction	9.A.09
	Electrical Items	147	Electric Hazards	9.C.08
	Plumbing	148	Water Quality and Access, Drowning	5.A.08, 5.A.09, 5.B.06, 9.A.01, 9.B.02, 9.C.05, 9.D.01, 10.D.02
	Fire Warning and Safety Systems	149	Fire Protection	9.C.11
	Maintenance of the Facility	149	Cleaning, Sanitation, and Disinfecting Frequency	5.C.01, 5.C.02, 9.C.06
	Maintenance of the Facility	150	Containers for Soiled Diapers	5.A.08
	Maintenance of the Facility	150	Integrated Pest Management (IPM)	9.D.08
	Maintenance of the Facility	150	Animals	5.A.09, 5.C.05, 9.D.08
	Maintenance of the Facility	151	Washing Mouthed Toys	5.C.03
	Maintenance of the Facility	152	Toxic Substances	9.D.09
	Maintenance of the Facility	152	Radon, Carbon Monoxide	9.C.11, 9.D.01
	Maintenance of the Facility	152	Asbestos	9.D.01, 10.D.02
	Transportation	153	Transportation	9.C.14, 9.C.15
	Transportation	154	Ratios During Transport	10.B.12
	Transportation	156	First Aid Kit	9.C.10
	Transportation	157	Passenger Safety Education	1.D.02, 2.K.03
Chapter 11. Caring for Children with Short-Term or Chronic Health Needs or Disabilities	Care of the Mildly Ill Child	160	Caring for Ill Children	10.D.01
	Special Considerations for Programs that Do Not Exclude Mildly Ill Children	162	Health Consultant	5.A.02
	Giving Medication in a Child Care Program	163	Medication Administration and Storage	5.A.11, 9.D.09, 10.D.01
	Common Illnesses and Chronic Health Conditions	168	Allergies	5.B.05, 9.D.07, 10.D.09

HYC Chapter	HYC Section Title	Page #	Topic Related	NAEYC Criterion
	Common Illnesses and Chronic Health Conditions	168	Asthma and Smoke-Free Facility	9.D.06
Chapter 12. Inclusion of Children with Special Needs	Inclusive Education: The Individuals with Disabilities Education Act	174	IFSPs and IEPs	3.A.01
	Preparing to Care for Children with Special Needs	175	Modifications and Adaptations for Children with Special Needs	2.A.08, 9.A.01, 9.A.03, 9.A.12, 9.B.01
	Modifying an Early Education Program to Accommodate Children	176; 178	Teamwork with Families and Specialists with Special Needs	3.A.01, 7.A.10, 7.C.06, 8.A.05, 10.B.10
	Medical Procedures	178	Instructions on Special Health Needs	5.A.01
	Medical Procedures	178	Special Feeding Needs	5.B.04
	Emergency Planning Considerations for Children with Special Needs	179	Medical Emergencies	10.D.09
	Resources to Plan Care for Children with Special Needs	180	Staff Training in Special Needs	6.A.12
Chapter 13. Child Maltreatment (Abuse and Neglect) and Administration of the Health Component	Child Maltreatment (Abuse and Neglect)	183	Mandated Reporting	10.D.03
	Child Maltreatment (Abuse and Neglect)	183	Staff Training on Abuse/Neglect	6.A.02, 6.A.03, 6.A.04
	How Programs Can Help Abused Children and Stressed Families	185	Linking Families with Services	7.C.02, 7.C.03, 7.C.05
	How Programs Can Help Abused Children and Stressed Families	186	Code of Ethical Conduct	6.A.01
	Preventing Maltreatment in Programs for Young Children	187	Background Checks	10.E.02
	Preventing Maltreatment in Programs for Young Children	188	Open Door Policy	7.A.11
	Preventing Maltreatment in Programs for Young Children	189	Behavior Management Policies	1.B.09, 1.B.10, 1.E.01, 1.E.02, 1.E.03, 1.E.04, 1.F.01, 1.F.02, 2.B.01, 2.B.03, 2.B.04
	Preventing Maltreatment in Programs for Young Children	190	Child Abuse Policies	10.D.03, 10.D.04
	Administration of the Health Component	191	Program Health Policies	10.D.01

References

American Academy of Pediatrics, American Public Health Association & National Resource Center for Health and Safety in Child Care and Early Education. 2011. *Caring for our children: National health and safety performance standards; Guidelines for early care and education programs.* 3d ed. Elk Grove Village, IL: American Academy of Pediatrics; Washington, DC: American Public Health Association.

Aronson, S.S., ed. Forthcoming. *Model child care health policies.* 5th ed. Elk Grove Village, IL: American Academy of Pediatrics.

Aronson, S.S., & T.R. Shope, eds. 2009. *Managing infectious diseases in child care and schools: A quick reference guide.* 2d ed. Elk Grove Village, IL: American Academy of Pediatrics.

Benjamin, S.E., A. Ammerman, J. Sommers, J. Dodds, B. Neelon & D.S. Ward. 2007. Nutrition and physical activity self-assessment for child care (NAP SACC): Results from a pilot program. *Journal of Nutrition Education and Behavior* 39: 142–49.

Benjamin Neelon S.E., E.M. Taveras, T. Østbye & M.W. Gillman. Preventing obesity in infants and toddlers in child care: Results from a pilot intervention (unpublished paper, 2012).

Centers for Disease Control and Prevention. n.d. Estimates of foodborne illness in the united states. Online: http://www.cdc.gov/foodborneburden/index.html.

Copeland, K., S.N. Sherman, C.A. Kendeigh, H.J. Kalkwarf & B.E. Saelens. 2012. Societal values and policies may curtail preschool children's physical activity in child care centers. *Pediatrics* 129 (2): 1–10. Online: http://pediatrics.aappublications.org/content/early/2012/01/02/peds.2011-2102.

Council on Sports Medicine and Fitness and Council on School Health. 2006. Active healthy living: Prevention of childhood obesity through increased physical activity. *Pediatrics* 117: 1834–42.

Institute of Medicine (IOM). 2010. *Child and adult care food program: Aligning dietary guidance for all.* Washington, DC: The National Academies Press. Online: www.fns.usda.gov/ORA/menu/Published/CNP/FILES/cacfpiom.pdf.

Kotch, J.B., & P. Isbell. The quality enhancement project for infants and toddlers 2000–2007. (unpublished paper prepared for the NC Department of Health and Human Resources, Division of Child Development, Raleigh, NC, final report, 2007).

McPherson, M., P. Arango, H. Fox, C. Lauver, M. McManus, P.W. Newacheck, J.M. Perrin, J.P. Shonkoff & B. Strickland. 1998. A new definition of children with special health care needs. *Pediatrics* 102 (1): 137–39.

Moss, B.G., & W.H. Yeaton. 2011. Young children's weight trajectories and associated risk factors: Results from the early childhood longitudinal study–birth cohort. *American Journal of Health Promotion* 25 (3): 190–98.

NAEYC. 2011. Code of ethical conduct and statement of commitment. Position Statement. Washington, DC: Author. Online: www.naeyc.org/files/naeyc/file/positions/Ethics%20Position%20Statement2011.pdf.

National Association for Sport and Physical Education. 2002. *Active start: A statement of physical activity guidelines for children birth to five years.* Oxon Hill, MD: AAHPERD Publications.

Olds, A.R. 2001. *Child care design guide.* New York: McGraw-Hill.

U.S. Department of Health and Human Services. 2008. *Physical activity guidelines for Americans.* ODPHP Publication No. U0036. Online: http://www.health.gov/paguidelines/pdf/paguide.pdf.

U.S. Department of Health and Human Services, Administration on Children, Youth, and Families. 2009. *Child maltreatment 2007.* Washington, DC: U.S. Government Printing Office. Online: www.acf.hhs.gov/programs/cb/pubs/cm07/cm07.pdf.

U.S. Department of Health and Human Services and U.S. Department of Agriculture. 2005. *Dietary guidelines for Americans.* Online: http://www.health.gov/dietaryguidelines/dga2005/document/pdf/DGA2005.pdf.

Index

A

Abdominal pain, 18, 83, 115
Abscesses, 25
Academy of Family Practice, 13
Activities, suggested
    child maltreatment, 193
    children with special needs, 181
    chronic illness, 159
    clinical health services, 124
    exercise, 94
    facility, 157
    health education, 109
    medications, 169
    mental health, 109
    nutrition and food, 87
    oral health, 109
    planning for emergencies, 62
    preventing infection spreading, 32
    preventing injuries, 52
    staff and consultants, 143
    transportation, 157
    using this manual, 4
Activity, physical. *See* Exercise
Administration of health component. *See* Policies and procedures
AIDS/HIV. *See* HIV/AIDS
Air. *See* Ventilation
Alkon, A., 142
Allergies (*see also* Food, allergies), 38, 70, 94, 121, 151, 169, 176, 180
American Academy of Pediatrics (AAP), 3, 6–9, 11–13, 15–16, 18–19, 22, 24, 30–32, 35–36, 38–39, 42, 47–49, 55–57, 62, 68, 70–71, 78, 80, 85, 87, 89–90, 92–94, 104, 111–13, 116, 119–22, 124, 127–32, 135, 137–38, 141–42, 145, 148–50, 157, 159–66, 169, 173–75, 179–80, 183, 185, 187
    Chapter Child Care Contacts, 139
    health care guidelines, 113
    health education standards, 106
    health education topics, 108
    Medication Administration Packet, 164, 169
    on immunizations, 25–26
    Pennsylvania Chapter, 26, 141
    training standards, 132
    WellCareTracker™, 121
American Association of Family and Consumer Sciences, 78
American Cancer Society, 78
American College of Emergency Physicians, 179
American Diabetes Association, 78
American Dietetic Association, 65, 78
American Gas Association, 31
American Heart Association, 38, 78
American Lung Association, 31
American Public Health Association, 65, 78
American Society of Heating, Refrigerating, and Air-Conditioning Engineers (ASHRAE), 31
Americans with Disabilities Act (ADA), 16, 127, 140, 163–64, 171, 179–80
    information available, 172
Anemia
    causes of, 81–82
    iron deficient, 66, 81–82
    milk and, 66, 73, 119
    screening for, 119
Aronson, S.S., 142
Art and Creative Materials Institute, 38–39, 41
Art supplies, 12, 39–41, 133, 176
Asbestos, 152
Asthma, 94, 113, 121, 159, 168–69, 180
ASTM International, 36, 42, 47, 49
Attention-deficit/hyperactivity disorder, 180
Autism spectrum disorder, 180

B

Back
    injuries, 133–34, 143
    protecting, 135–36, 147
    sleep issues, 136
Batteries, 40
Bedbugs, 11
Bedding (*see also* SIDS), 21, 38, 49–51, 146
Behavior problems. *See also* Mental health
    common problems, 102
    community resources, 105–6
    consulting professionals, 103–4
    lack of space, 144–45
    mental health and, 9, 101
    staff and, 141
    stressful situations, 101–2
    transportation, 156
    working with families, 102–3
Blood. *See* fluids, body
Body fluids. *See* fluids, body
Bottles, 66, 69, 72–73, 101
Botulism, 70, 79
Brain development, 2–3
Breastfeeding, 3, 8, 66, 68–72, 192
Bright Futures, 113, 116, 124
Bronchiolitis/bronchitis, 17
Bruises, 189
Building. *See* facility
Burns, 37, 189

C

California Childcare Health Program, 87, 122, 129, 141
Campylobacter germs, 19, 20–21
Car pools, 156–57
Carbon monoxide, 152
Cellulitis, 25
Center for Early Childhood Mental Health Consultation, 102, 104–5
Center on the Social and Emotional Foundations for Early Learning, 104–5
    pyramid model, 105
Centers for Disease Control and Prevention (CDC), 11, 13, 22–24, 26–27, 30, 66, 79, 91, 116, 118–20, 131, 128, 138–39, 141
Certified Playground Safety Inspectors (CPSI), 146
Check-ups. *See* Health care, preventive; Screenings
Chickenpox, 18, 24–25, 132, 135
Child Abuse Prevention and Treatment Act (CAPTA), 183–84
Child abuse. *See* Child maltreatment
Child and Adult Care Food Program. *See* Community and national resources
Child Care Law Center, 122, 180
Child Health Assessment form, 115
Child Health Insurance Program (CHIP), 111–13, 173
Child maltreatment, 182–91
    definitions, 183–84
    helping children and families, 185–87
    Hotline, 183–89
    in child care settings, 187–90
    incidence of, 183
    legal/ethical issues, 185–86
    mental health and, 101–2
    preventing, 182
    reporting, 82, 140, 182–83, 186–87, 189–90
    risk factors for, 185
    signs of, 82, 111, 132, 140, 183
    written policies, 185
Child Protective Services, 183
Child Welfare Information Gateway, 183–85, 189
Childhelp USA National Child Abuse Hotline, 183, 189
Choking, 37–38
Chronic illness. *See* Illness, chronic
CISP, 26
Cleaning, 19, 27–31, 130, 134, 144–45
    body fluids, 22–24
    carpets, 24
    diapers and changing areas, 12–13
    dishes, 151–52
    food service areas/equipment, 19, 21, 24, 36–37
    schedule, 12, 149–50, 157
    surfaces, 6, 22–23, 146, 152
    thermometer, 167
    toys, 21, 24, 151–52
Climbing apparatus, 42
Clothes. *See* laundry
CMV. *See* Cytomegalovirus
Colds, 15–17, 160, 167
Colitis, 70
Color Me Healthy Teacher's Guide, 94
Commission on Dietetic Registration, 65
Commodity Supplemental Food Program (CSFP), 77
Communal water tables, 147
Communication
    with doctors, 123, 164, 175–76, 179
    with families, 7, 55, 77, 102, 116–17, 123–24, 158-59
Community and national resources, 2
    CHIP, 111–13, 173
    children with special needs, 171, 180
    health, 140
    Medicaid, 111, 113, 116
    mental health, 105–6
    nutrition, 65–66, 75, 78, 85
Community nutrition resources
    CACFP, 65–66, 75, 78, 85
    WIC, 65–66, 75, 78, 85
Confidentiality. *See* Health care, confidentiality
Conflicting information, 3, 7, 123, 143
Conjunctivitis. *See* eyes
Consultants
    early childhood education, 138–39
    health, 96, 126, 128, 138–43, 162–63, 192
    mental health, 139
    nutrition, 65
Consumer Product Safety Commission (CPSC), 31, 35, 41–42, 46–47, 49–51, 146
Contact dermatitis, 168
Contagious diseases. *See* Diseases
Cooking. *See* Food, service; Snacks; Utensils
Copeland, K., 92

Coughing, 9, 15–16, 19, 115, 159, 167–68
CPR, 38, 46, 56, 62, 132
Cribs. *See* Bedding; SIDS
Croup/laryngitis, 17
Cytomegalovirus (CMV), 15–16, 132, 135

D

Daily health check, 158–60
    items to include, 159
Dairy Council, 78
Dehydration, 46, 92, 148
Dental health (*see also* Teeth), 96
    brushing, 8, 97–99, 107
    common problems, 100–101
    education, 99
    fluoride, 97–98
    nutrition and, 97
    preventive care, 99–100
    referral criteria, 100
    toothbrushes, 24, 99
Department of Health and Human Services (DHHS), 90, 116–17, 183, 185
    Dietary Guidelines, 67
Department of Public Health, 112
Development
    delays, 102, 105, 111, 171
    milestones of, 116
Diabetes, 66, 70, 159
Diapering, 9–12, 19, 32
    changing area, 12–13, 40–41, 48, 146, 150, 153
Diarrhea, 15, 18, 20–21, 24, 31, 70, 161, 168
Diets (*see also* Food)
    special, 81
    vegetarian, 81
Diphtheria, 24
Disabilities. *See* ADA; Special needs
Discipline, 132, 189
Disease
    control spread of, 7–13, 19–21, 27–31
    definition of, 7–8
    direct contact, 8, 21–22
    food-borne, 14, 78–79
    handling outbreaks, 192
    immunizations for (*see* immunization)
    infectious, 2–3, 6–31, 133, 158
    intestinal tract, 9, 19–21
    methods of spreading, 8, 17
    mild, 158
    noncontagious, 26–27
    preparation for outbreak of, 16–17
    reporting, 14, 20, 27
    respiratory tract, 9, 17, 19. 70, 167
    skin, 11, 45–46, 159, 168
    spread through blood, 22–24
    vaccine-preventable, 24–26
Disinfection. *See* Cleaning
Doctors
    communicating with, 123, 164, 175–76, 179
    written instructions from, 164
Documentation. *See* Records
Doors, 36, 145
Down syndrome, 180
Driving. *See* Transportation; Restraints, car seat
Drop-off/pickup, 153–55, 158–59, 191
Drowning, 46, 148

E

E. coli, 18
Ears (*see also* Screenings), 27
    hearing loss, 27, 118
    infection of, 25–27, 70
    preventing problems, 118, 131
Easter Seals, 155
Eating. *See* Feeding; Food; Food habits; Snacks
Eczema, 168
Edison Electric Institute (EEI), 31
Education. *See* Health, education
Electricity. *See* Wiring
Emergency
    contacts for child, 55–56, 155–56
    evacuation, 55, 58–59
    exit routes, 145
    fire (*see* Fire)
    natural disaster, 55, 59
    phone numbers for help, 56–58
    planning for, 140
    procedures, 55–56, 192
    security risks, 60–62
    special needs, children with, 55, 59, 176, 179
    transportation, 55, 155
Emotional health. *See* Behavior problems; Mental health
Environment, 144–57
    children with special needs, 175
    electrical items, 147–48
    equipment, 146–47
    fire safety, 55, 149, 156
    food service, 85–87, 146, 151, 161
    furniture, 146–47
    kitchen. *See* Food service
    maintenance of, 149–53
    noise levels, 147
    pest management, 10–11, 87, 92, 150, 153
    playground, 41–42, 146
    plumbing, 148–49
    space, 11, 145–46
    ventilation, 11, 19, 31–32, 144–45, 147, 149, 152
Environmental Protection Agency, 27–29, 46, 87, 152
    Design for the Environment, 149
    Public Information Center, 31
Environmental Rating Scales, 138
Epidemics, 14
Epilepsy. *See* seizures
Equal Employment Opportunity Commission, 127
Evacuation. *See* emergency
Exclusion. *See also* inclusion
    AAP recommendations, 6
    guidelines, 7–8, 11, 32
    infectious diarrhea, 21
    mental illness, 9, 101
    ill adults, 14–16, 161
    ill children, 14–16
    mildly ill children, 15, 160–62
    policies, 160–63
    recommended, 18
    symptoms not requiring, 16
Exercise, 4, 8, 88–94, 192
    appetite and, 79
    assessment of, 91
    children with asthma, 94
    modeling, 93–94
    national standards, 89–91
    obesity, 79–80, 88–89, 92
    outdoors, 89, 91–92
    structured, 90, 94
    teachers' views, 92–93
Extermination. *See* Pest control

Eyes
    conjunctivitis, 14–17
    impairment, 180
    infections in, 15
    screening, 117–19, 131

F

Facility, 144–57
    adaptations for children with special needs, 145
    electrical items, 147–48
    equipment, 146–47
    fire safety, 149
    food service, 85, 87, 146, 161
    furniture, 146–47
    kitchen. *See* Food, service
    lighting of, 61
    maintenance of, 149–53, 193
    noise levels, 147
    pest management, 10–11, 87, 92, 150, 153
    plumbing, 148–49
    safety checks of, 2, 35–41, 48–49
    separate areas, 11–12
    space, 11, 145–46
    ventilation, 11, 19, 31–32, 144–45, 147, 149, 152
Failure-to-thrive, 82
Families
    children with special needs, 172, 178
    communicating with, 7, 102, 116–17, 123–24, 158–59
    contact information, 155–56, 162
    health education, 107–8
    involving in food choices, 77
    involving in health screenings, 115–16
    notifying in emergencies, 55
    passenger safety education, 157
    permission from, 44–45, 57
    responsibilities of, 17, 153, 159–63, 179
    substance abuse, 184
Feeding (*see also* Food; Food habits; Snacks), 65, 192
    approaches to, 67–69
    children with special needs, 65, 83–85
    infants, 66, 69–74
    toddlers, 66–67, 74–75
Fever, 15–16, 18, 160–62, 165–67
Field trips. *See* transportation
Fiene, R., 142
Fifth disease, 16, 132, 135
Fire safety, 59, 149
    alarms, 149
    extinguishers, 55, 149, 156
First aid, 38, 130, 132
    choking, 37–38
    insect bites, 47
    kit contents, 31, 55–57
    seizures, 165–66
    while traveling, 156
"Five Rights" of medication administration, 164–65
Fluids, body, 6, 8, 16, 22, 31
    after exposure, 135
    cleaning, 149
    handling, 135
    preventing exposure, 22–24
Food (*see also* Feeding; Food habits; Snacks)
    allergies, 20, 79, 82–83, 168
    appetite, 75, 79
    brought from home, 78–79 , 192
    choking hazards, 37–38, 74
    choosing, 3

contamination, 14
equipment for preparing, 87
handling, 11, 36–37, 65, 70–72, 86–87, 130, 192
intolerance, 20, 73–74, 82–83
preparing, 3, 86–87
purchasing, 85–86
quantity, 66–68, 75
safety, 36–37, 70–72
service, 19, 21, 24, 36–37, 85–87, 130, 146, 151
sharing, 19
solid, 73–74
special needs, children with, 65, 83–85
storing, 3, 65, 70–71, 86
variety, 75
Food and Drug Administration, 26, 46, 164
Food habits (*see also* Feeding; Food; Snacks), 64–65
meals vs. grazing, 79–80
new foods, 73–75
reward/punishment, 77–78
salt, 80
starting solid foods, 73–75
weaning, 72–73
Forms. *See also* records
behavioral observation, 103
child health assessment, 115
emergency contact list for child, 55–56, 155–56
emergency phone list to get help, 56–58
injury report, 56–57
medication consent and log, 164
release of information authorization, 122
Furniture, 146–47

G

Garbage, 12–13, 87, 149–50
disposing of, 152–53
storing, 152–53
Giardia, 19–21
Gloves
disposable, 31, 37, 57, 135
Gross motor activities, 3
indoor, 35–36

H

Hand sanitizers, 9
Handwashing, 3, 6, 9, 19–21, 30–32, 107, 135, 148–49
poster, 10
Head Start, 94, 104, 116, 171
Headaches, 115
Health advocates, 126, 128–29
Health care. *See also* screenings
assessing, 110, 113–20
checkups (*see also* screenings), 110–14, 116–20
communicating with families, 123–24
confidentiality, 122, 192
coordination of, 113–14
education, 111–13, 117
preventive, 110–13, 120–23
primary provider, 113, 141
referrals for, 116
Health consultant. *See* Consultant, health
Health education, 96
for children, 106–7
for families, 107–8
for staff, 107–8
selecting topics, 108
Health histories, 6, 120–23

confidentiality, 122, 192
contents, 122
staff, 6, 131
Health Insurance Portability and Accountability Act, 122, 174
Health insurance, 110–11, 132
Health Resources and Services Administration, 179
Health team coordinator, 113–14
Healthy Child Care America Campaign, 139
Healthy policies, 14
Hearing. *See* Ears; Screenings
Heart disease, 66, 159
Height, 82, 118–19
Hepatitis A, 18, 20
Hepatitis B, 15–16, 22, 25, 71, 132, 135
Hepatitis C, 71
Herpes simplex virus (HSV), 22, 135
Hib, 17, 24–25
HIV/AIDS, 13, 15–16, 22, 71, 135
Hives, 168
Human papilloma virus (HPV), 22, 25
Hyperactivity, 83

I

Illness
chronic, 94, 113, 121, 159, 163–64, 168–70, 175, 180
common, 115, 158, 160–62, 165–68, 181, 192
legal rights, 175
mild, 160–62
Immunizations, 2, 4, 6, 8, 13–14, 17, 32, 110–11, 113, 191
adults, 6, 8, 17, 25, 131, 140
documentation, 192
legal exemptions, 13–14
recommended, 24–26
Impetigo, 18, 21
Inclusion, 96 (*see also* Exclusion)
benefits of, 171–73
carrying out, 173
of children with special needs, 170–71
of mildly ill children, 9, 101, 158, 160–62
policies, 160–63
Indiana University, 36
Individualized Education Programs (IEPs), 112, 174–76, 179
Individualized Family Service Plans (IFSPs), 112, 174–76, 179–81
Individuals with Disabilities Education Act (IDEA), 130, 173–75, 180–81
Infants
CPR, 38
increasing disease resistance, 8
lifting, 134
nutritional guidelines, 66
safe sleeping, 49–51
safety tips, 47–50
tummy time, 89
Infections, 6–31
controlling spread of, 6–12
ear, 25–27
respiratory, 9, 17, 19
tick-borne, 6, 8, 27
yeast, 27
Infectious diseases. *See* diseases
Influenza, 14, 25, 131
Injuries, 2–3, 111
back, 133–34, 143
child maltreatment, 189
preparing for, 54–55
prevention of, 34–52
records of, 56–57, 192

reporting of, 56–57
transportation, 144, 146
Insect bites, 11, 47
Institute of Medicine (IOM), 66
Intestinal tract. *See* Diseases, intestinal tract
Iron. *See* Anemia; Nutrition

J

Job descriptions. *See* Staff
Juvenile Products Manufacturers Association (JPMA), 47

K

Kitchen. *See* Cleaning; Food, service; Utensils

L

Labeling of Hazardous Art Materials Act, 38
Ladders, 42
Laundry, 12–13, 149–50, 153
Lead poisoning, 111, 119
screening, 119–20
Legal concerns/licensing
administering medications, 164
Americans with Disabilities Act, 16, 127, 140, 163–64, 171–72, 179–80
building codes, 145, 157
Child Abuse Prevention and Treatment Act, 183
child maltreatment, 185–87
children with special needs, 170–71
federal standards for infant sleep equipment, 51
Health Insurance Portability and Accountability Act, 122, 174
health records, 124
Individualized Education Programs (IEPs), 112, 174–76, 179
Individualized Family Service Plans (IFSPs), 112, 174, 176, 179–81
Individuals with Disabilities Education Act (IDEA), 130, 173–75, 180–81
injury/incidence reports, 56–57
licensing, 192
OSHA requirements, 22
reporting abuse, 182–83, 186–87, 189–90
reporting illnesses, 14
transportation, 154
Lice, 16, 18, 21
Lighting. *See* Facility; Security
Limping, 115
Lyme disease, 26
Lymphoma, 70

M

Mainstreaming. *See* inclusion
Maintenance workers, 130
Meals. *See also* Feeding; Food; Food habits
Measles, 18, 24–25, 135
German (rubella), 18, 24–25, 135
Medicaid, 111, 113, 116
Medical home, 111–13
components of, 112
definition of, 111
for children with special needs, 111–13
Medical procedures, 178–79
Medication
administering, 56, 140–41, 158, 160, 163–65, 178, 192
asthma, 168–69

side effects, 164
storing and labeling, 164
Meningitis, 14, 25, 70
Mental health, 96, 101–6, 112 (See also Behavior problems)
adult, 105
challenging behaviors, 101
common problems, 102
community resources, 105–6
consultants, 192
emergencies, 55
referrals for assessment, 103–5
stressful situations, 101–2
working with families, 102–3
Microwave ovens, 72
Milk, 64, 68
anemia and, 66, 73, 119
breast, 3, 8, 66, 68–72, 192
cow's, 68, 74
diarrhea and, 168
formula, 66, 68, 72–75
intolerance of (see Food, intolerances)
limiting, 81
low-fat, 68, 74, 80
Molluscum contagiosum, 16
Mononucleosis, 14
Montessori, Maria, 172
Mosquitoes, 6, 8, 26
Mouth. See Dental health; Teeth
MRSA infection, 16
Mumps, 18, 24–25, 135

N

Nap time, 9
National Academies Press, 67
National Agricultural Library, 78
National Association for Sport and Physical Education (NASPE), 90
National Association for the Education of Young Children (NAEYC), 11, 127, 132, 139, 180, 186
National Center on Birth Defects and Developmental Disabilities, 116, 180
National Dissemination Center for Children with Disabilities, 180
National Fire Protection Association, 52, 59
Risk Watch®, 157
National Heart, Lung, and Blood Institute, 66
National Highway Traffic Safety Administration, 153–54
National Program for Playground Safety, 42
National Recreation and Park Association (NRPA), 41, 146
National Resource Center for Health and Safety in Child Care (NRC), 132
National Safety Council, 136
National Sanitation Foundation, 151–52
National School Food Service Management Institute, 78
National Training Institute for Child Care Health Consultants, 85, 132
National Weather Service, 45–46, 91
Natural disasters. See Emergency
Nausea, 115, 167
Neglect. See Child maltreatment
Nemours Health and Prevention Services, 94
Nutrition, 64–87, 130, 132
calcium, 66–67, 82
consultants, 65
dental health and, 97
education, 75–78
guidelines, 66–67, 84–85
sugar, 8, 66–67, 80
Nutritional and Physical Activity Self-Assessment for Child Care, 91, 94
Nutritional practices, 3, 8

O

Obesity (see also Weight; Screenings), 65–66, 70, 79–80, 141
Observations. See Staff, observations
Oral health. See Dental health; Mouth; Teeth
OSHA (Occupational Health and Safety Administration), 22–23, 29, 132, 135, 152
Outdoor play, 19, 89, 91–92
safety, 41–42, 146

P

Parasites. See Lice; Pinworms; Ringworm
Parents. See Families
Parvovirus. See Fifth disease
Pedestrian safety. See Safety, pedestrian
Pediatric First Aid for Caregivers and Teachers, 38
Permission, parental. See Families, permission from
Personal items, 24, 98
Pertussis, 18, 24, 131
Pest management, 10–11, 87, 92, 150, 153
Pets, 177, 192
limiting exposure to, 10–11, 150–51
related diseases, 11, 151
Physical activity. See Exercise
Pinworms, 19–20
Plants, 39, 177
Playdough, 39
Playgrounds. See also Exercise
equipment, 42, 146
safety, 41–42, 92, 146
Pneumonia, 14, 17, 24–25
Poison Control Center at Children's Hospital of Philadelphia, 39
Poisons, 38–49, 87, 140, 144, 146, 152
Policies and procedures, 192
child abuse, reporting suspected, 82, 140, 182–83, 186–87, 189–90
child care assessment, 110, 113–20
child maltreatment, 191–92
cleaning and maintenance, 12, 149–50, 157
discipline, 189
emergency, 55–56, 192
health care guidelines, 113
health care, 163
health education standards, 106
healthy, 14
inclusion/exclusion, 160–63
medications, 163–65
training standards, 132
transportation, 153–57
Polio, 24–25
Potty chairs, 148–50
Power failure, 59
Pregnancy, 135, 151
Prevent Blindness America, 117–18
Preventive health care. See Health care, preventive
Primary care providers
children with special needs, 175–76
communicating with, 123, 164, 175–76, 179
Procedures. See Policies and procedures

R

Radon, 152
Rashes, 16, 18, 21, 169
Ratios (staff/child). See Supervision
Records
behavioral observations, 103
confidentiality of, 122, 141, 192
emergency information form for children with special needs, 179
enrollment/attendance/symptom record, 160
evacuation drill logs, 58–59
facility health policies, 191–92
health histories, 6, 114–15, 120–23, 131, 192
immunization, 110, 192
injury/incident reports, 56–57, 192
observation and symptom report, 159–60
transportation, 156
Rehabilitation Act of 1975, 171
Resources. See Community and national resources
Respiratory infections. See Diseases
Respite care, 112
Restraints, car seat, 44–45, 153–54, 156–57
seat belts, 157
Riding toys, 43–44
Ringworm, 16, 21
Risk management, 4
Rocky Mountain spotted fever, 26
Role modeling
animal interactions, 151
dental health, 99
healthy behaviors, 107
physical activity, 93–94
safe behaviors, 51, 132
Rotavirus, 24–25
Rubella. See Measles, German
Runny nose, 15–16, 19, 159–60, 167

S

Safe areas. See Security
Safe Building Alliance (SBA), 31
Safe Kids coalitions, 52
Safety, 34–52
checks, 35, 51–52
education, 36, 51–52
food, 36–37
infants and toddlers, 47–50
insect bites, 47
pedestrian, 44, 157
playground, 41–44
summer, 32, 45–47, 91–91
supervision, 51
transportation, 44–45
water rules, 46
winter, 31–32, 47, 91–92
Salmonella, 18–21
Sanitization. See Cleaning
Scabies, 18, 21
Screenings, 4, 110–14, 116, 191
anemia, 119
hearing, 118, 131
height and weight, 118–19
lead, 119–20
urine, 119
vision, 117–19, 131
Seat belts. See Restraints, car seat
Security. See also Safety
fences/gates, 61
lighting, 61
parents/guardians access, 60–61
planning, 60–62, 192

risks, 60–62
safe area, 60
Seizures, 159, 165–66
Separation of children by ages (*see also* Exclusion), 20, 133
Sexually transmitted diseases (STDs), 22
Shaken baby syndrome, 34, 50, 183, 189
Sheltering-in-place, 55
Shigella infection, 18–21
SIDS (sudden infant death syndrome), 34, 49–51, 70, 140
    defined, 50
Sinks, 146, 148–50, 153
Skin diseases. *See* Diseases, skin
Sleep, 8, 192
    back issues, 136
    bedding, 21, 38, 49–51, 146
    SIDS, 34, 49–51, 70, 140
Slides, 42
Snacks, 64, 75
    nutritious, 76
Sneezing, 9, 19
Snow. *See* Safety, winter
Social Security Act of 1997, 111
Society of Nutrition Information, 78
Space, 11, 145–46
    behavior problems and, 144–45
    for children with special needs, 145
    for mildly ill children, 160–63
Special needs, children with
    adaptations for, 159, 175–78
    child maltreatment, 183–85
    emergencies and, 179
    feeding, 65, 83–85
    immunizations, 131, 140
    inclusion of, 170–81
    medical procedures, 178–79
    numbers, 160
    overprotection of, 176, 178
    peer acceptance, 177–78
    pregnant women and, 151
    resources for, 180
    space for, 145
    staff and, 132, 141, 173, 178
    substitutes, 137
    training staff, 132
    transporting, 154–56
Staff, 126–43
    and children with special needs, 134, 141, 173, 178
    background checks, 187–88
    benefits of inclusion, 172–73
    breaks for, 135, 137–38
    directors/supervisors, 127–28, 191
    disabled, 127
    excluding, 135–37
    food service personnel, 130
    hazards for, 127
    health assessments, 105, 130–32
    health education, 107–8
    health/safety concerns, 127–33
    hiring and retaining, 127–33
    infectious disease risk, 135
    job descriptions, 127
    maintenance, 130
    mental health, 105
    observations by, 102, 114–16, 177
    occupational risks, 133–35
    pregnancy, 135
    records, 192
    recruiting, 127–33
    responsibilities of, 127
    supervising, 191
    teachers, 129–30
    training of, 132, 141
    transportation, 130
    turnover of, 32, 61–62, 133
STDs. *See* Sexually transmitted diseases
Strep throat, 18, 113
Stress. *See* Mental health
Sudden infant death syndrome. *See* SIDS
Sugar, 8, 66–67
Summer. *See* Safety, summer
Sun safety, 45–46
Sunburn, 45–46, 92
Sunscreen, 45–46, 92
Supervision, 42, 51
    of staff, 188–89
    sleeping arrangements, 50
    staff-to-child ratios, 163
    toddlers, 50
    transportation, 154–56
Supplies, 56, 59
    labeling, 152
    storing, 87, 149–50, 152
Swelling, 115, 168, 189
Swings, 42

T

Technical Assistance Center on Social Emotional Intervention, 105
Teeth, 2
    brushing, 98–99
    decay of, 73
    dental care, 99–100
    dental hygiene, 8
    fluoride, 97–98
    healthy foods and, 97
    injuries to, 100–102
    preventing illness, 4
    teething, 167
Temperature taking, 159, 166
Tetanus, 24
Thrush, 16
Ticks, 6, 8, 27, 151
Title V, 112
Toys
    chests, 39
    mouthed, 39–40, 151–52, 167
    riding, 43–44
    safety, 38–39, 47–48
    sanitization of, 24
Transportation, 44–45, 144, 153–57, 192
    children with special needs, 154–56
    emergency procedures, 155
    legal requirements, 154
    passenger safety education, 157
    safety rules, 154
    staff, 130
    supplies, 155–57
Traumatic brain injury, 34, 36, 50, 183, 189
Tuberculosis, 18, 131

U

U.S. Department of Agriculture (USDA), 66–68, 78, 85, 90, 151
    Food and Nutrition Service, 67, 77
    MyPlate guidelines, 84–85
U.S. Department of Education
    Disability and Business Technical Assistance Centers, 127
    Office of Special Education Programs, 180
U.S. Department of Justice, 171–72
U.S. National Health and Nutrition Survey (NHANES), 66
United Way, 141
University of North Carolina at Chapel Hill, 91
    National Training Institute for Child Care Health Consultants, 139
Urinary tract infections, 70
Urine screening, 119
Utensils, 36–37, 151–52
    children with special needs, 176–77

V

Vaccinations. *See* immunizations
Vegan diet. *See* vegetarian diet
Vegetarian diets, 81
Ventilation, 11, 19, 31–32, 144–45, 147, 149, 152
Vision. *See* Screenings
Vomiting, 18, 115, 167, 168

W

Water, 8
    plumbing, 148–49
    safety, 46, 148
    tables, 147
Weight (*see also* Obesity; Failure-to-thrive), 118–19
Whooping cough. *See* Pertussis
Windows, 60–61, 145, 149
Winter. *See* Safety, winter
Wiring, 37, 147–48
Women, Infants, and Children (WIC). *See* Community and national resources
World Health Organization, 111

Y

Yeast infections. *See* Infections

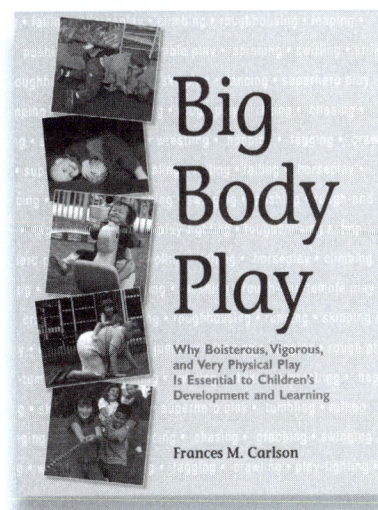

Big Body Play: Why Boisterous, Vigorous, and Very Physical Play Is Essential to Children's Development and Learning
Frances M. Carlson

"Big body play"—the sometimes rowdy, always very physical running, climbing, tagging, jumping, and wrestling that most children love and many adults try to shut down—*can* and *should* be an integral part of every early childhood setting. This book explains the multitude of benefits of big body play for young children's development. Also learn how to organize the physical environment, set rules and policies, and supervise the play.

Item #: 241

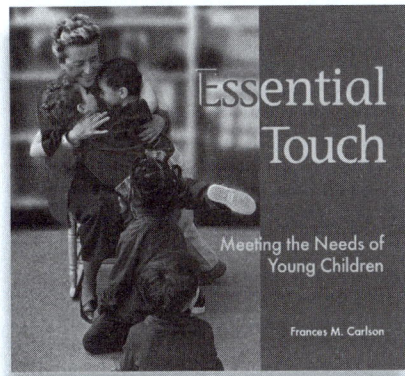

Essential Touch: Meeting the Needs of Young Children
Frances M. Carlson

Experiences of touch in all its forms—whether nurturing touch from adults, tactile explorations of the environment, or physical interactions with peers—are essential to high-quality early care and education. Learn why touch is essential to young children's development and how it can be incorporated safely into early childhood settings, from the infant program to the primary classroom.

Item #: 799

Preschool Learning Centers (10-Poster Set)

These colorful, laminated posters are based on the popular *TYC* feature Revisiting Learning Centers. Each of the 10 posters in this set is 11"x14" and suitable for framing or posting in the classroom. Titles and labels are in both Spanish and English.

Item #: 4160

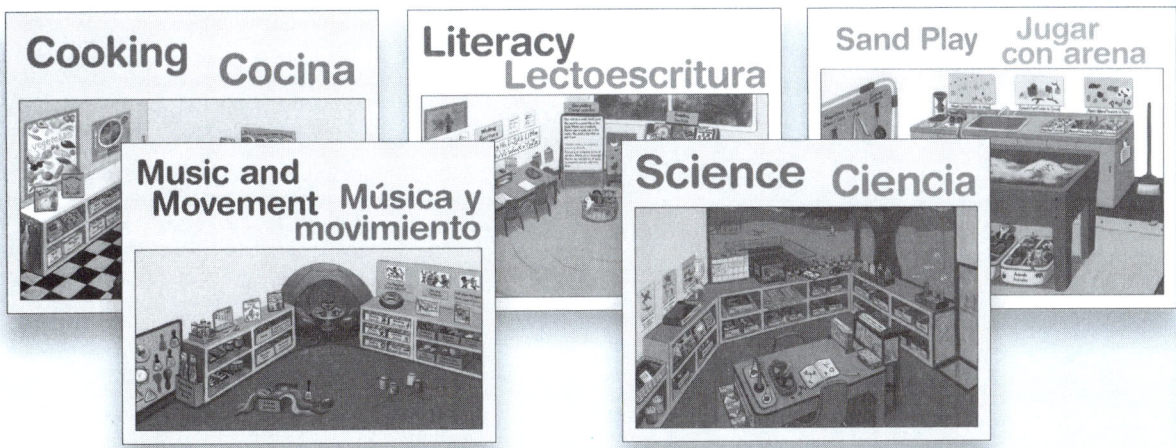

For a complete listing of resources, please visit www.naeyc.org/store or call 800-424-2460.

More Resources Available through NAEYC